COMPLETE MANUAL THERAPY

Chiropractic and Physical Therapy in One Approach

COMPLETE MANUAL THERAPY

Chiropractic and Physical Therapy in One Approach

CHARLES A. OLIVER, DC, MPT, OCS

Founder/Director, Comprehensive Chiropractic & Physical Therapy
San Antonio, Texas

Author: Charles A. Oliver, D.C., M.P.T., O.C.S.
Photographs: Mark Langford, Mark Langford Photography Inc.

Printed in the United States of America

ISBN: 978-0-692-00786-0

Library of Congress Control Number: 2010921480

Dedication

To my wife, Trish, thank you so much for your love, patience and support.

To Kara, a father could not ask for a better daughter. I am so proud of you as a student, an athlete, and a budding actress. You are so wonderful.

To Lauren, the greatest little girl in the whole world. All I can say is that you have the sweetest disposition of anyone I have ever *met. Please, please stay this way. You are so wonderful.*

To my parents, Alex and Kathy Oliver. Thank you for your unconditional love and support for all of these years. Mom, as a mother of three boys let me apologize for all of the missed birthdays and Mother's Days you have had to endure. We love you.

Acknowledgments

I WISH TO GRATEFULLY ACKNOWLEDGE THE GREAT MINDS WHICH CREATED AND DEVELOPED the chiropractic and physical therapy professions. This book would not be possible without them. I also wish to recognize the brilliant men and women who have added so much to each profession—from the time of each field's infancy up until today. These innovators have made each of us more effective practitioners by sharing new techniques, principles, and approaches with the world.

Lastly, I want to thank my past professors and instructors. Each of you has shaped the way I practice today. To the great faculty of Parker College of Chiropractic, I commend you for teaching your students not only the practical applications of chiropractic but also the physiology, neurology, and endocrinology behind the science, philosophy and art of chiropractic. To my past seminar instructors, including Brian Mulligan, Evan Mladenoff, John Iams, Ron Hruska and Ken Humber—thank you for teaching me so many techniques to help my patients. To others I have never met but whose genius has changed the way I practice: B.J. Palmer, John F. Grostic, George Goodheart, David Walther, D.D. Palmer, John Upledger, Vladimir Janda, Karel Lewit, Geoffrey Maitland, F.M. Alexander, Thomas Hanna and Lawrence Jones—thank you. Finally, to my mentor when I was a young physical therapy student, Tom Turturro, P.T. Tom, your vast knowledge is only overshadowed by your impeccable character. I consider it an honor to know you.

Contents

About the Author

CHARLES A. OLIVER, DC, MPT, OCS BEGAN HIS CAREER AS A PHYSICAL THERAPIST, EARNING his Master's of Physical Therapy degree from the University of Texas Health Science Center at San Antonio. While in private practice, Dr. Oliver received the Orthopedic Clinical Specialist designation from the American Physical Therapy Association Board of Physical Therapy Specialties.

Always striving to learn more treatment methods to help his patients, Dr. Oliver closed his physical therapy practice so that he could attend Parker College of Chiropractic. Following graduation, he and his family moved to San Antonio, where he founded Comprehensive Chiropractic & Physical Therapy. In private practice as a chiropractor and physical therapist, Dr. Oliver utilizes the principles outlined in this text to provide his patients with "the best of both worlds."

For further information on the author's practice or for any other information, he may be contacted at:

Comprehensive Chiropractic & Physical Therapy
930 Proton Rd., Ste. 104
San Antonio, TX 78258
(210)545-1810
www.chiropracticandpt.com

1 The Complex Body

IN THE 1960'S DR. ROBERT BECKER INTRODUCED THE WORLD TO A BRAND NEW CONCEPT: the use of electrical therapy in healing non-united fractures. From a practical standpoint, this was a remarkable invention in that it provided orthopedic surgeons with an effective method for helping fractures heal which otherwise would not heal on their own. From a philosophical standpoint, Dr. Becker's innovation was even more impressive. After all, it had essentially bridged the gap between modern medicine and energy-based therapies.

Dr. Becker recounts his story and details the science behind energy medicine in his bestselling book, *The Body Electric.*[1] This is considered a landmark text by many, and it is certainly a very interesting read. But I must say my favorite passage from it does not have anything to do with energy, healing, or physiology. It is more philosophical than those topics. It is a description of just how complicated the body is, and how no person or profession can fully understand it. He writes: *"Unfortunately, no approach is a sure thing. In our ignorance, the common denominator of all healing—even the chemical cures we profess to understand—remains its mysteriousness. . . Physicians can offer no reason why one patient will respond to a tiny dose of a medicine that has no effect on another patient in ten times the amount or while some cancers go into remission while others grow relentlessly unto death."*[1]

Indeed, it is the body's complexity which causes it to behave so "mysteriously" as Dr. Becker describes. It is also the reason why brilliant thinkers like him and many others have earned a place in the spotlight—because there is always room for new ideas, methods and techniques in the healthcare field. In a sense the body "demands" these innovations because there are still so many unsolved problems. This is also the reason why the healthcare field draws so many great minds: there is always something left to figure out. There is always one more mystery, one more unanswered question.

Besides having the power to humble the greatest minds in the world, the body's complexity is evident when we consider the vast number of professions that make up the "healthcare field." To best appreciate this notion just compare it with other fields. For instance, ask yourself the following questions: "How many professions specialize in accounting?" "How many professions specialize in auto repair?" Or, "How many professions specialize in teaching?"

The answer to these questions is one. There are not "alternative" accountants, auto mechanics, or teachers available to serve the public. Nor is there a need for them. Even in the fields of law and engineering where there are specialists there is hardly a fraction of the number of specialists needed in the medical profession.

For the manual therapist the challenge is even greater. He has to work on arguably the most complex system of the entire body. Don't believe it? Just consider how many healthcare professions treat the musculoskeletal system. To list a few:

1. Chiropractor.
2. Physical therapist.
3. Osteopath.
4. Massage therapist.
5. Occupational therapist.
6. Orthopedic surgeon (and its many subspecialties).
7. Neurosurgeon.
8. Neurologist.
9. Pain specialist (anesthesiologist).
10. Family practitioner
11. Pilates instructor.
12. Yoga instructor.
13. Muscle activation therapist.
14. Acupuncturist.
15. Reflexologist.
16. Reiki practitioner.

17. Physiatrist.

18. Podiatrist.

19. Rolfer.

20. Feldenkrais practitioner.

21. Alexander Technique practitioner.

And this is only a partial list! There are many other professions in the alternative medicine field which specialize in treating the musculoskeletal system. Moreover, some of the professions listed above even have multiple approaches within them. For instance, in chiropractic medicine alone there are almost two hundred different approaches!

Now compare the number of practitioners working with the musculoskeletal system with those working in other aspects of the healthcare field. How many practitioners specialize in treating the urogenital system? What about the digestive system? The cardiovascular system? Even a structure as complicated as the eye has only two practitioners—the ophthalmologist and the optometrist—dedicated to it. Even if we concede that each of the systems mentioned is complex in its own rite there must be a reason why the musculoskeletal system has so many practitioners. The answer? Its complexity!

DIFFERENT TREATMENTS, SIMILAR RESULTS

Besides looking at the number of practitioners available to treat the musculoskeletal system, we can also learn about the body's complexity by studying its response to treatment. For instance, just consider the fact that different forms of treatment often create a similar physical response. This tells us a great deal. This is especially apparent when we consider how treatment from different practitioners—often utilizing completely different treatment methods—can each affect a positive change.

To illustrate this concept consider the following scenario: 12 patients with low back pain visit 12 different healthcare practitioners, including: a physical therapist, a chiropractor, a physiatrist, a family practitioner, an osteopath, a reflexologist, an acupuncturist, a podiatrist, an ergonomics specialist, a movement therapist, a massage therapist, and a fitness trainer. Each patient is examined with a different method and receives a different treatment. The physical therapist believes that muscle imbalance is responsible for the patient's problem and prescribes stretching exercises to improve flexibility. The chiropractor finds subluxated vertebrae in the thoracic and upper cervical spine and performs adjustments to restore normal motion.The physiatrist finds trigger points within the erector spinae and injects them. The family practitioner notes excessive muscle tone in the lumbar paravertebrals and prescribes anti-inflammatories and muscle relaxants.The osteopath detects tender points in the quadratus lumborum and performs strain-counterstrain to reduce muscle hypertonicity. The reflexologist finds tender points on the rearfoot that correspond to lumbar spine pain and then massages these points. The acupuncturist believes energy flow along a specific meridian is blocked and uses needles or digital pressure to restore normal flow along the affected meridian. The podiatrist notes excessive pronation during gait and fits the patient with orthotics to reduce abnormal stress on the low back. An ergonomics specialist finds the patient's workstation promotes forward head posture and prolonged lumbar flexion, and then makes changes to reduce these stresses.The movement therapist notices the improper way the patient rises from a chair, and teaches him the proper way to utilize his body during this motion.The massage therapist finds the iliopsoas and lumbar paravertebrals are tense and massages them until normal muscle tone is restored. The fitness trainer believes core weakness is causing lumbar instability and places the patient on a thorough program of core strengthening/retraining. Now imagine that in each of these cases the result was the same.The patient felt at least 70% better and was satisfied with the results.

The fact that each person consulted a different medical professional is not odd. What is odd is that each person improved despite substantial differences in the treatment received.This scenario is not hard to believe.We all know a person who needs a massage once-in-a-while to stay loose. Or, maybe he needs to have his anti-inflammatory prescription refilled to feel like normal. Possibly, he may need an acupuncture session to feel "like new" again. But how can this be? How can approaches so different from one another actually help fix an identical problem?

The successes of these different treatment approaches only serve as further evidence of the complexity of the human body. More importantly, they illustrate how different factors play a role in our patient's health.This is further proof that our patient's symptoms rarely have only one cause and only one solution. For instance, in the previous example we see how the body is influenced by four important physical factors.While each factor is important on its own accord, it is easy to understand how even a "simple" problem such as low back pain can be influenced by changes made to a patient's mechanical system, nervous system, movement pattern scheme, and energetic system.A brief introduction to each of these factors follows.

INTRODUCTION TO THE FOUR PRIMARY FACTORS

Of the aforementioned "factors" influencing the musculoskeletal system, most familiar to those in the traditional medical field is the mechanical system. We were trained to rely on the mechanical system to explain almost all forms of orthopedic dysfunction. This goes for conditions ranging from structural insults (i.e. torn supraspinatus tendon) to those due to faulty biomechanics (ex. plantar fasciitis). In short, we were taught that almost every musculoskeletal problem can be attributed to problems involving the mechanical system. This logic even extends to problems seemingly involving only the nervous system. For instance, common diagnoses such as carpal tunnel syndrome, cubital tunnel syndrome, and cervical radiculopathy are each considered simple cases of mechanical compression upon a neurological structure.

Treatment under the mechanical philosophy is simply to restore normal biomechanics and/or structural symmetry. This involves techniques such as stretching, strengthening, or the application of orthotics to improve biomechanical status. Or, it may include surgical repair or excision in order to recreate normal structure. In essence, practitioners relying on the mechanical system use their knowledge of anatomy combined with the laws of physics to make diagnostic and therapeutic decisions.

The nervous system has an equally important role in physical function and dysfunction. In normal function, the nervous system works on a voluntary and involuntary basis to relay messages from the brain to the rest of the body. When dysfunctional, it perpetuates problems through muscle spasm, holding patterns, and complicated reflexes. While the chiropractic profession already considers the nervous system as the "master system," most manual therapists utilize the nervous system to help their patients even when they do not realize it. For instance, during manipulation, mobilization, massage, and sustained pressure the nervous system is influenced to as a great a degree as any structural component. Typically, this is through inhibition of excess tone. However, in other instances we affect change by facilitation of inhibited muscles.

A person's movement pattern schema is the third factor to be evaluated and treated in musculoskeletal disorders. Simply put, this topic is centered on the way we move. This can relate to intentional, voluntary movements or it can refer to unintentional, involuntary movements. For instance, the way a person walks, lifts, or even breathes may be dysfunctional and thus put extra strain on the system. This strain then causes symptoms for the patient and/or perpetuates symptoms already present. With this in mind, altering the way these activities are performed reduces muscular and articular strain and conserves valuable energy.

Last but not least is the effect of energy upon our system. While many of us in the West do not fully understand energy-based approaches, they are gaining in popularity and general acceptance. Practitioners of these methods hold that proper energy flow is responsible for almost every function of our body—down to that of our cells. Slowly but surely, modern research is proving many of these theories true. This has not gone unnoticed by large policy-making entities such as the World Health Organization (W.H.O.). In fact, the W.H.O. has stated that acutherapy is an effective treatment for the following diagnoses as well as many others:[2]

- Headaches
- Migraine Headaches
- Trigeminal Neuralgia
- Bell's Palsy
- Polio
- Meniere's Syndrome
- Neurogenic Bladder Syndrome
- Intercostal Neuralgia
- Tennis Elbow
- Sciatica
- Back Pain
- Rheumatoid Arthritis
- Acute Bronchitis
- Bronchial Asthma
- Constipation
- Diarrhea
- Duodenal Ulcer
- Common Cold
- Toothache
- Gingivitis

For the purpose of this text we will limit our discussion to basic acupressure and reflexology techniques which are meant to be used on musculoskeletal disorders. However, due to the understandable reluctance of many practitioners to stray from traditional techniques, a lengthy discussion is included to describe the science behind energy medicine as well as its proven efficacy. This is evidence-based research which hopefully will help the skeptical reader become more open-minded and in the end, more effective.

The example given above also demonstrates the differences in focus of the various professions. While some professions treat exactly at the site of symptoms, others treat a distant structure. This may be superior or inferior to the patient's symptoms. It may be superficial or it may be deep. It may even be on the opposite side of the body. As with treatment via different "factors," success occurring by treating different regions proves a valuable point. It illustrates the countless connections the human body has engrained within it. From a clinical standpoint, this means that there are many, many ways a patient can end up with a certain musculoskeletal problem. It also means that there are many, many avenues by which a patient can be treated.

SIMILAR TREATMENT, DIFFERENT RESULTS

Another indication of the body's complexity is seen in the day-to-day management of our patients. All of us have patients who improve right away. Other patients take a long time to get better. Then there are those people who do not improve no matter what we do for them. Sometimes these results are predictable. But many times they are not.

We often treat two people with seemingly identical problems who respond completely differently to our treatment. For instance, imagine treating two people who present with the same subjective and objective findings. Treatment involving a gentle mobilization in the direction of the limitation (a direct approach) leads to quick improvement for one person while the other person reports no change. For this second person we try several different mobilizations and find that going in the opposite direction of the limitation (an indirect approach) is the most successful one.

Take another example. Let's say this time two "identical" patients report tremendous improvement after the same manipulation. One returns a week later reporting 95% improvement and does not need to follow-up after her second visit. The other returns in two days noting only 15% improvement since the manipulation, and must return 2–3 days per week for the next 2 months. This person's chiropractor told her that the frequency and duration of her treatment was necessary because she kept "falling out of alignment." Now, while there are valid reasons why adjustments do not hold indefinitely, why would one person's body require continued treatment while the other person was back to normal after two adjustments?

These two cases reinforce one of the central themes of this text: the body does not always behave as we believe it should (at least when we look at it with a narrow perspective). No matter how well a patient fits into a theoretical framework, how skilled the practitioner, or how "right" the technique is, the body has the last say. It determines how it will respond despite everything else. In actuality, its response to a given treatment overrides any argument based on theory or philosophy. In fact, at times it almost *seems* to defy logic.

One of the ways manual therapists have responded to the body's unpredictable nature is by developing new approaches with which to treat it. In some cases this is to fill a void left by existing philosophies. In other cases it is to help a patient whose problem has gone unresolved using existing techniques. In any event, every approach was created because the existing approaches at the time did not fix every problem. That is still the case today. Despite a great number of fascinating techniques at our disposal, there is still not a single approach which fixes every problem. Likewise, there is not a single profession which can fix every problem. Consequently, limiting one's practice to a single approach or the teachings of only one profession inherently impedes a person's therapeutic potential.

RANDOM OR CALCULATING?

While the previous section was written as though the body randomly "chooses" a path towards wellness or dysfunction this is certainly not the case. It only seems that way sometimes. But it *always* acts rationally. It is a finely-tuned, calculating machine that responds to what it is presented with—usually with more sophistication than we give it credit for. Paradoxically, the more confident the practitioner is that his treatment will help the patient, the more random the whole process seems when the patient does not respond. But again, this is not due to haphazard behavior on the part of the body. Instead, it is the body responding to the stimulus it is presented with.

What makes the body's behavior appear random is a narrow-scoped treatment regimen. This applies to the four factors, first and foremost. In other words, if we are treating only 1 of the 4 factors it is easy to be unsuccessful and not understand why. In addition to this, there are other stressors we will discuss later in the chapter which can influence the body in a similar manner. Once again, if we do not address these stressors the body will not respond as we would expect and the person does not improve. Conversely, by addressing all stressors we can minimize the seemingly random behavior of the body and see consistent patient improvement.

In the following examples we examine the rehabilitation process in the presence of multiple forms of treatment. This allows us to do several things. First, we get to see how the body responds to different factors and treatments separately. This helps explain why some "ideal" patients fail our treatment but flourish under another's care. Second, we are able to see how factors can act in a summative manner, whereas the examples given before tested each factor in isolation.

In this instance the patient is a 50-year-old computer programmer with neck pain of 5 months duration. Highlights of his subjective examination are as follows:

1. There was no apparent cause for the symptoms. There was neither trauma nor change in occupational or leisure-related activities.
2. The nature of the pain is best described as a burning sensation.
3. The location of the pain is on the right side of the neck at the junction with the thorax.
4. The pain typically comes on around 3 o'clock each workday. On weekends the pain does not arise until almost 8 o'clock and is of less intensity.
5. The patient's job involves sitting and working on a computer for most of the day.

Scenario #1. Let's assume this man first goes to a physical therapist for treatment. After speaking with him for several minutes the therapist begins formulating a hypothesis to explain the cause of his symptoms. She delves deeper into his work environment and finds his workstation is poorly designed and thereby adds tremendous stress to his cervico-thoracic junction. She also concludes that the placement of the computer mouse and phone force the patient to use his right upper extremity in an improper fashion. This overworks his upper trapezius and levator scapula. Next, she performs her evaluation and notes the following:

1. Tightness/tenderness of the right upper trapezius, levator scapula, scalenii, and sternocleidomastoid.
2. Postural dysfunction including forward head displacement and "rounded shoulders."

3. Bilateral pectoralis minor tightness and scapular retractor weakness.
4. Cervical range of motion is mildly limited into left sidebending and bilateral rotation.

As expected, the objective findings correlate with the patient's subjective exam. This strengthens the therapist's hypothesis that the patient's neck pain is due to postural dysfunction exacerbated by poor work habits. Now all that needs to be done is to implement corrective treatment.

The therapist devises a rather thorough treatment plan to address all factors contributing to the patient's symptoms. This includes making changes to his work environment in order to put his entire body in a less-stressful position. It also includes corrective exercises and manual therapy to improve the dreadful forward-head, rounded shoulders posture. Last but not least, it involves direct treatment of symptomatic tissues to reduce pain and inflammation.

From the physical therapist's perspective this sounds like an excellent treatment regimen. Not only is the symptomatic area being addressed, but it appears that the causes for the patient's problem are being corrected as well. So, with the treatment plan in place all we have to do is wait for changes to start happening.

Unfortunately, after six weeks of intensive therapy the patient reports only minimal improvement. But how can this be? This appeared to be a textbook case of postural strain. And treatment to address this as the cause was certainly thorough. At this the therapist ran out of explanations. She was left believing that his pain would not go away because his muscles were irritated each day at work and that as long as he worked he would have pain. She also reasoned that this, combined with growing older, more deconditioned and possibly slightly arthritic had left him virtually unable to be helped.

Fortunately for the patient he did not stop looking for help. After his last visit with the therapist he decided to try reflexology. Despite not understanding how "massaging" his feet could help his neck pain, the patient was thrilled to note great improvement after just two sessions. He was completely symptom-free after 8 sessions and discharged himself from care.

Scenario #2. Let's take this same patient but completely reverse the outcomes. This time he sees a reflexologist first and has absolutely no relief. In contrast, the physical therapist's treatment does the trick. He reports some improvement right away and after several weeks of therapy is symptom-free.

Scenario #3. Let's say this same patient first goes to see the physical therapist. After four weeks of therapy he is making improvement but does not appear to be on track to becoming symptom-free. Without quitting therapy he begins seeing the reflexologist as well. This addition to his treatment regimen causes substantial improvement immediately. In fact, within one week he is symptom-free.

Scenario #4. For the final scenario let's reverse scenario #3. This time the patient goes to see the reflexologist first. After four weeks of treatment he is definitely improved but does not appear to be improving at a rate which suggests he will be "fixed" with his current regimen. Without quitting reflexology sessions he begins seeing the physical therapist. Pain relief comes quickly with this addition and he is pain-free within one week.

Discussion. These scenarios speak volumes. They illustrate not only the complexity of the human body but also the shortcomings of individual professions and single approaches. They also open our eyes to the possibility that the way we view our patients' symptoms is somehow not complete. This relates to the way we try to identify the cause of the problem. It also relates to the way we address the issue believed to be at fault.

Scenario #1 exemplifies the great power each of the four factors has on the body. In this particular case we witnessed the power of the energetic system. We saw that it can be powerful enough to work by itself in isolation when nothing else does. For those of us trained under the traditional medical model it opens our eyes to the power of such a subtle force. However, highlighting the efficacy of the energetic system is not the intention of this scenario (we will present scientific research on energy medicine's efficacy later in the text). Instead, it is just a vehicle to show the reader how much dominance one factor can have in a patient's case. When such a factor is not addressed or utilized in treatment, the patient will not significantly improve under our care. This is why it is imperative all practitioners working on the musculoskeletal system are cross-trained in all factors. For this reason each of the four factors is discussed at length in chapters that follow.

Scenario #2 is identical to Scenario #1 with the exception of the outcome. Once again the power of each individual factor is displayed. In this case we could assume that the patient's symptoms were caused primarily by mechanical strain based on the response to treatment (which intentionally reduced this strain).

In such a case removing impediments to energy flow would not be successful as long as the patient's body is under great mechanical stress for 40 hours per week.

In scenarios #3 and #4 we see that sometimes a patient's symptoms involve more than one factor. Consequently, more than one factor must be utilized in treatment. In this example a combined approach of mechanical and energetic treatment led to symptom resolution. The reason the patient improved in this case is simple—treatment addressed all factors involved in creating and perpetuating the problem. This principle not only applies with this case but also with cases involving three or four factors.

One of the unknowns in this case is what the results would be if each treatment approach was applied in succession instead of in combination. While there is probably no perfect answer to this question, one can speculate that there is a synergistic effect when treatments are used together. They can simultaneously reduce pain, reduce neuromechanical stress upon the system, and improve the flow of energy. This is akin to "breaking up the pain-spasm-pain cycle." With all systems of the body in better working order, the body is less likely to go into a neurological holding pattern or continue to use a mechanical compensatory mechanism. In essence, it is allowed to "reboot" with a clean slate.

Common to all 4 scenarios is what we are trying to achieve with each one. That is, we are trying to bring the patient's pain down to the other side of the symptomatic threshold. In scenarios #1 and #2 all we had to do to achieve this was address one dominant factor. When that factor was eliminated or sufficiently reduced in intensity, the patient's symptoms diminished and then disappeared as the symptomatic threshold was crossed.

In scenarios #3 and #4 we had to "bombard" the patient's system with treatments comprised of different factors in order to drop symptoms below the threshold. In real life it is more common to see these scenarios than #1 and #2. This is especially true in chronic cases or in those arising insidiously. That is because of the body's complexity. For instance, in cases where only one factor is affected, the body has the energy reserves needed to repair and correct itself. Consequently, minor insults to one of the factors do not typically progress to becoming a chronic problem. On the other hand, a severe trauma such as a torn ACL is considered a major insult to the mechanical system. In this case the body is not capable of repairing itself even if the body's other three factors are functioning normally. While the treatment in this case is done by a surgeon instead of a manual therapist, the repair itself still works on a mechanical basis as assumed.

It is implied in each of the scenarios that all other conditions affecting the patient's problem directly and indirectly remain equal and unchanged. For instance, in scenario #1 it is implied that all other matters in the person's life remain unchanged and the only addition is the reflexology treatment. However, let's consider a slight twist on this scenario. What if the patient became ill, began working longer hours, or was forced to work in an even less favorable ergonomic position at the same time reflexology was started? Would the outcome have been the same? Probably not. Moreover, if his outcome was not the same, does it necessarily negate or minimize the role of the energetic system? No, it would not.

These are also the implications for scenario #3. With the addition of reflexology to the mechanical treatment, we assume the patient's success is due to the practitioner meeting all of the body's needs and eliminating all causative factors. Once again, what would have happened if there was an increase in negative stressors to the patient as he began combined mechanical/energetic treatment? If he did not improve does it totally negate the influence of the mechanical and energetic systems? Of course not. It only opens our eyes to the fact that there are other variables influencing the body's ability to repair itself.

The same reasoning stands when a patient improves. There may be countless other matters perpetuating a patient's symptoms that are removed just as treatment is initiated. Of course, without being aware of all of these things the practitioner assumes the treatment is responsible for the improvement. For example, we often hear patients note that they felt better while they were away on vacation. Is this entirely because work-related mechanical/postural stress was eliminated? It is almost impossible to tell. That is because this stressor was not subtracted in isolation. It was subtracted along with many other stressors when the patient went on vacation. Getting the kids ready each morning, carrying the baby into daycare, the morning commute—all of these things and more ceased their attack on the body's balance. At the same time, the patient was enjoying herself and felt elated to be out of town.

The examples above introduce the other important influences on the body: the secondary factors. Like the primary factors, the secondary factors have the power to create problems, perpetuate problems, or be utilized in treatment. Included in this category are all factors that influence the body but are not directly treated with manual therapy. Take an activity the patient performs each day, for instance. If it is performed repetitively, asymmetrically, or improperly it automatically places stress upon the system and should be addressed. This could be the way the person sits, drives, or even sleeps. Besides these mechanical stressors, this category also includes factors affecting the person's overall health including their emotional, nutritional and biochemical status. There are many secondary factors which can prevent a patient from responding to care, just as there are many primary factors which can do the same. Therefore, understanding and addressing all of them is vital to success. Please see Chapter 8 for further discussion of these factors.

A COMPLEX BODY, A COMPLEX APPROACH

The more we know about the body the easier we can understand how it can falter and how it can be helped. We also begin to realize that things which once seemed like "random" events are not random at all but instead are by-products of the body's complex nature and the things it is exposed to. Indeed, as more research is done we are beginning to see that most medical problems are not a chance occurrence but instead are the results from a knowable cause.

Understanding this concept is vitally important to the practitioner. Overall, it means that most problems are not the result of a random error which we cannot affect. Instead, there is a cause which we *can* affect. That means we have the potential to affect the patient in a greater way than most of us imagine. It also means that we have few excuses when a patient does not improve. Therefore, we have a greater responsibility to the patient to help them because we can. Their body is not carrying out some random action which is out of anyone's control. Instead, it is acting in response to the stimuli it is presented with.

Detecting and addressing these stimuli is our job. In some cases these causative factors are obvious and at other times they are subtle. Sometimes there is a single cause and other times there are multiple causes. Sometimes the cause is near the site of symptoms. Other times the cause is far away.

Overall, this is not an easy task. Cases arising from an insidious onset require time and perseverance to find all of the causative factors. Cases due to trauma can present similar difficulty when practitioners only consider the area directly affected by an injury and forget to look outside this region.

To achieve the goals of both finding and treating *all* factors responsible for the patient's problems we need to take a brand-new approach to patient examination and treatment. We cannot limit ourselves to the theories and techniques of a single profession. After all, why should we when no profession boasts a 100% success rate? From the examples given previously it is obvious why this statement is true. The body is just too complex to be explained by a single theory. Likewise, it cannot be "fixed" by an approach or profession which limits its scope to a single factor or region of the body.

That is why we must be *inclusive*, rather than *exclusive*, when treating the musculoskeletal system. We must include all possible ways the body can be helped. To exclude or omit beneficial treatments from a "comprehensive regimen" is only courting disappointment and failure.

To begin applying these principles we must first look at the entire wellness/dysfunction process in a new way. Instead of trying to attribute the cause of a symptom to one primary or secondary factor we must consider the influence of all of them. This includes not only how a stressor from each group creates dysfunction but also the way in which all stressors affect the whole.

The method proposed here for doing this is called the Complete Manual Therapy approach. In short, it is a way of viewing the wellness/dysfunction process as a balance between positive and negative. For our purposes it allows us to visualize the numerous ways the body can be helped and harmed by different factors. It also helps us understand how the body as a whole operates and the harmful results which occur when its operation is disrupted. By doing this we begin to see how many problems arise and are perpetuated by mechanisms we previously never considered. Therefore, it provides an excellent framework by which we can apply treatment to eliminate negative influences and amplify positive ones.

We must also understand the many factors which influence the body. These were mentioned earlier in this text in reference to the things which cause symptoms and the physical methods by which problems are addressed. They are presented in greater detail in later chapters along with examples of their clinical relevance. For the four primary factors this discussion includes a look at not only their influence on a local level but also the way they can influence distant parts of the body. Examples of the latter are excellent tools to help demonstrate the body's interactions and connections while also illustrating how treatment distant to the site of symptoms can be effective. At the same time these examples help the reader recognize patterns and assist him/her in treating outside the site of symptoms.

2 The Wellness Continuum

ONE OF THE MAJOR CONCEPTS INTRODUCED IN CHAPTER 1 IS THAT THE BODY IS INFLUENCED BY many different factors. We also discussed how these factors (or stressors) affect the entire individual. We saw that in some cases it took the influence of a single factor (or stressor) to create dysfunction and symptoms. At other times it took several stressors working in unison to breach the symptomatic threshold.

When we consider the influence of these stressors upon the system, we begin to see the musculoskeletal system's function in a new perspective. Specifically, we realize that the body's attempt to maintain musculoskeletal balance is not unlike its attempts to maintain balance internally. That is, the body has an incredible ability to heal itself as well as ward off disease and illness. This process is known as homeostasis—a guiding premise utilized by physiologists and medical doctors the world-over.

Per Guyton, homeostasis is the "maintenance of static, or constant, conditions in the internal environment. Essentially all the organs and tissues of the body perform functions that help maintain these conditions." He further points out that each of the one hundred trillion cells in the body "benefits from homeostasis, and in turn each cell contributes its share toward the maintenance of homeostasis." Where some of this interplay is lost "all the cells of the body suffer. Extreme dysfunction leads to death, whereas moderate dysfunction leads to sickness."[3]

While we do not often consider the musculoskeletal system as playing a large role in system-wide homeostasis, there is no doubt that the concept of homeostasis applies to it as well. As with the internal system its goal is to maintain a stable environment despite numerous challenges. For example, it must deal with countless factors threatening to disrupt its optimal biochemical state. It must deal with altered nerve flow interfering with afferent and efferent input. It must deal with circulatory problems threatening the need for adequate blood flow into and out of its thirsty joints and muscles. It must deal with structural asymmetries placing excessive stress upon sensitive joint surfaces. It must deal with occupational factors forcing muscles to work and ligaments to be stretched for hours on end.

These factors are just a few of the countless stressors challenging our musculoskeletal system—from both the inside and the outside environments. In fact, the body must constantly monitor, regulate, and act upon these stressors in order to maintain a healthy musculoskeletal system and avoid breakdown. When the body is unable to maintain balance under this model dysfunction results and symptoms ensue. To prevent this, it uses its reserves to maintain, repair, or even compensate for any abnormality. This process acts as a "buffer" to low-grade problems in the short term because it can keep these abnormalities at a level below the symptomatic threshold. It is with the passage of time, the addition of other stressors, or the weakening of the homeostatic system as a whole that these problems pass through the symptomatic threshold and we recognize their existence.

THE WELLNESS CONTINUUM MODEL

An excellent way to view the progression from homeostasis to disease is the wellness continuum model. Within this model we are able to see how the body slowly goes from a healthy, balanced state to one of dysfunction, illness, and disease. We are also able to better appreciate the factors which disrupt homeostasis in the first place. Thus, the wellness continuum model provides an excellent framework to understand "pathology" so we may interrupt it and restore a balanced, homeostatic environment.

To begin, let's examine the progression seen with typical chronic disease processes. A problem (internal) begins and is undetected by lab studies. As it progresses, it affects laboratory values to the extent that the physician recognizes it as a problem. With further progression the patient begins to notice symptoms. Eventually this alters the organ's function, leading to organ failure and either death or organ transplant surgery (see Figure 2-1).

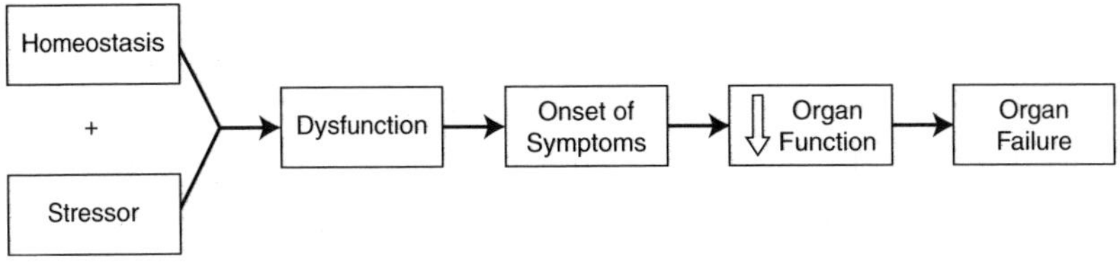

Fig. 2-1

Many musculoskeletal problems begin in a similar fashion. Imagine a subtle weakness or asymmetry causing disproportionate strain on a joint surface. This goes unnoticed by the person and is initially undetectable by x-ray or MRI. Over time this causes degenerative changes visible on x-ray as well as localized pain. As the problem progresses it leads to chronic pain, advanced degenerative changes, and diminished functional ability. At this point, surgical intervention is indicated (Fig. 2-2).

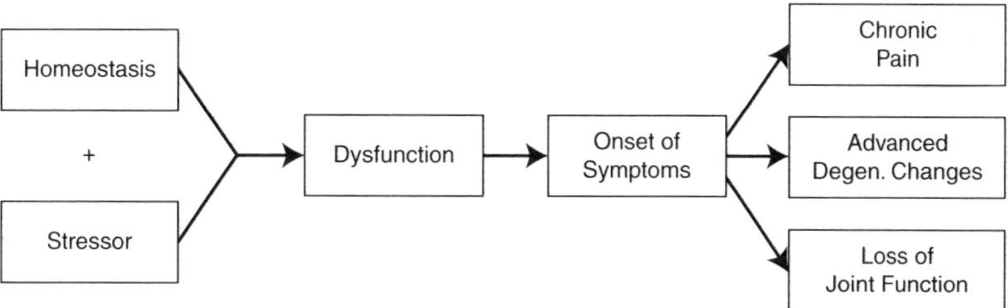

Fig. 2-2

In each of these cases we see how a problem begins and initially goes undetected. At this point the body is still trying to maintain order and function near optimal levels. Slowly it begins to lose this battle and the problem becomes detectable by lab or imaging studies despite the patient often remaining asymptomatic. Then, a long time after the actual start of the problem the person begins to complain of symptoms because the symptomatic threshold is breached. From this point on the disease/dysfunction progresses and function is lost and symptoms continue to worsen. The end point is complete failure in either organ or joint function.

Now that we have described the basic progression from a healthy, balanced state to a dysfunctional, diseased state, let's explore the way traditional and alternative practitioners view the process. This gives us further insight into how the disease process starts, its results, and effective modes of treatment.

TRADITIONAL MEDICINE

For the purposes of this text, the term "traditional medicine" is used to indicate the traditional medical system in the United States and Europe. This includes medical doctors of all specialties as well as physical therapists, occupational therapists, and all others under the medical doctor. For the most part this has been the dominant approach in the West and continues to be the system most patients follow.

Under the traditional model, homeostasis is viewed on a system-by-system basis. In this sense, each organ is considered to function almost independently of the other organs of the body. Therefore, each organ works to achieve homeostasis on its own. There are even different specialists assigned to each organ—the nephrologist, the hepatologist, the pulmonologist, and the cardiologist.

Examination under this model begins by scanning the different systems for problems. When a problem is detected it is looked into further. This usually involves further diagnostic tests so that an exact diagnosis can be reached. It is also done so that baseline quantitative values can be established.

Let's use cardiovascular disease as an example to better understand this process. In the case of cardiovascular disease it is common practice to focus a great deal of attention on the results of the disease. These results are evident both in labwork as well as imaging studies (angiogram). Consequently, both of these tests are used to determine the presence and extent of cardiovascular disease. They are also used as reliable markers to determine the progression or regression of pathology.

Treatment under this model is focused on reducing the "results" of the disease process. In the case of abnormal lab values medication is prescribed. This is done to bring total cholesterol and HDL and LDL levels back into a statistically "normal" range (Please note that these three markers are chosen here for their popularity; there are other equally important markers of impending heart disease). In advanced cases of cardiovascular disease an angioplasty or cardiac artery bypass graft is performed. These are mechanical ways of reducing the effects of the disease process (Fig. 2-3).

We see a similar means of addressing low back pain under this model. In this case the person presents with the primary complaint of low back pain. Judging by the nature and location of the patient's symptoms the practitioner begins to categorize the patient's problem: back pain of mechanical origin. Orthopedic tests or imaging studies such as x-ray, MRI, or EMG are performed in order

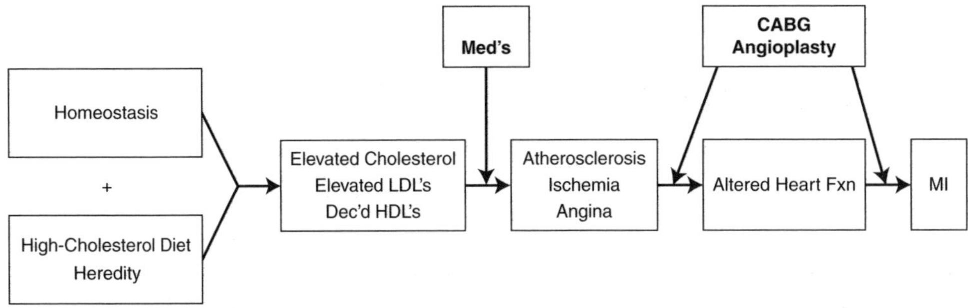

Fig. 2-3 Traditional medical approach to heart disease.

to ascertain the location and extent of pathology (of course, any abnormality visible by X-ray or MRI is a result of a long history of dysfunction with the exception of recent trauma). From this the patient's complaint is reduced to a mechanical problem involving a specific part of the musculoskeletal system.

Treatment is focused on reducing the major effects of the patient's problem. This is usually pain, inflammation, reduced mobility, and limited function. To do this the medical doctor prescribes pain medications and anti-inflammatories. The physical therapist utilizes different methods but often works on the same part of the spectrum. Modalities are utilized to reduce pain and inflammation. Exercise, massage, and mobilization are implemented to the involved tissues to improve motion and enhance function (Fig. 2-4).

In each of these cases we see that treatment is administered in a similar fashion. In both, the treatment is applied more heavily to the effects of the "disease/dysfunction" process near the end of the continuum. We also see that treatment is limited in its extent. In the case of cardiovascular disease, treatment is limited to the cardiovascular system. In the case of low back pain treatment is a little less limited, influencing the neurological and mechanical systems by reducing pain, inflammation, and restoring mobility.

This way of viewing and addressing the homeostatic process is consistent with traditional medicine's view of disease. Simply put, the allopathic model places the utmost importance on the disease process. Under this model the disease is often looked at as an entity which attacks at will when and where it wants to. Little importance is placed on the strengths or weaknesses of the body in this process. Consequently, treatment focuses directly on the disease. This is to either attack and eliminate it or to reduce its harmful effects. Less stress is placed on finding the cause in non-infectious processes (or non-traumatic musculoskeletal complaints).

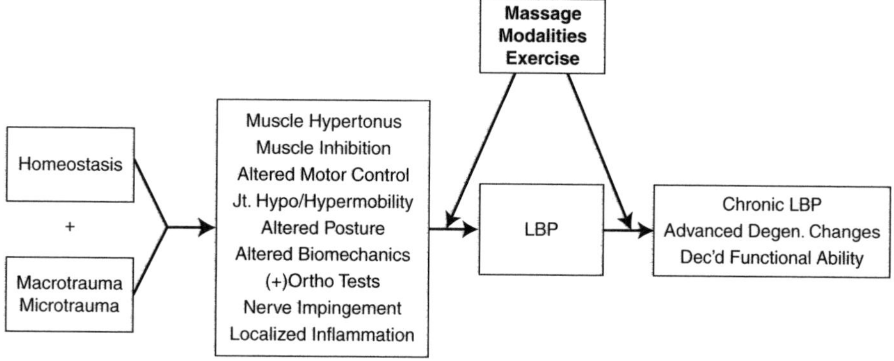

Fig. 2-4 Traditional medical approach to low back pain.

ALTERNATIVE APPROACH

Most professions which do not fall under the traditional approach are considered "alternative." This includes chiropractors, naturopaths, and homeopathic practitioners among many others. Virtually all professions practicing "energy-based" medicine fall under this heading as do those practicing traditional Eastern medicine. The origins of osteopathy come from this paradigm as well, although most osteopaths practicing today do so with an allopathic/traditional mindset.

Unlike the traditional model, the alternative approach does not view homeostasis on a system-by-system basis. Instead, it considers homeostasis as a process involving the entire body. Within this model the organs and systems of the body influence one another. More importantly, this concept holds that the condition of the whole can affect that of its parts and vice versa. Examination and treatment adhere to this concept; the health of the entire person is considered even when the person's symptoms seem to exist independent of the rest of the body.

In fact, the inherent healing ability of the body is of the utmost importance under this approach. Philosophies from different professions all converge on this point. For instance, in chiropractic medicine there is the belief of an Innate Intelligence which strives to maintain the body in a state of health. For this reason treatment focuses on removing barriers to this natural process. This is done by correcting vertebral subluxations, which interfere with the healing process either directly through nerve interference (efferent and afferent function) or indirectly through reflex mechanisms and autonomic dysfunction.

Osteopathic medicine holds a similar viewpoint. An important principle in osteopathy is that "the body has the inherent capacity to defend itself and repair itself."[4] Treatment, therefore, is meant to assist the body's natural healing ability.[4] Renown osteopath Philip Greenman adds,[5] "the goal of the physician should be to enhance all of the body's self-regulating mechanisms to assist in the recovery from disease."

In Eastern medicine the body is thought to contain ch'i, or a "life force." This life force flows through the body in meridians, providing energy to all structures and systems. Disease is believed to occur when the flow of ch'i is disrupted. For this reason treatment is directed at restoring the normal flow of ch'i in order to allow the body to restore balance on its own.

Wellness guru Dr. Andrew Weil classifies these approaches as Hygeian in nature because they assume "the body has a natural ability to resist and deal with agents of disease."[6] Treatment under this tenet is inside-out by nature. It strives to strengthen the body and let it fight off illness and disease instead of trying to attack the problem from the outside-in.

Consistent with this mode of thinking is a different view of disease. Alternative practitioners consider disease as the result of dis-ease (or lack of ease) of the body. Therefore the disease process is *not* random at all. It is the *effect* of disruption of the body's normal healing mechanisms. Moreover, because the disease is an effect, a cause exists which should be treated. Consequently, the goal of the alternative medicine practitioner is to find the cause which disrupted homeostasis. With this in mind let's look at how alternative medicine would address the same cases of cardiovascular disease and low back pain (See Fig. 2-5).

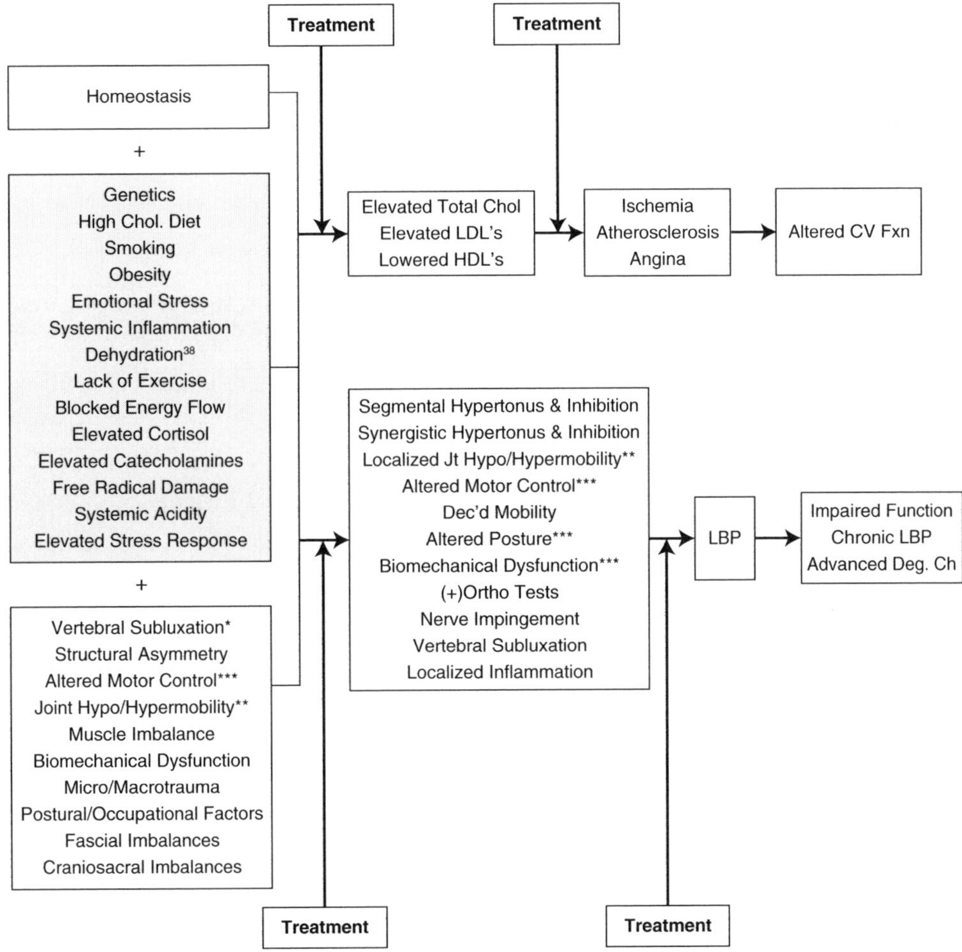

Fig. 2-5 The Alternative Medical approach to cardiovascular disease and LBP.

As the reader can see, the alternative medicine practitioner places a greater emphasis on treating at the start of the continuum. This especially relates to the patient's overall health, including their nutritional habits, emotional status, and other lifestyle factors which can be altered (although not often recognized by traditional approaches). For the manual therapist working in this role treatment also includes addressing any mechanical, neurological or energetic issue which could impact the health of the individual.

This diagram also illustrates the common ground two seemingly unrelated ailments share. Surprising, isn't it? More than just surprising in the author's opinion. It is educational. It answers many questions we have about the progression from a state of wellness to one of sickness, dysfunction, and disease. It also gives rise to three concepts we can use to look at the wellness-dysfunction continuum in a different way. Let's discuss these concepts further and explore the implications each has for the manual therapist:

"The musculoskeletal system does not operate independently of the internal system"

Instead, the musculoskeletal system is subject to dysfunction from negative biochemical factors just as the internal system is. That is, factors we normally consider as affecting only the internal system—dehydration, acidity, emotional stress, hormonal imbalance, deficient blood flow, and systemic inflammation can create or perpetuate musculoskeletal problems. This fact creates a direct link between the patient's overall health and his musculoskeletal function.

For example, diminished peripheral blood flow due to smoking, diabetes, or autonomic dysfunction reduces nutrient flow to thirsty joints and muscles. Likewise, excessive production of the catabolic hormone cortisol promotes breakdown of bone, muscle and cartilage.[7] Systemic inflammation helps perpetuate peripheral inflammatory processes. Excess bodyfat imposes an added mechanical strain on the system, thereby causing increased tension in some areas and excessive compression in others. Additionally, because bodyfat produces inflammatory substrates, obesity worsens the inflammatory state as well. These are just a few ways the overall health of a person affects the body's ability to heal the musculoskeletal system. Consequently, these factors may halt our best efforts at rehabilitation.

"There are common causative factors which disrupt homeostasis, thereby leading to the signs and symptoms of a disorder and then to the final stages of disease"

In fact, these same factors are implicated in many, many other problems besides just CVD and LBP. That is because they disrupt the body's normal balance. For this reason, they are frequently targeted by alternative medical practitioners regardless of the patient's chief complaint. This common starting ground makes the practitioner's job easier by providing several issues to focus on.

Just as there are many harmful lifestyle-related factors there are also many beneficial choices patients can make. The reader will find that these recommendations counter the ill-effects of the negative factors. Some of the more common suggestions are listed in Fig. 2-6.

1. Drink plenty of water (spring water, preferably).
2. Eat lots of fruits and vegetables.
3. Avoid saturated and trans fats.
4. Limit caffeine and alcohol intake (or eliminate them altogether).
5. Limit stress.
6. Exercise regularly.
7. Do not smoke.
8. Sleep at least 7–8 hours each night.

Fig. 2-6 Universal recommendations for overall well-being.

Of course, this is only a partial list. What is fascinating is that while each one has been suggested for a long time, the reason why each is believed to be beneficial has changed as our knowledge grows. For instance, we have always been told to eat plenty of fruits and vegetables. For some time this was just to get fiber. Or maybe it was for certain vitamins and minerals. Or maybe because it was a lower-calorie alternative to meats and heavy gravy. Most recently this thinking has focused on these foods' phytochemical and antioxidant properties as their most beneficial quality. Another valid theory looks at systemic acidity as the major cause of most diseases, pointing out that fruits and vegetables are alkalizing and that this is the reason to eat them. Whatever the case, there certainly seems to be specific "rules to live by" according to almost every alternative medical approach. It just so happens these rules overlap and help counter the common causative factors listed previously.

"The body tends to 'default' to certain problems when homeostasis is disrupted"

With all of these causes in common, and working with the premise that the body reacts in a specific manner when homeostasis is disrupted, wouldn't it be true that certain conditions such as LBP and CVD are found together? Well, yes it would. And, by the way, yes they are. According to Hestbaek et al.,[8] there is a positive association between LBP and cardiovascular disease. Their literature search also proved a positive relationship between LBP and angina pectoris/ chest pain, LBP and intermittent claudication, LBP and unspecified cardiovascular disease, and between LBP and atherosclerotic changes.

As expected, research has also proven that there are positive associations between LBP and many other problems.[8] These include respiratory disorders, gynecological disease, irritable bowel syndrome, allergies, and constipation. Additionally, three studies found patients with LBP have more nonback morbidities than controls.

As implied, the results of these studies are not surprising. *When homeostasis is disrupted by certain factors the body follows a common pattern as a response.* The physiological results of this response are predictable, and it is for this reason that treatment applied at the start of the wellness continuum has such widespread benefit.

This phenomenon helps explain why there are numerous approaches which appear to be able to cure almost everything. That is because they treat factors which have devastating effects upon homeostasis. For example, consider some of the results of systemic inflammation:[9,10] allergies, asthma, Alzheimer's disease, depression, immune system compromise, obesity, hypertension, headaches, heart disease, diabetes, and osteoarthritis among others. Seaman expands on this, noting that many muscle and joint pain syndromes are inflammation-based. Additionally, he points out that the intervertebral disc and synovial joints are especially prone to inflammation-based pain due to their high content of phospholipase A2, an enzyme capable of promoting the production of proinflammatory eicosanoids.[11]

Excessive acidity is believed to be an equally harmful factor. Experts believe it can cause:[12] allergic tendencies, angina, immune system compromise, depression, irritability, poor function of most endocrine glands, low back pain, neck stiffness, migrant joint pain, nerve pain, acute sensitivity to pain, tendonitis, headaches, as well as many other problems. As is the case with systemic inflammation, dietary changes to reverse the factors causing systemic acidity will lead to improvement in all related diseases/disorders.

Free radical damage is another major causative factor linked to all chronic diseases of modern times. It appears this involves "a final common pathway to cell injury in such varied processes as chemical and radiation injury, oxygen and other gaseous toxicity, cellular aging, microbial killing by phagocytic cells, inflammatory damage, tumor destruction by macrophages and others."[13] Free radicals also create inflammation, thereby magnifying their system-wide destructive capacity. They do this in several ways, including the production of arachnidonic acid from cell membranes and by enhancing the production of various cytokines such as tumor necrosis factor.[11] Again, as with the previous two theories, treatment to address this problem leads to improvement in the countless sequelae associated with this process.

The examples above also reinforce how different stressors result in similar disorders/diseases in the long run. The fact the body has countless diseases and disorders it could succumb to, but instead usually acquires one of a select few is quite amazing. But what does this mean? Are our bodies just predetermined to fail in a predictable sequence? Or, are some of our systems just poorly designed in the first place? The answer to both of these questions is a resounding no. Instead, most of these "diseases" are really nothing more than the changes the body has made in an attempt to regain homeostasis. We will detail many of these changes and the prime suspect in this mystery in the next section, The Stress Response.

The Stress Response

We have all heard that too much stress is bad for us. In fact, most healthcare workers will concede that it leads to an increased risk of heart disease and hypertension. We may even go so far as to tell our patients to relax because stress tends to tighten the neck muscles. But are we really giving it enough credit for what it is responsible for? Not hardly.

As early as the 1930's Hans Seyle began connecting chronic stress with disease. An endocrinologist, Seyle focused most of his attention on studying the effects of stress on the endocrine system. He developed a concept called the General Adaptation Syndrome, or GAS, to describe the body's response to stress. This syndrome has three stages: the alarm reaction, the stage of resistance, and the stage of exhaustion.

The alarm reaction is characterized by the stimulation of the adrenal gland to secrete epinephrine and norepinephrine. This occurs with the first exposure to stress, which can take countless forms. Besides stress as we normally think of, it may include virtually anything that challenges the body's well-being. This may be **physical exertion, mental exertion, emotional disturbance, trauma (recent or long ago), fatigue, exposure to heat or cold, or pain**[*1]. The alarm reaction is unavoidable despite our best attempts. Fortunately, it is usually short-lived.

* The word 'pain' in this context refers to nociception which the patient IS and IS NOT aware of. Keep in mind Melzack and Wall's Gate Control Theory which emphasizes the modulatory effects of mechanoreception upon pain coming into the CNS. Understanding this concept is imperative to understanding how joint dysfunction creates/perpetuates/accentuates pain and the physiological cascade resulting from it.

The resistance stage is the second phase of the GAS. It occurs after the alarm reaction, as the body prepares to take on the stressor for a prolonged period of time. It is in this stage that adrenal hypertrophy begins and adrenal hormone imbalance ensues.[14] As time goes on, this imbalance worsens and the person's health begins to suffer.[14]

When the adrenal glands can no longer function at this level they become depleted. This marks the exhaustion stage. This stage is witnessed in patients suffering from chronic health problems, long-term nutritional deficiency, and long-term emotional problems.[14]

These stages, of course, are just a broad overview of the stress response. They serve to demonstrate the general progression from the onset of stress to its final stage. However, it is what occurs during the stress response which is so vital in helping us understand why the process is so harmful. Components of the stress response are as follows:[3,7,15]

1. Increased catecholamines.
2. Increased heart rate.
3. Increased vasoconstriction.
4. Increased arterial pressure.
5. Increased blood lipid levels.
6. Increased blood cholesterol levels.
7. Increased rate of blood coagulation.
8. Increased protein degradation of muscle and connective tissue.
9. Increased blood glucose concentration.
10. Insulin resistance.
11. Increased feeling of stress, fear, anxiety, and depression.
12. Decreased short term memory, ability to concentrate, and learn new material.
13. Decreased serotonin levels; increased noradrenaline levels.
14. Increased sensitivity of sensory systems including those for pain.
15. Decreased cellular immunity (with chronic stress).
16. Decreased anabolic hormones like growth hormone, testosterone, luteinizing hormone, etc.
17. Bone loss, muscle fiber type changes.
18. Increased cortisol.

Fig. 2-7 Physiological changes with the stress response.

Of course, in the short term the "fight or flight" response is necessary for survival. It provides us with things like increased energy and enhanced blood clotting ability in order to survive a predator's attack. This was more important to our survival long ago when we were out in the wild, running for our lives or attempting to fight off animals trying to hunt us. In the modern era we still need the stress response—just with less frequency than our ancestors did.

Therein lies the problem—although we don't need the stress response for true survival as often as our forefathers did, we tend to turn this response on far too often. For many of the people around us this response is obvious. They are noticeably anxious, worried, and upset all the time. But what about the people who appear calm and collected? Are they stressed as well? Yes, they are too. Maybe less stressed than others, or just better at hiding their stress. But in this day-and-age everyone is under stress in one form or another.

Actually, it almost seems that our entire society is geared to stress us out. And what do we do about it? We worry. We worry over our careers. We worry about finances. We worry about the safety of our family. We worry about the possibility of war with another country. We worry about the weather. We worry about the planet. We worry about crime. We worry about people less fortunate than us. These examples are just a few, and they only cover internal strife. What about external strife? How are our interactions with others? Do you have a boss that does not appreciate you? Or maybe a co-worker that resents you? An old friend that stopped calling you? All of this is almost too much to handle. Then you find out your mother-in-law is coming to live with you!

Besides using the stress response too frequently, many authors agree that much of the harm comes from being unable to shut the stress response off. Levine,[16] for instance, points out that the actual "fight or flight" our ancestors engaged in burned off the hormones and nervous energy produced by the response itself. This cleared these substances from our system so we could go back to resting and digesting. In the modern era, however, our "battles" are usually more civilized ones. There is no fight to the death nor sprint away from our enemies to burn off the adrenaline we have running through our systems. Instead, after conflict we just sit at home or work "brewing" in our own hormones, rehashing the issue over and over in our minds.

Now let's refer back to Fig. 2-7 to see the physiological changes associated with chronic stress. Do they look familiar? They should. They are the building blocks of disease—specifically the most common diseases of our time. Seyle called diseases resulting from chronic stress the "diseases of adaptation."[17] In Figure 2-8 below we see how each change in physiology is paired with its long-term result:

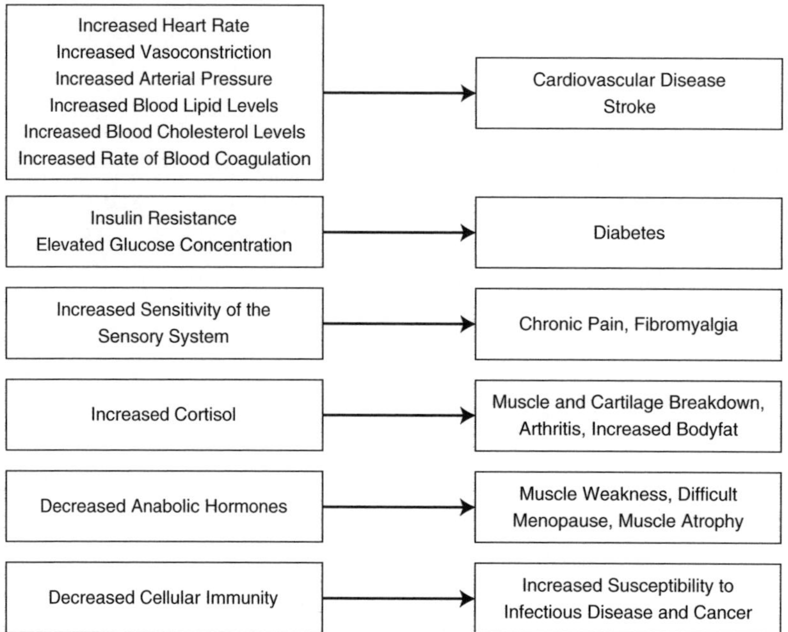

Fig. 2-8 The long-term results of chronic stress.

These findings are consistent with researcher's estimates that the stress response is responsible for causing up to 80% of all diseases.[18] They are also consistent with the assertion that there is something driving the body to "default" to certain diseases instead of falling victim to all established diseases in a randomly-distributed manner. Again, please note that the stress response is triggered by more than just emotional stress. It is a process that is triggered by *disrupted homeostasis.*

The Musculoskeletal Stress Response

Just as the body seems more prone to several internal diseases/conditions, the musculoskeletal system is more susceptible to certain problems of its own. For one, there are certain bodyparts affected more often by dysfunction than others. Just consider the frequency with which we all treat low back, neck, knee, or shoulder pain. Compare this with the relative infrequency of sternocostal, sternoclavicular, or ulnohumeral complaints.

Besides specific regions of the body being more problematic, there are even certain tendons more prone to strain than others. When we think of tendonitis we immediately think of the quadriceps, supraspinatus, and wrist extensors. Very seldom do we treat tendonitis of the serratus anterior or rectus abdominis.

Likewise, certain muscles are affected by chronic strain more than others. Of these, the hamstrings, piriformis, and lumbar paravertebrals seem especially prone to irritation. On the other hand, we do not treat strains of the tensor fascia lata or lower trapezius with the same regularity. Why is that? With an almost limitless potential for failure, one assumes the body would randomly fall victim to injury with no predisposition of one bodypart over another.

It is the author's contention that the reason for this discrepancy is the same as we described for the internal system. Simply put: *when homeostasis is disrupted the stress response is activated.* This leads to an inherent imbalance within the system, making certain bodyparts more vulnerable to breakdown than others.

This response in the musculoskeletal system is largely neural instead of hormonal. It causes altered posture, heightened sensitivity to pain, muscle hypertonicity, muscle inhibition, balance problems, and altered motor control—all in a very predictable pattern. In fact, it is this "common pattern" of dysfunction which we all treat with remarkable frequency.

This goes for gross, visible changes in posture as well as the most minute changes in motor control. Unfortunately, we often treat just a single part of this pattern, or at most the end results of it. That explains why there are so many musculoskeletal disorders resistant to anything greater than short-term improvement. Without treating the entire pattern—and its causes—it is no surprise many problems never go away completely.

Probably the greatest neurological explanation for the musculoskeletal stress response and the common pattern resulting from it is the startle response. In fact, this reflex is even at the center of two prominent approaches in movement therapy: Somatic Technique and the Alexander Technique. Thomas Hanna, the founder of the Somatic Technique, placed great importance on the startle response.* He believed psychological influence led to the activation (or over-activation) of this reflex along with the Landau reflex. This over-activation results in a specific postural pattern as well as

* Technically, Hanna referred to this reflex as the withdrawal response, although he mentioned it was also called the startle response. We will use the term 'startle' because it is used more often by researchers. Additionally, some authorities refer to the withdrawal response (Goddard, Sally. Reflexes, Learning and Behavior. Fern Ridge Press. Eugene, OR. 2002) as the most primitive form of the startle response. It involves "freezing" in the face of stress instead of protective muscle contraction.

inappropriate movement patterns. Over time this leads to chronic pain and loss of normal function.

It is interesting to note that Hanna considered this reflex as the outward manifestation of the stress response. In fact, he was probably the first person to make this connection. He also believed that the musculoskeletal changes (especially its effects on respiration) caused other problems, including cardiovascular disorders.

F.M. Alexander, the creator of the Alexander Technique, also believed the startle reflex played an important role in creating dysfunction. He held that this reflex created what he called "The Downward Pull." This is described as the unseen force acting to pull the base of the occiput downwards. It then leads to shortening of the entire spine, which Alexander believed was very harmful. Consequently, teaching patients to inhibit this force is of top priority in AT treatment.

But what exactly is the startle response? Simply put, it is a reflex ingrained within us for survival. It becomes active when we need to fight or escape from a dangerous situation. Unfortunately, it also becomes active when we are afraid or under stress. This is primarily due to neurological mechanisms, as mentioned previously. But it is also affected by humoral factors. Norepinephrine, an important neurotransmitter utilized by the sympathetic nervous system, has been shown to help activate the startle response.[19] This connection is very important to the manual therapist; it is one more way the stress response can maintain and amplify itself within the body.

The activation pattern of the startle reflex has been measured thoroughly. Its sequence is as follows: within .014 second after activation (such as hearing a car backfire), the jaw muscles contract. Twenty milliseconds after this, the eyes and brow contract. Only five milliseconds later, the trapezius raises the shoulders and the head goes forward (EMG studies also confirm strong sternocleidomastoid contraction). Thirty-five milliseconds later, the elbows flex and the forearms pronate. This chain-reaction continues down the body, contracting the abdominal muscles, thereby pulling the rib cage inferiorly and halting respiration. Next, the knees bend and point inward and the ankles roll the feet inward.[19] Hanna summarizes these reactions under what he calls The Red Light Reflex:[17]

1. Closing of the eyes.
2. Tensing of the jaw and face.
3. Pulling forward of the neck.
4. Elevation of the shoulders.
5. Flexion of the elbows.

6. Clenching of the fists.
7. Flattening chest.
8. Tightening of the abdominals.
9. Contraction of the diaphragm and breath holding.
10. Contracting perineum, including the sphincters of the anus and urethra.
11. Contracting gluteus minimus which internally rotates femurs.
12. Thigh adduction.
13. Contraction of the hamstrings to bend knees.
14. Flexion and supination of the feet.

Besides the startle reflex, there is another well-studied protective response which influences our "hard-wiring." It is the flexor withdrawal reflex, or nociceptive flexion reflex. Like the startle reflex, the flexor withdrawal reflex is characterized by a dominant flexion pattern. This pattern is so common and so inconspicuous that it is seen in the clinical setting virtually every day. All it takes is for the practitioner to firmly palpate the sensitive hand or foot of a patient and watch his or her extremity draw up into flexion. As we learned in school, this is an involuntary reflex designed to prevent tissue damage. The classic example of this reflex is withdrawing the hand from a hot stove (via excitation of the upper extremity flexors and inhibition of the extensors.) Another example is the person about to be bitten by a snake, who withdraws his foot and lower extremity while extending the opposite limb to maintain support (via excitation of the ipsilateral flexors and contralateral extensors and inhibition of the ipsilateral extensors). Indeed, all of this is an ingenious invention on the part of the Creator.

Unfortunately, as with the startle reflex, the flexor withdrawal reflex often overstays its welcome. That is, it serves its purpose in the short-term by preventing, or at least minimizing, tissue damage. However, the pattern of flexor facilitation and extensor inhibition often remains to some extent. This residual activity alters posture, changes joint function, and frequently causes pain.

Applied Kinesiologist and chiropractic neurologist Walter Schmitt discusses the importance of the withdrawal reflex in maintaining dysfunctional patterns for decades after trauma.[20] These patterns, he points out, can cause local or distant problems throughout the entire body. In his clinical experience he reports that when these patterns are eliminated, the person often becomes asymptomatic instantaneously.

In his lecture series, Schmitt illustrates the neurological pathway by which nociceptive afferent activity activates the flexor withdrawal reflex while also ascending to the hypothalamus and exciting the sympathetics. Indeed, this is an important part of the "bridge" between the autonomic nervous system, the endocrine system, and the musculoskeletal system.[20] *This connection is integral to understanding the musculoskeletal stress response.*

The clinical findings associated with hypersensitivity/hyperactivity of these reflexes are visible across the spectrum of neurological disorders. This ranges from cases of true neurological injury to minor functional alterations. All in all, we see the emergence of a "default" pattern when the nervous system's function is disrupted. This creates a common ground very important to the clinician. Even more importantly, it illustrates how the nervous system has the power to alter structure and function, thereby leading to many common musculoskeletal disorders.

Let's begin this discussion by first looking at two neurological disorders which share great similarity with the startle and nociceptive withdrawal reflexes. The first condition in this group is that of organic brain injury. This can be due to factors including trauma, stroke, or complications at birth. It creates flexor synergies characterized by the following:

Upper extremity [21]

1. Downward-rotated scapula (the glenoid is facing inferiorly)
2. Posterior rotation of the rib cage (the abdominals are too weak to anchor the rib cage)
3. Elevation of the scapula
4. Internal rotation and hyperextension of the humerus
5. Forward head carriage, scapular protraction and humeral horizontal adduction (at times to guard against falling backwards)
6. Elbow flexion
7. Pronation of the forearm
8. Wrist flexion and ulnar deviation
9. Finger flexion
10. Thumb adduction

Lower extremity [21]

1. Elevation and anterior rotation of the pelvis
2. Retraction of the pelvis

3. Hip flexion, internal rotation, and adduction
4. Knee flexion or hyperextension (genu recurvatum frequently occurs in an effort to bring the center of gravity over the plantarflexed ankle)
5. Equinovarus of the calcaneus
6. Midfoot supination
7. Forefoot adduction

The second "disorder" in this group is much less-involved than this one, though it still signifies some level of neurological dysfunction. It is the pattern of muscle imbalance well-documented by pioneering researchers such as Vladimir Janda. In this pattern we find that patients display facilitation of the postural muscles (mostly flexors) and inhibition of the phasic muscles (mostly extensors). This results in the Upper and Lower Crossed Syndromes, a common postural pattern familiar to all manual therapists.

This pattern is very consistent despite the fact authorities attribute it to several different causes. According to Janda, emotional factors play an important role in activating this pattern. He points to the strong relationship between the limbic system and the neck muscles in particular as a direct means whereby our emotions can affect the musculoskeletal system.[22] Another belief is that the muscle imbalance begins as a result of faulty posture and is then reflexively "ingrained" into a consistent pattern. Pain is yet another explanation; it creates facilitation of both the extensors and flexors at a segmental level. However, due to the ability of the postural muscles to endure prolonged contraction, they outlast and eventually inhibit the phasic muscles.[5] This pattern is summarized as follows:[5]

Upper Crossed Syndrome:

Muscles Prone to Tightness:

1. Upper trapezius.
2. Levator scapula.
3. Sternocleidomastoid.
4. Pectoralis major and minor.
5. Scalenii.
6. Flexors of the upper extremity.

Muscles Prone to Weakness:

1. Middle and lower trapezius.
2. Serratus anterior.
3. Rhomboids.
4. Supraspinatus.
5. Infraspinatus.
6. Deltoid.
7. Deep neck flexors.
8. Extensors of the upper extremity.

Lower Crossed Syndrome:

Muscles Prone to Tightness:

1. Iliopsoas.
2. Rectus femoris.
3. Tensor fascia lata.
4. Quadratus lumborum.
5. Short thigh adductors.
6. Piriformis.
7. Hamstrings.
8. Lumbar erector spinae.

Muscles Prone to Weakness:

1. Gluteus maximus, medius, and minimus.
2. Rectus abdominis.
3. External/internal obliques.
4. Peroneals.
5. Vastus medialis/lateralis.
6. Tibialis anterior.

Now take a moment to compare and contrast these two disorders with one another and with the startle response and nociceptive flexion reflex. There is an undeniable *common pattern* which exists, involving not only each bodypart but also the body's posture as a whole. This common ground should be surprising given the fact that each reflex and condition has a different explanation for its cause: emotional stress, pain, brain damage, and faulty posture. This is just more evidence that a musculoskeletal stress response exists when homeostasis is disrupted—in one way or another.

Bolstering this philosophy further are several studies which clearly detail the progression from 'disrupted homeostasis' to a component of the pattern we have described above. Not only do they reinforce the concept of a common pattern, but they also give us better perspective into motor control problems. Specifically, they help answer many questions we have regarding the role of motor control as being either the cause or the effect of our patients' problems. Besides doing all of this, these studies also give us further clues as to the many factors which can disrupt homeostasis, thereby turning the pattern on. Below are some of these studies in summarized form:

1. Tecco et al. studied the effect of anterior cruciate ligament injury on the cervical and masticatory musculature.[23] At rest, the patients in the experimental group displayed higher surface EMG activity of the anterior temporalis, masseter, sternocleidomastoid and lower trapezius compared to control subjects. INTERPRETATION: A stressor which creates pain and/or instability will cause activation of specific muscles involved in the common pattern.
2. Tecco et al. studied the effect of anterior cruciate ligament injury on the cervical lordosis.[24] They found subjects in the study group had significantly high craniocervical angulations compared with control subjects. INTERPRETATION: A stressor which creates pain and/or instability will cause mechanical changes throughout the body. This mechanical change is consistent with activation of the common pattern, specifically activation of the suboccipitals.
3. Pierrynowski et al. studied the gait patterns of women with fibromyalgia compared with controls.[25] They found the normal-speed walking pattern of women with fibromyalgia was similar to that of the controls' fast walking pattern. Most notably, this required greater recruitment of the hip flexors during gait. INTERPRETATION: Another example of over-utilizing a facilitated muscle. This could be one more reason why direct treatment to relax the hip flexors may not work.

4. Ekholm et al. found that activation of receptors in the knee joint capsule facilitated flexor motoneurons and inhibited extensor motoneurons.[26] This pattern is replayed by several studies which show that experimentally-induced knee joint effusion causes atrophy of the quadriceps (especially the vastus medialis) but spares the hamstrings. INTERPRETATION: Pain and swelling cause the knee to go into a flexed posture as expected. This also substantiates the importance of treating the cause of muscle weakness instead of just its results. For example, in patellofemoral dysfunction, some clinicians are very focused on improving the strength of the vastus medialis without questioning why it became inhibited. When we understand that this inhibition is part of the common pattern, it shifts our focus to the true cause of the problem.
5. Jull et al. compared the strength of the deep neck flexors in patients with neck pain of insidious onset with those suffering with pain secondary to whiplash.[27] The results were the same: both groups of patients had reduced strength of the short neck flexors and heightened activity in the sterno-cleidomastoid during cranio-cervical flexion testing. INTEPRETATION: The finding of deep neck flexor weakness and increased SCM activity in both groups is consistent with the common pattern. It also opens up the possibility that the weakness/atrophy can be a result of injury, rather than just act as a causative factor. Consequently, attempting to rehabilitate this muscle in isolation is less likely to be as effective as treating the cause of its inhibition (segmental dysfunction, spasm, pain, inflammation).
6. Abbott studied the effect of Mulligan's mobilization with movement on shoulder range of motion in patients with lateral epicondylalgia.[28] He found that patients with lateral epicondylalgia had reduced shoulder external rotation compared with controls. After treatment with the mobilization with movement technique, the patients showed increased external rotation range of motion bilaterally. INTERPRETATION: The pre-test findings of decreased external rotation are consistent with what is expected as part of the common pattern. Treatment to reduce elbow pain/dysfunction led to a reduction in the common pattern's influence unilaterally and contralaterally; this demonstrates the global effect of nociception on the system and the widespread improvement when this input is removed.

The common pattern evident from the descriptions above is very important to the manual therapist. In the context of this chapter it serves to illustrate that the condition of the musculoskeletal system is directly connected to that of the internal system. This makes it vulnerable to dysfunction by anything which disrupts the body's homeostasis. Additionally, its existence proves that there is a driving force behind many of the clinical findings we encounter. This helps establish the need for a more holistic approach to musculoskeletal medicine.

So, what are the exact neuroanatomical connections responsible for both (a) the synergistic patterns the body defaults to and (b) the clear relationship between the autonomic nervous system and these synergies? They are the mesencephalic reticular formation (MRF) and the pontomedullary reticular formation (PMRF). The MRF increases flexor tone on the contralateral side and excites the intermediolateral (IML) cell column bilaterally.[29] Thus, it is the connection which explains how musculoskeletal changes occur concomitantly with visceral ones under sympathetic stimulation.

The PMRF counters the actions of the MRF. It inhibits flexor tone and IML activity ipsilaterally. This influence on the flexors means that it reduces tone in the anterior musculature above the T6 level and the posterior musculature below T6.[29] In other words, the PMRF counters the patterns discussed so far while the MRF drives them.

Because the common pattern has a tremendous role in causing and/or perpetuating the majority of orthopedic problems it should be addressed with all patients. In this chapter we only discussed its effects on the body on a global scale. In Chapter 9 we look into this pattern in greater detail to examine its implications for each region of the body. There, we will see that many professions and approaches converge on individual findings, but that their attempts to explain these findings are often very different. This impacts patient management, as one could imagine. In the majority of cases it results in failed treatment because only a small fraction of the pattern—the symptomatic part—receives attention.

It should go without saying that these principles are most valuable to the clinician in chronic cases and in those of insidious onset. Obviously, in acute cases due to a specific trauma, this model does not play as important a role because the cause of the disorder is known and is most likely limited to a single region and primary factor. Nevertheless, because the body needs to be working optimally in order to repair itself optimally, one can understand how holistic treatment enhances the rehabilitation process. In addition, because all cases of pain and dysfunction initiate the stress response, it is in the patient's best interest to do everything possible to halt the progression of this harmful cascade. Further discussion of the healing process and optimal management strategies are presented in the next chapter, Complete Manual Therapy.

3 Complete Manual Therapy

In the preceding chapter we introduced several important concepts including the homeostatic process, the wellness continuum, the stress response, and the common pattern. This was to lay the foundation for a new method of viewing the patient with musculoskeletal dysfunction. The author has taken the liberty to name this system Complete Manual Therapy.

Briefly, the central theme of this approach involves applying our knowledge of the homeostatic process to the patient's problem in order to achieve the optimal outcome. This includes the incorporation of all concepts previously discussed into patient examination, assessment, and treatment. It also includes several other theories described later in this chapter.

Let's begin our discussion by first looking at how traditional and alternative approaches treat the body. As discussed in Chapter 2, we know these approaches work at different ends of the wellness continuum. But they also use different methods, treat different stressors, and have a different overall philosophy. Due to the body's complexity they are both effective at treating many conditions. Conversely, because neither approach is comprehensive, each is prone to failure at other times.

Understanding how each approach succeeds and fails is important to the manual therapist. It removes some of the doubt she may have about the effectiveness of her work. It also removes the notion that the patient's response to treatment is random, or at times "anyone's guess." Instead, it outlines the mechanisms by which a patient improves when he improves. It also outlines the mechanisms by which a patient fails treatment when he does not respond. Let's begin this overview by looking at the traditional medical approach.

TRADITIONAL APPROACH

The traditional medical approach tends to look at the end result of dysfunction as the most important thing to be treated. This applies to most medical or musculoskeletal conditions; the condition itself is treated while the "entire" person is not. For this reason traditional medical intervention is applied at the end of the wellness continuum instead of at the start.

The traditional model of assessment and treatment has many strengths. Most notable is its ability to address trauma or acute infection. It also has many positive applications for the manual therapist. The most powerful of these is in treating problems of acute onset, such as those due to a specific sprain or strain. Very often, these isolated incidents can occur without the great summative effect of many factors as we see with chronic cases and those of insidious onset. Instead, some of these problems only have a single factor which needs to be addressed. This is where the traditional approach thrives.

Let's use the case of a patient presenting with low back pain to illustrate this. This time we will assume his pain is due to a recent fall. Upon examination the patient appears to be in good overall health and displays no other objective findings except a tight and tender right quadratus lumborum. This corresponds to the exact mechanism of injury. Treatment is applied locally, consisting of modalities, massage, and light stretching. The patient excels with this treatment and is symptom-free within a few visits (Fig. 3-1).

This example is simplified, of course. Not included in the diagram are *all* sequelae of trauma, including the results of the stress response. Instead, in this example it is assumed that these factors are playing just a minor role compared with the local effects. This is why treatment works so well in this case.

This approach is successful in managing many other cases as well. For instance, treating a postural issue resulting from either mechanical or neurological stress can be very beneficial. It results in improved biomechanics for the neck, shoulder, low back, etc., thereby helping decrease symptoms in each area. The

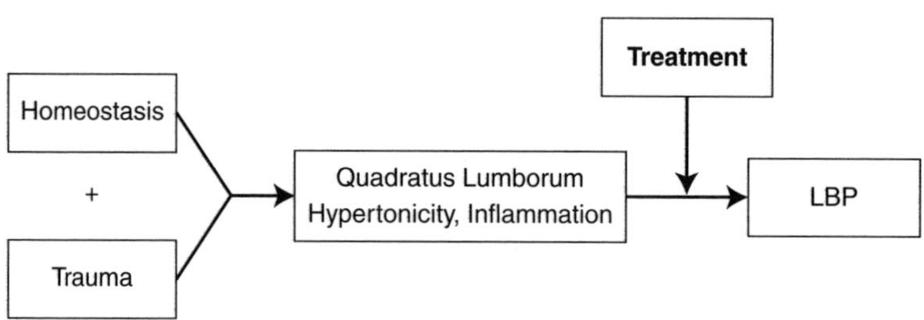

Fig. 3-1 Traditional approach to low back pain.

extent to which this treatment is beneficial is often unknown. It depends on what factors are driving the pattern. If it is created by a continuous insult to the system, it is unlikely that local treatment will be useful. If, on the other hand, the patient's posture is due to a resolved trauma or another cause that is long-gone, then this treatment will have long-lasting benefit.

In addition to the benefits listed above, this approach has the important distinction of being able to directly interfere with the many reflexes and feedback loops within the body. Simply put, these are the ways problems feed-back into the system. They allow certain problems to perpetuate and aggravate themselves while creating other problems by disrupting homeostasis (Fig. 3-2). Because these feedback loops are so important (and destructive), they are discussed in detail below.

A simple example of this feedback loop is the pain-spasm-pain cycle. In short, this is a theory wherein pain begets muscle spasm, which worsens pain, which worsens muscle spasm, which worsens pain, etc. Mostly through chemical irritation and reflex activity, this cycle seems to continue indefinitely until something stops it. This is where gentle manual therapy and modalities are so helpful. Local treatment helps to "break the cycle" by bringing the patient's pain level and/or muscle spasm down enough to shut it off.

Buskirk has done an excellent job outlining the many consequences of pain, as well as detailing the mechanisms by which it works.[30] Among the effects of pain are increased sympathetic nervous system activity, which then results in visceral dysfunction and immune system compromise. Also included are the activation of nociceptive, or nocifensive reflexes he states "involve both specific segmental responses and often multisegmental attempts to minimize the noxious input by removing stress from the affected nociceptors. In some cases, the injured muscle will be shortened by action of its synergists or of those fibers

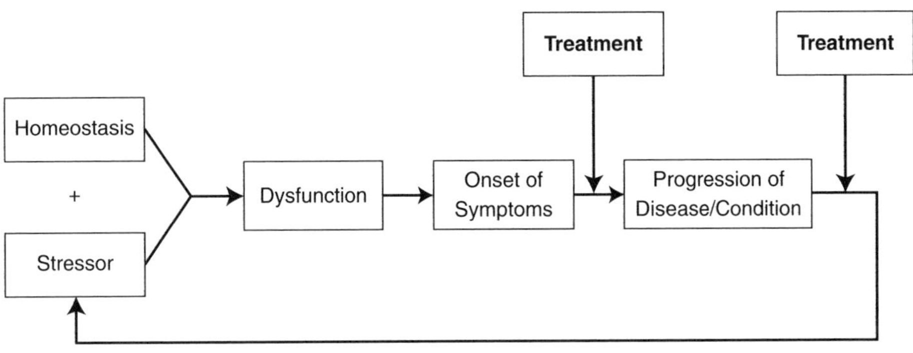

Fig. 3-2

within the muscle that are not traumatized." He goes on to state that other muscles, including those overlying the injured one, will contract in a nocifensive reflex in order to "minimize the noxious drive at the spinal level."

Buskirk asserts that this protective mechanism is the reason why treatment should be neurologically-based instead of mechanically-based. That is because direct stretching increases nociception and worsens the guarding. Instead, techniques which modulate neural activity should be used. He considers the osteopathic techniques of strain-counterstrain, muscle energy, and high-velocity, low-amplitude manipulation as good options to achieve this.

Myofascial trigger points are yet another way an unresolved dysfunction can feed-back into the wellness continuum. That is because they often exist on their own once the stimulus which created them is gone. This causes aberrant neurological input (such as pain) from the muscle they reside in. They can also cause activation or development of other trigger points through reflex mechanisms. Travell and Simons describe many of these connections in their text.[31]

Myofascial trigger points have even been shown to alter movement patterns. Lucas et al. found that trigger points in the scapular rotator muscles not only changed local muscle activation patterns, but they also changed distal activation patterns.[32] Therefore, allowing trigger points to remain activated will cause even more problems by altering motor control patterns. In turn, this alters normal biomechanics and places added stress and strain on surrounding joints and soft-tissues. It also reinforces muscle imbalances by recruiting the hypertonic muscles at the expense of the inhibited ones (This causes many problems. An important one is atrophy of phasic muscles like the multifidi). Segmental motor control is replaced by a pattern of "en-bloc" recruitment, which further deprives mechanoreceptors of vital afferent input. Examples of altered movement patterns and their widespread effects are detailed in Chapter 6.

Altered posture perpetuates itself through the mechanisms described previously. Therefore, even though the original stimulus for its development is gone, it will continue. It will also cause other problems by interfering with normal mechanoreceptor input. Or, it may cause mechanical strain on a related joint, thereby creating a disorder such as patellofemoral dysfunction or impingement syndrome.

Surgical scars are another important dysfunction capable of adding into the "cycle." This is because they "affect soft tissue in all its layers from the skin to the subcutaneous tissues, the superficial and deep fascias, the muscles, and even the tissues of the abdominal cavity."[33] By this involvement, scars can send nociceptive input back into the system. They also create mechanical shortening which leads to guarding, altered posture, etc. Unfortunately, in many cases, the patient does not complain of pain at the site of the scar. We see this frequently with appendectomy and Cesarean section scars. Because the patient does not perceive the pain at the surgical site, the scars are rarely treated. This allows the scar to interfere with function for months, years, or even decades before it is finally (if ever) addressed. Lewit describes how gentle manual treatment of the scar can be extremely effective in treating many musculoskeletal conditions.[33]

The examples listed above are just a few of the many ways dysfunction feeds back into the system to either perpetuate itself or disrupt homeostasis (See Fig. 3-3). But why does this occur in the first place? After all, it seems quite contradictory to say that the body is a complicated machine capable of healing itself and then infer it is responsible for perpetuating its own problems. The answer to this dichotomy goes back to the reason we have the stress response in the first place: survival. Our ancestors needed protection from predators and adverse living conditions. We saw this on a grand scale when we dissected the stress response and its effects on the internal environment. We discussed it on an equally great scale when we detailed the speed of the startle response. Even on a smaller scale, we discovered protection was the key when we read Buskirk's research on the nocifensive reflexes.

These reflexes fit into the homeostatic process as positive feedback mechanisms. Guyton described this mechanism as one which feeds back into the system, creating a vicious cycle.[3] He notes that there are only a few beneficial uses for this form of control including childbirth, nerve signaling, and blood clotting.

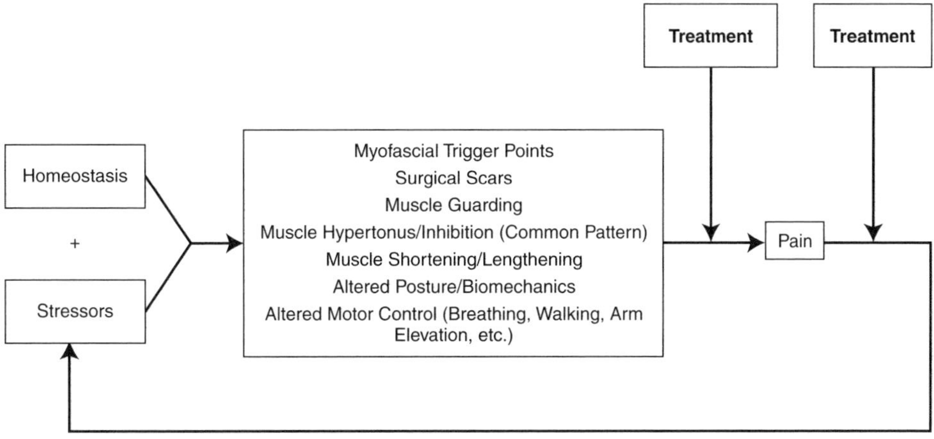

Fig. 3-3

Otherwise, he considered positive feedback as something which did not lead to stability but rather "to instability and often to death."[3] In the case of musculoskeletal dysfunction death is not the end-result, fortunately. However, this cycle certainly helps pave the way to chronic pain.

ALTERNATIVE APPROACH

As we discussed in Chapter 2, the alternative medical approach works under the philosophy that the body is extremely adept at the maintenance and repair process. Consequently, it is believed that the body can heal itself if the obstacles to healing are removed. For this reason, treatment is applied on the left side of the wellness continuum, geared at removing these obstacles and allowing the body to heal itself.

By treating at the start of the wellness continuum, the chosen intervention is often able to have widespread benefit. That is because the cause of disrupted homeostasis is altered, thereby stopping a cascade of effects. A good example of this is seen in a research report out of Sweden. Leboeuf-Yde et al studied the responses of 1504 patients being treated by chiropractors for musculoskeletal problems.[34] These patients were asked if any *non*-musculoskeletal problems improved (after their previous visit) on their own without being intentionally treated. Twenty-three percent of respondents (342 of 1504) reported at least one positive change. This percentage was directly related to the number of areas of the spine manipulated. For patients adjusted in just one area of the spine, only 15% reported a positive change. For those adjusted in 4 areas this number rose to 35%. Most of the improvements patients noted were related to respiratory function* (26% of positive responses) and digestive function (25%), though many patients reported improved vision (14%) and circulation (14%) as well.

Of course, due to the nature of the study we cannot make powerful assertions as to exactly how chiropractic manipulation helped reduce these symptoms. What is known, however, is the fact that treatment applied at the start of the continuum (to a vertebral subluxation) led to changes in various symptoms appearing at the end of the continuum (Fig. 3-4). This is consistent with alternative medicine's assertions that treating the body—and removing impediments to optimal function—will allow it to fight disease, restore normal function, and

---

* The study's researchers eliminated cases where the adjustment helped improve rib cage elasticity directly).

heal itself. It also reinforces the belief that musculoskeletal problems (especially those emanating from the spine) can lead to visceral problems.

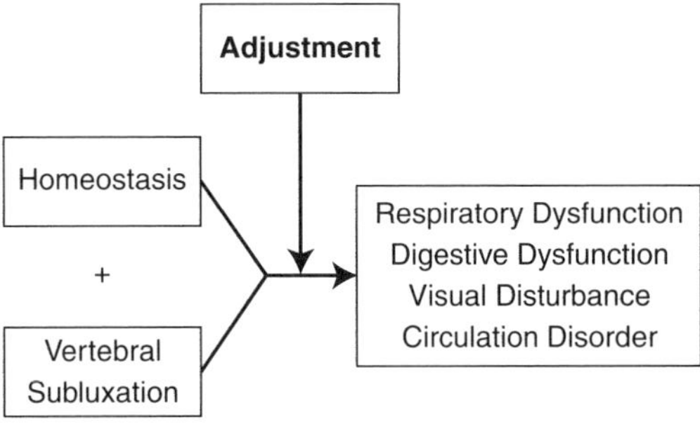

Fig. 3-4

With these principles in mind, let's look at an example of how the alternative approach works. Take a patient suffering with low back pain as we discussed in Chapter 2. Imagine he goes to see a chiropractor who determines his most significant finding is a subluxated atlas. This problem will create great interference in the nervous system, even if it is not painful, due to the rich supply of mechanoreceptors in the area. With this in mind, by addressing the subluxated atlas, it is possible to affect the patient's low back pain as well as the muscle hypertonus, muscle inhibition, lumbar hypomobility, inflammation, and altered motor control coexisting with it. If there are no other perpetuating factors this treatment can eliminate the patient's symptoms and be a long-term solution (Fig. 3-5).

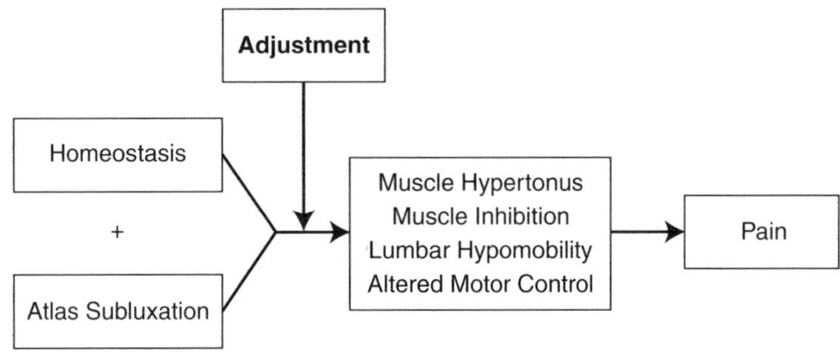

Fig. 3-5

Of course, this is a very simplified case of low back pain. It is also a simple, stream-lined approach to treatment. A more thorough approach to back pain is to address all stressors we outlined in Chapter 2. If we did, the same chart would appear as it does below (Fig. 3-6). Indeed, this would be a powerful, comprehensive regimen with the power of restoring homeostasis and reducing back pain in the process. Do you think a similar program might be helpful to patients

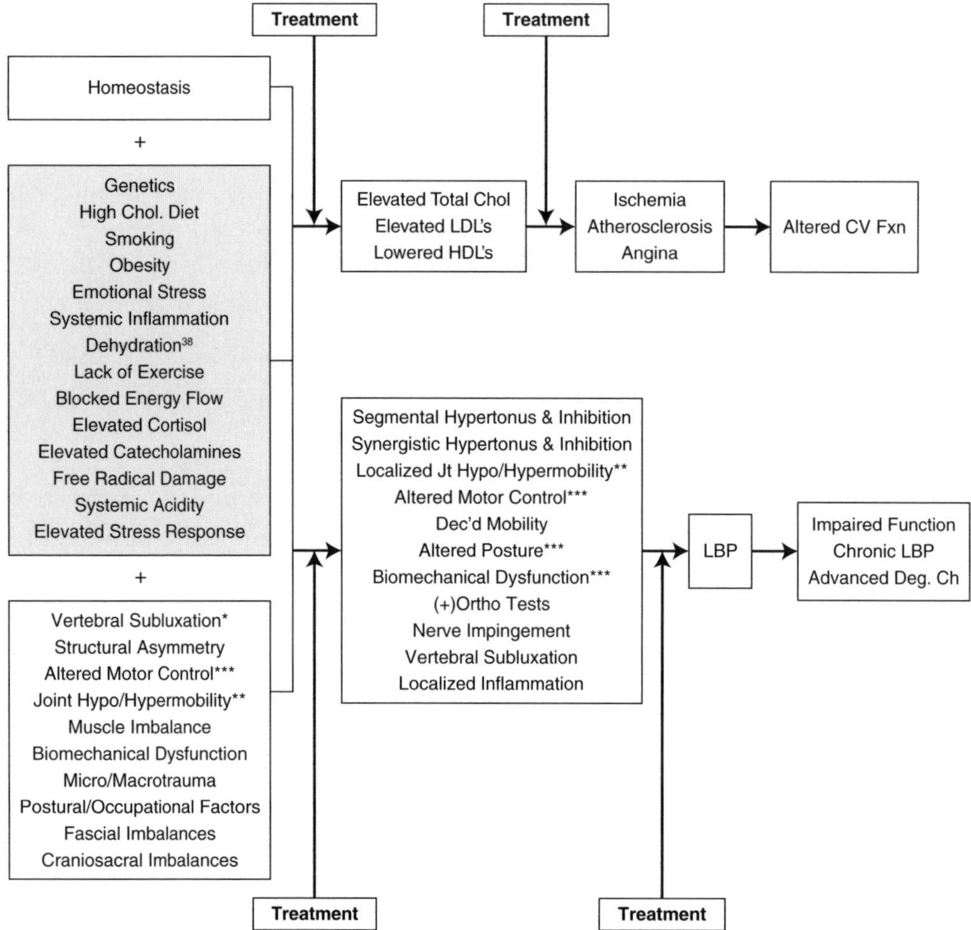

*Included as LBP cause only, although some believe a somatovisceral relationship exists, whereby cardiovascular problems can result from spinal dysfunction
**Referring to hypomobility or hypermobility anywhere in the body
***Indicates that these factors can be the cause or result of altered homeostasis

Fig. 3-6 The alternative medicine approach to low back pain.

with heart disease? Certainly. In fact, it *already* has been proven to be incredibly successful by renowned cardiologist Dean Ornish, M.D.

In his landmark study published in the Journal of the American Medical Association, Dr. Ornish proved that it was possible to actually reverse heart disease with lifestyle changes.[35] His program was *thorough*, to say the least. Instead of just asking his patients to make slight changes to their diets and begin an exercise routine, he forced his patients to take this to the extreme. Their dietary fats and sugars were slashed while their intake of fruits and vegetables were increased exponentially. Stimulants like coffee were discontinued. Smoking was not allowed. Exercise was performed daily. Oh, and that's just part of it. His other major focus was on addressing what he believes to be the underlying cause in most cases of heart disease—the patient's emotional status. For stress reduction, the patients performed meditation, yoga and breathing exercises for up to one hour per day! And to get to the "heart" of the matter, the patients attended a support group as well (the reader is urged to read Dr. Ornish's book, *Dr. Dean Ornish's Program for Reversing Heart Disease*, for the complete intervention.)[36]

In the author's opinion, Dr. Ornish should be applauded for his work. He was not satisfied with the current treatments for heart disease and knew it that there were more effective methods to be found. He also had the drive to find the real causative factors behind heart disease. To do this, he had to look far "outside the box" to recognize the role of the mind and emotions in heart disease. In addition, he was open-minded enough to implement several alternative methods by which to treat it. Bravo!

All of these interventions had one thing in common, of course. They all brought the patient back closer to homeostasis. When this occurs, disease is either prevented or the patient has at least embarked on the road to recovery. In this regard, the dietary changes Dr. Ornish implemented would have greatly benefited the patients' overall health even if they did not have heart disease. That is because this diet, while probably implemented to be "heart-healthy" over 15 years ago, does much more than just help the heart. In addition, it is rich in anti-oxidants, counters systemic inflammation, and is alkalizing. Together, these healthy qualities help with almost all conditions. (By the way, Dr. Ornish performed a similar study in 2005 to examine the effects of his program on patients with prostate cancer. He found that his program led to a drop in PSA levels over the course of one year, whereas the control group PSA levels rose. He also demonstrated something even more impressive. The blood from the experimental group was able to kill cancerous cells with a 70% success rate, whereas blood from the control group only had a 9% success rate.[37] How about that for the healing power of the body!)

In short, we see that treatment addressing *all* factors disrupting homeostasis has an incredible effect on the entire system. This reduces or eliminates the stress response. It leads to improvement in the patient's biochemical, neurological, mechanical, energetic and movement pattern status. Subsequently, the "building blocks of disease" can be eradicated, as can the "building blocks of musculoskeletal dysfunction."

Despite the great benefit from this treatment approach there is one important disadvantage. This is due to the many feedback loops mentioned previously. These reflexes allow the results of dysfunction to feed-back into the process, thereby perpetuating and aggravating the pathology. This short-circuits many of the efforts made at the start of the continuum.

THE APPROACH

Now that we have discussed the principles of homeostasis (and the wellness continuum), it is time to discuss the proposed method of treatment, Complete Manual Therapy. Simply put, this system is a comprehensive approach to manual therapy utilizing all of the concepts previously mentioned in order to restore optimal physical function. In some cases it uses traditional methods of treatment. In other cases it uses alternative methods. Most often, though, it utilizes the best of both worlds for maximum efficacy.

We begin this discussion by describing *what* the approach treats. For the most part, this includes the primary and secondary factors stressing the body. Following this, the general method *how* Complete Manual Therapy addresses these factors is presented. This includes a basic framework for integrating the treatment principles provided. This helps the clinician organize and implement a thorough regimen to address any and all sources of stress.

THE PRIMARY AND SECONDARY FACTORS

The Primary Factors

In the Complete Manual Therapy approach it is important to address the four primary factors. That is because each of them (mechanical, neurological, energetic, and motor control) has the power to create and/or perpetuate musculoskeletal dysfunction on its own. More often than this, however, we see them working in conjunction with one another to cause musculoskeletal problems. In either case, the involved factors must be addressed to restore homeostasis.

Unfortunately, there are few (if any) professions or approaches which address all four factors. In fact, some of them treat only one or two. Their frequent success with this limited approach confirms the notion that involvement of a single factor can lead to musculoskeletal dysfunction. At the same time, their inability to succeed with a significant percentage of patients signals the inadequacies of this limited approach. It is for this reason that all factors must be addressed.

The Secondary Factors

As with the primary factors, all of the secondary factors are addressed in the Complete Manual Therapy approach. This is because these stressors also have the power to create and perpetuate musculoskeletal dysfunction. Again, it is unfortunate that there are very few (if any) professions or approaches which address all of these factors. Failing to treat a problematic secondary factor stressing the system results in sub-optimal outcomes in the same way ignoring a primary factor does.

APPLICATION

In order to effectively combine all concepts presented thus far, we must lay out a thorough plan of action. That way, we can be sure all primary and secondary factors are addressed with each patient. This ensures all stressors causing or perpetuating the patient's problem are eliminated.

The first thing we will do is separate the treatments into whether they treat the patient's problem directly or indirectly. Treatments addressing a problem directly are used to create a knowable change at the area of involvement. Most often, this change occurs with one of the four primary factors. Sometimes direct treatment is applied locally. Other times it is applied distant to the involved area. As long as the results of treatment are known to affect the involved region in a physical manner, they are considered direct treatments.

Treatments addressing a problem indirectly are different. They are not utilized to create a knowable change at the area of involvement. Instead, they are known to benefit the system as a whole, thereby benefiting the involved bodypart indirectly. As with direct treatment, this therapy can be near or distant to the site of symptoms. Examples of this approach are often seen in chiropractic—especially at times when people report somatic improvement outside areas neurologically or mechanically connected to the treated area. Or, as reported previously, when patients report improvement in visceral function when the adjustment was intended to benefit the musculoskeletal system.

Needless to say, classifying all treatments with 100% accuracy is not as important as including them in the first place. That is because each treatment addresses factors with the power to create or perpetuate symptoms. In most cases there are numerous factors playing a role in the patient's symptoms. This is especially true in subacute or chronic cases, or in those of insidious onset. But it is also true when there is a dominant factor responsible for the patient's problem. In a case like this it is obviously important to treat this factor as a top priority. However, it is also important to remember that the entire body is connected. Therefore, the clinician has the power to speed-up the healing process by eliminating all of the body's stressors and helping it function at its potential.

The general outline behind Complete Manual Therapy is presented below. Included under each subheading are specific examples of direct and indirect treatment to help the reader distinguish between the two. Additionally, further discussion is given to the wellness continuum and the role each factor and treatment plays in it.

DIRECT TREATMENT

Primary Factors

Direct treatment via the primary factors consists of those treatments we know are beneficial to the patient in a specific fashion. This includes anything with a known effect on a mechanical, neurological, energetic, or movement pattern basis.

Locally: Treatment is applied directly to the affected area. It has a great effect on pain and even removes a cyclical effect. Our goals are to decrease pain, normalize muscle tone, normalize motion, etc.

1. Joint mobilization/manipulation of the affected area or in the immediate vicinity in order to increase mobility, improve normal function (on many levels), and restore structural symmetry.
2. Soft tissue techniques including massage and myofascial release to relax muscles, increase blood flow, and remove adhesions. Trigger point therapy to eliminate myofascial trigger points in the symptomatic area that are causing pain.
3. Strengthening/facilitation exercises to address muscle imbalance, influencing both the neurological and mechanical systems. This also helps stabilize hypermobile areas.
4. Stretching of tight structures to address muscle imbalance, influencing both the neurological and mechanical systems.
5. Modalities to reduce inflammation, pain, and possibly to increase elasticity of tight tissues.
6. Movement pattern retraining—this involves techniques related more to movement than to postural re-education. Additionally, it relates in many ways to specific muscles' activation/inactivation and recruitment patterns. A common way this is used in physical therapy is teaching patients to "turn-on" certain muscles while performing a given task. For example, teaching a patient with shoulder impingement to contract his lower trapezius during arm

elevation leads to better scapular positioning and stabilization. This improves leverage for the rotator cuff muscles and lessens mechanical strain and pain. These techniques also help re-program the system over time to allow for prolonged improvements in leverage, symptom reduction, and diminished mechanical strain.

7. Neurologically-based techniques such as strain-counterstrain, functional technique, and positional release therapy, each of which is intended to reduce excessive muscle tone. Muscle energy techniques fall into this category as well because the primary way they benefit the patient is by influencing the nervous system and causing relaxation of the muscle being stretched.
8. Taping techniques applied to the affected area to alter structure, improve circulation, and/or influence the nervous system.

Distant: These techniques are applied away from the symptomatic bodypart and are known to benefit the symptomatic area by reducing mechanical strain, normalizing neural function, decreasing pain, etc.

1. Manual treatment to normalize structure. This is through manipulation, mobilization, and specific stretching/strengthening which improve structural symmetry thereby resulting in reduced mechanical strain on an affected bodypart. For instance, correcting pelvic asymmetry can restore symmetrical scapular positioning, thereby reducing impingement symptoms. Another good example of this is seen in Chiropractic Biophysics, an approach which places great importance on restoring the normal cervical lordosis. This is believed to improve the normal curvature of the rest of the spine.
2. Manual therapy to normalize joint motion along the kinetic chain can reduce problems at distant areas suffering from mechanical compensation. For example, we all know what happens when talocrural dorsiflexion is limited: the body must get extension from somewhere else. It may try to pronate even further, which causes breakdown of the midtarsal joint. It may force the 1st MTP to dorsiflex beyond 65 degrees. Or, it may cause knee hyperextension. It may even cause increased hip extension, anterior pelvic tilt and excessive lumbar lordosis at the end of stance phase in order to maintain a fairly-normal gait pattern. Because of this, restoring normal motion in an articulation like the talocrural joint can have predictable benefit to any of these joints if they are symptomatic. Dysfunction in any of these joints can

influence one another in a similar way; whether it is in the sagittal, coronal, or transverse plane (or a little of all three).

3. Orthotics to improve structural symmetry of the entire kinetic chain.
4. Proprioceptive training to improve balance and overall stability. This is mostly a neurological process, as the nervous system is forced to recruit stabilizing muscles at reflex speed in order to maintain balance.
5. Treatment to normalize neural function. In this section this approach is limited to those treatments which work along the course of a specific nerve or a nerve root distribution by affecting innervated soft tissues or joint structures. For instance, treatment via manipulation/mobilization often results in improved neural tone in the extremities. Remember that this relationship can run in the opposite direction as well, from the periphery to the center.
6. Energy techniques such as reflexology or acupressure which involve pressure applied distant to the affected bodypart but are intended to reduce pain in a specific area.
7. Movement therapies which have a widespread affect. For instance, practicing the primary control in Alexander Technique results in a lengthening of the entire spine. Doing this while arising from a seated position has been shown to reduce low back pain. Another example is teaching a patient with a pattern of femoral internal rotation, genu valgus, and excessive pronation to walk, arise from sitting, and ascend stairs with attention on maintaining the knees facing forward (instead of going into valgus). This leads to decreased anterior pelvic tilt, reduced lumbar facet compression, and less pain. It also reduces pronatory stress in the lower limb.

Secondary Factors

As with treatment via the primary factors, the goal of addressing the secondary factors is to reduce pain and strain on the affected bodypart. Many of these stressors are related to static posture; they are the things we spend the majority of our day and night doing. Then there are dynamic stressors, including repetitive motions performed at home and on the job. Simply put, for each stressor it is important to maintain structural symmetry to reduce aberrant strain on the affected bodypart.

Also note that some of these stressors are the cause of the patient's problem, or at least a partial cause. In other cases, the person's dysfunction (along with the ensuing common pattern) may have worsened their posture. So, we do not always know if we are treating the cause, the effect, or both. In any event, reducing strain on the affected bodypart will benefit the patient's condition. Below are common stressors addressed directly in Complete Manual Therapy.

1. Standing posture. Deviation in any of the three planes creates a strain pattern throughout the body. The practitioner can use his/her knowledge of biomechanics to minimize these asymmetries and reduce stress on the affected bodypart by teaching the patient to assume a different standing posture. Further discussion of standing posture is presented in Chapter 8.
2. Sitting posture. Changing a person's sitting posture can have marked effects on their condition. This is for two reasons. For one, most people sit way too long each day. Second, it can be incredibly stressful on the spine and upper extremities when an improper posture is assumed. Again, the practitioner can use his/her knowledge of biomechanics to reduce stress on the affected bodypart. Please see Chapter 8 for further discussion.
3. Sleeping posture. The position a person sleeps in can easily aggravate his condition, so the patient must be questioned thoroughly on this topic in order to minimize stress on the affected bodypart. Please refer to Chapter 8 for a detailed review of postural faults and treatment options.
4. Driving position. Like sitting, driving puts the spine and shoulders in a very awkward position if it is done improperly. Chapter 8 details the asymmetrical posture associated with driving.
5. Repetitive occupational tasks. These stressors may vary widely, depending on the person's job. A thorough history is necessary to ascertain what tasks are performed over and over, as well as the exact form used during these tasks. From there, the clinician can work to lessen strain on the affected bodypart by changing the way the patient performs these tasks. Additionally, he or she needs to evaluate the rest of the kinetic chain to be sure the rest of the body is moving as it should so that force is widespread and not localized to one bodypart over another. In Chapter 6 this concept is discussed further.
6. Repetitive tasks at home. The things a person does at home over-and-over can also irritate his or her condition. Remember to question the patient thoroughly to find out what he does at home that irritates his condition so that his form/technique can be altered. In some cases, even teaching the patient to break up a time-consuming task into smaller tasks is beneficial. These concepts are presented in greater detail in Chapter 8.

INDIRECT TREATMENT

Primary Factors

Indirect treatment via the primary factors involves those treatments we know are beneficial to the patient in general (and thus his condition), although there is not a direct connection between the given intervention and the patient's area of complaint. This creates a category of techniques which help balance the entire system in a mechanical, neurological, energetic, or motor control-wise fashion.

Mechanically, this treatment includes anything which restores structural symmetry or mobility. In chiropractic, for instance, it is believed that restoring normal structure in one area of the spine will improve structure elsewhere, because the entire vertebral column is connected. Likewise, in orthotic therapy, we may assume that correcting excessive pronation/supination can have beneficial effects for the entire body, even up to the temporomandibular joint. This is because everything is connected.

Myofascial release practitioners perform what seem to be "miracles" using this model. They attribute their success to the continuity of the fascial system. Indeed, the fascial system envelops every structure of our body so it makes sense how these miracles occur. Craniosacral practitioners work in this realm as well, influencing the fascial system enveloping the body's most important component, the CNS. Of course, they also influence the nervous system to a great extent with their techniques.

Neurologically, we must implement treatment with the goal of normalizing the function of the entire nervous system. Most of this is in regards to normalizing afferent input, as this is what feeds back upon the system and helps create the stress response and associated guarding patterns. Special emphasis should be placed on areas with high mechanoreceptor/proprioceptor innervation and/or dural connections, such as the upper and middle cervical spine, pelvis, coccyx, temporomandibular joint, and the feet. Methods to assess and treat these areas are presented later in this text.

The patient's movement patterns can also have marked effects on homeostasis thereby making it impossible for the body to heal itself. A common movement pattern disorder is dysfunctional breathing. This dysfunction can sometimes occur insidiously, though many experts believe it is a result of pain, emotional stress, or some other factor which causes a "guarded" pattern of breathing. This causes local problems, of course. But is also causes problems for all living tissues due to relative hypoxia. This results in obvious local and systemic problems.

Fortunately, it is possible to restore normal breathing and even normal pulmonary function in the majority of patients. Again, this is just one more way we can positively affect the system and its capacity to heal. Just imagine doing every technique in the book on a patient without adequate oxygen flow going to the tissues! Would one *expect* him to get better?

The energy-based techniques have an important role here as well. That is because they can enhance the overall healing capacity of the body. Studies point to their ability to stimulate the release of endorphins and enkephalins, both of which are powerful natural pain killers. They are also able to stimulate the parasympathetic nervous system, which promotes all phases of the rest and digest process. Practitioners already use these principles to enhance function of the endocrine and circulatory systems before treatment, which we can do as well.

Secondary Factors

Indirect treatment of the secondary factors involves addressing any stressor which can impact the body's overall healing ability. It also includes treating any secondary factors not covered under 'direct' treatment if there is not a known connection between the stressor and the patient's condition.

Emotions. During our discussion of the stress response in Chapter 2 we outlined the devastating effects stress has upon the body. We listed the chronic diseases stress leads to, and we described the way it also creates musculoskeletal dysfunction. In other words, emotional stress—from anger to sadness to loneliness to anxiety—plays an important role in the formation of dysfunction and disease. It also causes a change in autonomic balance, often favoring sympathetic dominance. This causes numerous changes including reduced tissue perfusion. The corresponding drop in vagal tone favors inflammatory conditions, as mentioned later in this chapter. These findings, along with countless other negative sequelae, make this topic one the manual therapist should be well-versed in so that he can provide optimal care. Please see Chapter 22 for a thorough discussion of this important topic.

Diet. A person's diet is directly related to their overall health, so it is not surprising that it can cause or perpetuate musculoskeletal disorders. This may be by creating systemic inflammation or acidifying the body. In other cases, a person's diet is not so much toxic as it is deficient in vital nutrients. This disables the body's healing mechanisms, thereby stalling or preventing the repair process. Please see Chapter 8 for further discussion of dietary factors.

Sleep Quantity. Besides the physical position a person sleeps in, it is also very important to consider the quantity of sleep a person gets. This is important to the health of the individual and vitally important to the healing process. Please see Chapter 8 for further details on the effects of sleep deprivation.

Dehydration. As mentioned previously, dehydration has devastating effects on the entire body, including the musculoskeletal system. Batmanghelidj reports dehydration has many causes, including the stress response.[38] It can also occur due to inadequate water intake, or the intake of diuretics such as caffeine and alcohol. He also states that many prescription medications are to blame for dehydration.

Interestingly, dehydration is believed to also cause the stress response instead of just resulting from it. Because of this relationship, the list of musculoskeletal disorders attributable to dehydration is not limited to just those tissues requiring copious amounts of water to function. Instead, by triggering the stress response, dehydration creates many other musculoskeletal problems.

Lack of Exercise. Few people get the right amount of exercise our bodies need to function optimally. In fact, most people not only fall short of the recommended amount of exercise—they do not come anywhere close. This is unfortunate, as regular exercise is proven to benefit almost every system of the body. This ranges from improved cardiopulmonary function to enhanced insulin sensitivity to improved mental health. In fact, studies show that regular exercise can be as beneficial as prescription drugs at controlling anxiety and depression.[7]

One of the many ways exercise helps us is by burning up the norepinephrine released in the stress response so that it is not allowed to circulate in our systems for a prolonged period of time. In addition to this, exercise causes the release of endorphins. This reduces pain and improves mood.

Neurologically, researchers point out that the barrage of afferent mechanoreception exercise provides helps to modulate noxious stimulation. It also helps to "feed" the cerebellum, drive the cerebral cortex, and has countless roles in modulating central nervous system function. Please consult Chestnut for further details on the neuroanatomy and neurophysiology behind these benefits and many others.[39]

Last but not least is exercise's benefit to the joints. Repetitive motion helps lubricate the joints, maintains mobility, increases circulation, and helps maintain strength (of osseous and soft tissues). This is absolutely necessary to avoid the devastating effects of immobilization.

Standing, Sitting, Sleeping, Driving Postures and Repetitive Motions. For these stressors we will use assessment and treatment principles similar to those described in the previous section. The only difference is our intention. That is, we will not entirely rely on the mechanical benefit of enhanced posture or improved form. Instead, we will consider all effects on the health of the individual including respiration, energy expenditure, proprioception, etc.

By treating the body with these indirect methods we are striving for a slightly different goal than we were under the direct approach. In this case we are working more closely with the concept of "holism." We are also trusting the healing power of the body by assuming that it can remove dysfunctions on its own once the factors disrupting homeostasis are eliminated.

Treatment under this premise takes place at the start of the wellness continuum. This leads to widespread improvement—especially when a stressor is able to affect the health or function of the musculoskeletal system. This was discussed earlier when we noted that dehydration can lead to disc and synovial joint damage because both of them need water to function properly.

The other important way treatment at the start of the continuum has widespread effects is by addressing stressors which trigger the stress response. In this case, we can see how diet, sleep deprivation, and dehydration can cause even more widespread problems. Consistent with the rest of this text, remember that any treatment which reduces or eliminates the stress response is of great benefit.

SAMPLE CASE

Now that we have dissected the elements of the Complete Manual Therapy approach, let's see how it can be used to treat a common musculoskeletal problem: insidious-onset low back pain.

Low Back Pain. As we have discussed previously, insidious-onset low back pain can be caused and perpetuated by a number of different primary and secondary factors. In this example we will examine and address *all* factors (as noted later in the chapter there are reasons why we would not perform all treatments on the same visit.) Please note that in this example, treatment is detailed with the assumption that there is dysfunction present; this is obviously not always the case in the real world.

DIRECT APPROACH

Primary Factors

Local:

1. Joint mobilization/manipulation of hypomobile lumbar/pelvic joints.
2. Soft-tissue techniques to reduce tone/increase mobility of painful muscles: quadratus lumborum, lumbar erector spinae, iliopsoas, gluteals. This includes trigger point work, massage, and myofascial release among others.
3. Therapeutic exercise to increase strength/facilitate weak muscles in the lumbar region. This involves many "core" muscles, such as the multifidi, transversus abdominis, and rotatores.
4. Therapeutic exercise to increase flexibility of the psoas, erector spinae and hamstrings.
5. Modalities to reduce pain and inflammation.
6. Acupressure applied to points on the low back.
7. Movement therapy to reduce strain on the low back. This includes teaching the patient to stabilize his low back during certain activities. It also involves showing him how to accentuate or diminish the amount of lumbar lordosis during a specific activity.
8. Strain-counterstrain/positional release technique to reduce tone of tender low back muscles.
9. Taping of the lumbar spine.

Distant:

1. Joint mobilization/manipulation to restore structural symmetry and mobility to the entire spine with the intention of lessening strain on the lumbar region.
2. Mechanical therapy along the kinetic chain. This involves gait analysis and evaluation of the lower extremities to investigate for asymmetries/movement

restrictions. Address any abnormality with an intervention to reduce strain on the low back. This may include fitting the patient for orthotics, performing manual therapy including joint mobilization/manipulation, or implementing therapeutic exercise. Instructing the patient to consciously correct postural faults, such as excessive hip internal rotation and anterior pelvic tilt may help as well.

3. Proprioception/balance training to increase strength and stability of the entire spine. According to Janda, this form of therapy is effective at strengthening inhibited muscles at reflex speed. This benefits the lumbar spine for obvious reasons; the more stable each joint is, the easier it is for the joint to remain in the neutral position.
4. Acupressure or reflexology applied to points known to reduce lumbar pain and inflammation.
5. Movement therapies involving the entire body often benefit the lumbar spine. One technique proven to help the low back is the arising-from-sitting drill taught in the Alexander Technique. Although this technique is primarily focused on maintaining proper head and neck posture, it can often help reduce low back pain by changing alignment and muscle recruitment.
6. The patient's dynamic activities (at home, work, and play) need to be evaluated. Again, treatment in this context is focused on reducing strain on the low back. For everyday activities treatment is relatively straightforward. For complex movements such as throwing or running, effective therapy is more complicated. We must spend more time dissecting the patient's form in order to find overt biomechanical errors. We also must come up with effective solutions to help reduce stress on the affected bodypart without hindering the person's performance. Please see Chapter 6, Movement Pattern Considerations for further discussion of these mechanical principles.
7. Stretching/strengthening exercises addressing muscle imbalance in the rest of the spine which could be placing greater stress on the low back.

Secondary Factors

The patient's standing, sitting, sleeping, and driving postures must be assessed and treated as necessary to reduce mechanical strain on the low back. Remember that the low back tends to go into excessive lordosis with most people while standing. The opposite occurs with sitting; most people lose their lordosis completely when sitting in an average chair. Specific ways to address these static postures are presented in Chapter 8, The Secondary Factors.

INDIRECT APPROACH

Primary Factors

1. Any mobilization/manipulation to restore normal mobility/symmetry to the spine and pelvis.
2. Any manual technique to optimize proper mechanoreceptor input into the central nervous system. Special attention should be paid to areas with high mechanoreceptor innervation and dural connections, such as the upper cervical spine. Other important areas are the middle cervical spine, pelvis, coccyx, TMJ and feet.
3. Techniques designed to restore normal mobility to the soft tissues of the body (esp. fascial and neural/meningeal). Prime examples of this are the approaches of craniosacral therapy and myofascial release. These techniques are revered for their ability to help conditions distant to the area being treated by either mechanical or neurological influence.
4. Breathing retraining.
5. Acupressure or reflexology to points corresponding with improved immune and endocrine functioning. This enhances the body's overall healing ability.

Secondary Factors

1. Dietary advice. Focus on having the patient avoid pro-inflammatory and acidifying foods. Replace these with fresh fruits and vegetables (Note: there are many more dietary interventions that could be included in this discussion, but we are limiting these due to differences in the readers' respective scopes of practice. Because these two topics are well-publicized and thoroughly researched it is believed all practitioners can implement these simple ideas into their practice).
2. Advise the patient to drink an adequate amount of water each day. Many authorities agree that 8-eight ounce glasses are sufficient. Remember to

educate the patient in the things which cause dehydration, including caffeine, alcohol, some prescription medications, and hot weather among others.

3. Advise the patient to get close to 8 hours of sleep each night.
4. Advise the patient to stop smoking.
5. If the patient is obese, advise him or her to lose weight. This benefits the lumbar spine mechanically. It also reduces the systemic inflammation produced by adipocytes.
6. Assess the patient's emotional status. Stress, fear, anxiety, as well as other emotional factors can play a role in the development of the person's problem as well as its continuation. Please see Chapter 22 for further discussion.
7. Advise the patient to begin a gentle, non-impact exercise regimen 3-5 times per week, 20-30 minutes per session. This is so that the patient receives all the benefits of exercise as detailed previously. Please note that this exercise program should not aggravate the patient's symptoms. For the low back this means that an exercise requiring prolonged flexion like bicycling is not a good idea. On the other hand, walking is regarded by many as an excellent activity for the lumbar spine.[40] Take caution in implementing a new exercise regimen, however. It should start out relatively short in duration (according to the patient's tolerance) and with less frequency than listed above. (Note: some clinicians believe that patients with elevated cortisol levels should not begin an exercise program until this problem is resolved. Therefore, if the patient has this disorder, proceed with caution. See Stressed Out Headed for Burnout by Mladenoff for further information.[41]
8. Make changes to the patient's posture and form as indicated, even when a direct link between this and their presenting problem is not clear. Reducing strain upon the entire system will help the body repair the problematic area.

EFFECTS OF TREATMENT

Now let's examine how this treatment fits into the wellness continuum. As we see in Figure 3-7, treatment is implemented throughout the continuum. Going from left-to-right, we start by addressing the numerous stressors which disrupt homeostasis. These are varied in the way they influence the body, but each can lead to low back pain and must be addressed.

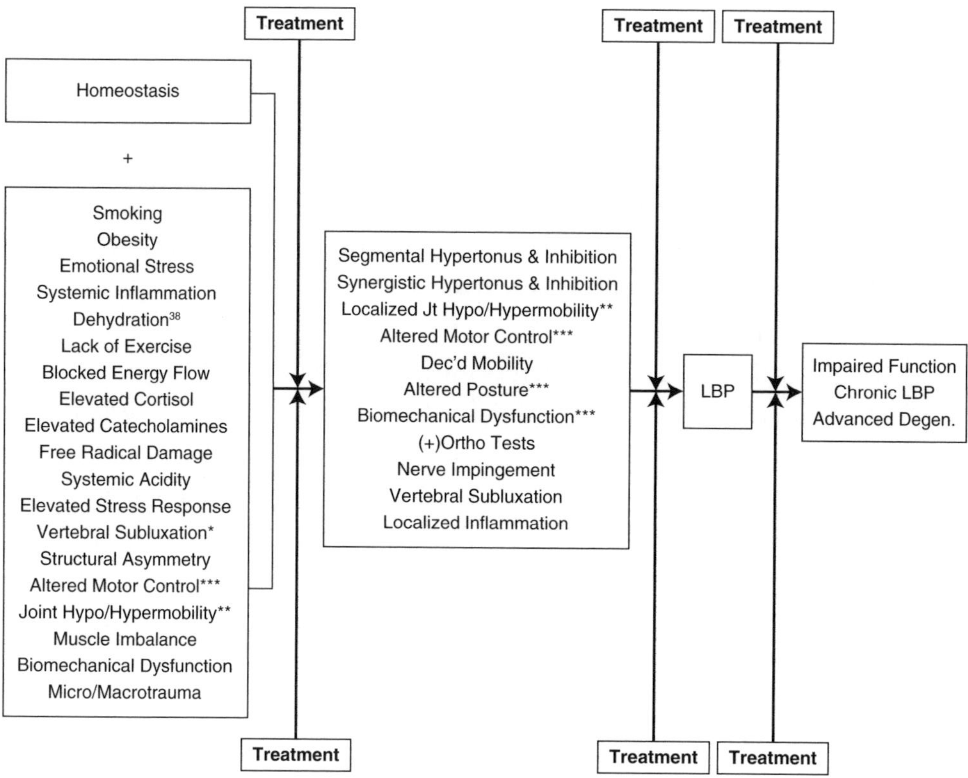

Fig. 3-7

Treatment is also carried out on the right side of the continuum. There, we treat many of the problems resulting from disrupted homeostasis and some problems due to the actual onset of low back pain. Remember, many of these factors have the ability to feed-back into the entire process, thereby perpetuating the main problem even if the original causative factors are addressed.

A brief summary of the effects of treatment is as follows:

1. Reduction in low back pain and local inflammation. Less positive feedback into protective muscle guarding patterns as well.
2. Restoration of normal tissue tone.
3. Reduction of common pattern intensity. This greatly reduces strain on numerous joints and soft tissues in the low back and throughout the entire body. Please see Chapter 9, The Common Pattern for a thorough discussion.
4. Improved hydration.
5. Lessened postural stress on the low back.

6. Increased strength of intrinsic/extrinsic muscles; enhanced stability.
7. Improved mobility osteokinematically and arthrokinematically.
8. Improved structural symmetry.
9. Reduction in sympathetic nervous system dominance; reduced circulating cortisol and epinephrine levels.
10. Less emotional interference; less hormonal involvement and diminished startle pattern.
11. Normalized energy flow throughout the body.

This is a good summary of the goals of Complete Manual Therapy. In actuality, we can summarize these goals even further: remove all obstacles interfering with a balanced, healthy state of homeostasis. This allows the body to heal itself and regain optimal function. As discussed previously, one of the most important ways it does this is by reducing the stress response and the presence of the common pattern. In fact, by modifying these processes we are able to make a quantum-leap in our ability to treat the musculoskeletal system. Instead of treating a single factor and getting a single improvement, we are treating multiple factors and getting an exponentially greater result. So, the result of treatment is not just the sum of all we do. It is much more. That is because the stressors to homeostasis have the power to create *so* many negative effects. They cause structural dysfunction, neurological dysfunction, movement pattern dysfunction, biochemical dysfunction, circulatory dysfunction, respiratory dysfunction, etc. This affects the system in a progressive manner, as we see with the wellness continuum. But it also creates problems due to different feedback mechanisms. This keeps the patient's problem going and going.

It is worth noting that some of the factors listed can play a sort of "double-duty." That is, they are capable of creating the stress response but they may also result from it. Two such factors are systemic inflammation and dehydration. This relationship only helps the process perpetuate itself; consequently, it underscores the importance of addressing these stressors. It also underscores how important it is to address all potential stressors.

PATIENT MANAGEMENT

The example above was provided to illustrate how the Complete Manual Therapy approach can be used to treat a common musculoskeletal problem. What it did not cover was the way in which treatment is applied, including the sequence of treatment application, progression, etc. These are all important points which can impact the patient's response to therapy.

In Complete Manual Therapy we are addressing all factors influencing the patient's system, so it is important to prioritize treatment according to methods we normally use. This relates to the mechanism of injury (insidious or traumatic), the stage of injury (acute, subacute or chronic), the irritability of the condition (low or high), and most importantly, the physical findings. Taking all of these factors into consideration we can decide what treatment should be applied initially as well as the intensity and quantity of treatment. Of course, in acute, irritable cases we would be judicious in our treatment selection so as to not aggravate the person's condition. In cases of traumatic onset we would be equally selective, especially if the injury was recent and the amount of overall involvement was relatively localized.

In chronic, non-irritable cases of insidious onset, treatment is more aggressive and comprehensive from the start. That is because many factors played a role in creating the person's symptoms. In addition to this, other factors became dysfunctional as the problem affected the entire system and more time passed. In a case like this, clinical judgment must come in again. We cannot bombard the patient's system with every manual therapy technique in existence because this will aggravate his condition. This can occur due to the force or pressure being applied, which may create a local inflammatory response. Moreover, even if local irritation is not an issue, treating too many areas at once is just too much for the system to handle.

On the other hand, we do not want to do too little. If only one area of the body is treated, or perhaps just one primary factor is addressed at a time, what about the other areas/factors involved? They often perpetuate the patient's problem through a myriad of reflexive pathways and other mechanisms. This quickly negates any positive result stemming from a limited treatment regimen. In further support of a comprehensive approach is the article previously mentioned, *"The Types and Frequencies of Improved Nonmusculoskeletal Symptoms Reported After Chiropractic Spinal Manipulative Therapy."*[34] In this study there was a direct relationship between the number of areas of the spine/pelvis manipulated and the number of unexpected, non-musculoskeletal improvements noted by patients: 1 area = 15%, 2 areas = 22%, 3 areas = 32%, 4 areas = 35%. With all of these things in mind, I believe we must resort to balance and sound clinical judgment. A good rule of thumb is 'not too much, not too little, and observe the patient's progress closely.'

Dealing with the secondary factors is entirely different. They can and should all be addressed immediately to reduce stress on the system without fear of exacerbation. For instance, a patient is not going to have a flare-up because he is put on an anti-inflammatory diet full of antioxidants. Nor is he going to feel worse because he is no longer slouched forward for eight hours per day at work. Drinking an adequate amount of water does not put a person into a tailspin either. Neither does handling stress in a more beneficial manner. Removing these negative stressors only benefits the system and should be done from the start.

GLOBAL VS. LOCAL TREATMENT

One of the most important aspects of patient management is determining where the patient's problem is—or at least where the causes of the problem lie. The clinician must ask himself, "Is this a local problem, a global problem, or does it involve a little bit of both?" This can certainly be a difficult question to answer if we are not methodical in our examination. Typically we find most clinicians are adept at examining and treating a problem locally. Many are also good about looking at adjacent structures to see if they are causing a problem. But the same cannot be said for problems stemming from global dysfunction. This is because there are just so many things to either miss or forget to look for—not to mention that some of the most influential parts of the body are just plain neglected by many of us.

For all of the reasons mentioned above, a quick screen has been developed to help the clinician gauge the overall state of the body and determine how much influence *it* is having on the patient's symptoms. Accompanying each step in the exam is a quick explanation as to why each component is assessed and exactly how it relates to the system as a whole. The way the common pattern manifests itself is also described in several of the tests. This helps expedite the exam and provides a good way to document progress as treatment ensues. The screen is as follows:

Gait analysis. A person's gait reflects the overall state of the locomotor apparatus from a mechanical, neurological, and movement pattern standpoint. Deficits in virtually any system will show themselves when an individual walks.

Postural analysis in sitting and standing. Mechanical dysfunction and neurological dysfunction manifest themselves in one's postural pattern. Expect to see the typical flexed posture, with upper and lower crossed syndromes. Most evident in this pattern is forward head carriage, upper cervical extension, lower cervical hypolordosis, coxa varum, genu valgum, and excessive pronation. In addition to this pattern look for other asymmetries including head tilt/rotation, high/low shoulder, scoliosis, and pelvic obliquity.

Observation of the patient's sit-to-stand pattern. As described in Chapter 6, this simple movement is performed incorrectly by the majority of patients. Expect to see excessive cervical and lumbar extension coupled with genu valgus. See Figure 6-3.

Observation of a miniature squat. By having the patient squat halfway to the floor we can examine for breakdown throughout the entire lower body. We expect to see "squinting patellae" with internal rotation of the femurs, genu valgus, and excessive pronation as part of the common pattern. Keep in mind that hypermobility is often present when we see significant breakdown in all three areas.

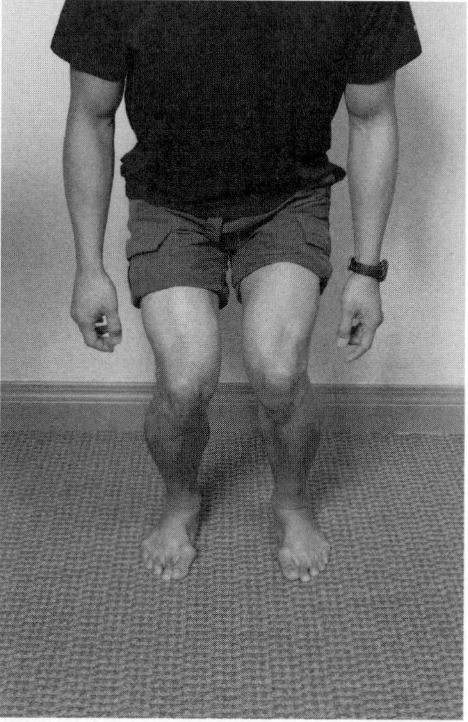

Fig. 3-8 Miniature squat demonstrating 'miserable malalignment'.

Observation of the quality and depth of respiration. Mechanical, neurological, and movement pattern disorders often manifest as paradoxical breathing. This stresses the structures at the cervicothoracic junction and ultimately results in decreased oxygen perfusion to all tissues.

Romberg test. This is a classic test to scan for neurological dysfunction. Very quickly we can test the patient's cerebellum, vestibular system, and dorsal column/medial lemniscal pathways for lesions. The patient will sway or deviate to the side of lesion in this test. With this information we can apply treatment to stimulate the appropriate region (Fig. 3-9).

Fukuda's marching in place test. This is another test to scan for neurological dysfunction. Again, we are testing the cerebellum, vestibular system, and dorsal column/medial lemniscal pathways for lesions. In this test, a positive result is when the patient turns to one side while marching in place with the eyes closed. The side to which the person turns is the lesioned side. As with the Romberg test we can use this information to stimulate the appropriate side (Fig. 3-10).

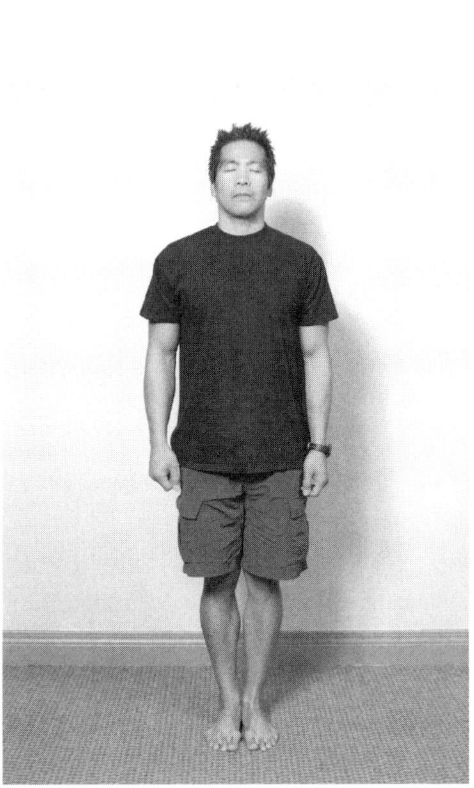

Fig. 3-9 Romberg test. Observe for subtle deviation towards the lesioned side.

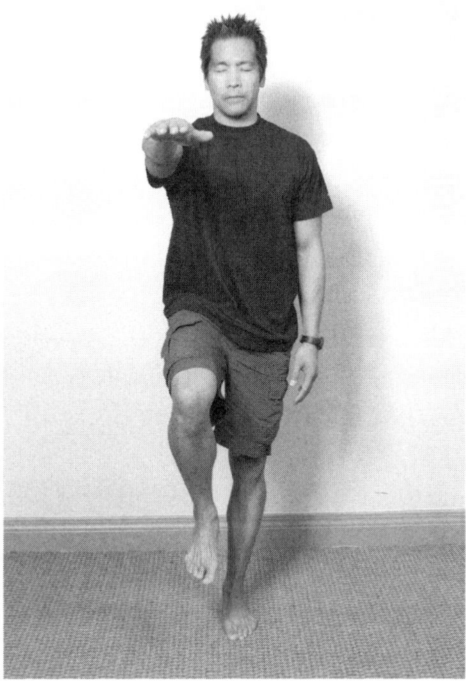

Fig. 3-10 Fukuda's marching in place test. Have the patient march in place, raising the ipsilateral arm as each leg elevated. After a few cycles have him close his eyes and continue for 30 seconds. Rotation of the body to one side indicates a lesion on that side.

Upper Cervical examination. In Chapter 11 the importance of the upper cervical spine is discussed in detail. Suffice it to say that it is arguably the most important region of the body and has more influence over the health of an individual than any other area. For these reasons it must be examined with every patient. Please see Chapter 11 for its examination and treatment.

Middle Cervical examination. Mechanical and neural stressors often place the mid-cervical spine in a hypolordotic postural pattern. This robs the CNS of vital mechanoreception (the C4-5 level of the spine has the greatest concentration of mechanoreceptors anywhere in the body), puts tensile stress on the spinal cord, and causes compensations in the rest of the spine. This means that dysfunction here can lead to system-wide problems. Specific assessment and treatment techniques are presented in Chapter 11.

Temporomandibular examination. The TMJ has tremendous influence on the nervous system; when it is not working properly neither is the rest of the body. This relationship is best described by Fonder in his article the Dental Distress Disorder. In a nutshell, Dr. Fonder's research shows a distinct connection between malocclusion and numerous chronic health disorders. He points out that the sympathetic nervous system is the mediator of these disorders, as it is activated due to the aberrant firing of high numbers of proprioceptors and mechanoreceptors in the joint complex. Examination and treatment techniques for the TMJ are presented in Chapter 12.

Pelvic girdle examination. The pelvis plays a very important role in the health of the individual. Mechanically it functions as the base of the spine. This means that it influences the rest of the spine on a mechanical level and can cause and/or perpetuate dysfunction in this regard. Similarly, the pelvis' mechanical alignment can affect the lower extremities, thereby compromising all related joints below the waist.

In addition to this, the pelvic girdle appears to have an equally strong neurological influence on the entire system. Several approaches have capitalized on this relationship and treat the pelvis as a means to treat the entire body. Two examples are craniosacral therapy and sacrooccipital technique, where the pelvis is treated along with the rest of the craniosacral system. Its clinical significance does not stop here. Just consider the Logan Basic approach, wherein the primary treatment is manual release of the sacrotuberous ligaments. Yes, balancing these ligaments is intended to balance the body altogether.

The work of others, including Dvorak and Dvorak supports the idea that the pelvic ligaments have global neurological influence.[42] These authors illustrate how different points along the course of the sacrotuberous and sacrospinous ligaments correspond to different levels of the spine, and how these areas can be treated to help the corresponding spinal segments.

One more author deserving mention on this topic is Dr. Henri Gillet. He is known as one of the original developers of the motion palpation adjustive technique. He was also the leader of a chiropractic research group in Belgium which contributed a vast amount of material to the chiropractic profession. One of the group's biggest contributions was the discovery of several "spinal fixation complexes."[43] These involve patterns wherein patients demonstrate a group of subluxations—seemingly unrelated—which exist together on a consistent basis. The pelvis is involved in most of these complexes, and dysfunction of different pelvic ligaments is described as a specific causative factor. For this reason, Gillet and his group suggest specific ways to stretch these ligaments. Please see Chapter 15 for further details.

The pelvis' influence on the body's movement pattern schema cannot be forgotten either. The presence of the lower crossed syndrome and all of its corollaries help set in motion a chain of dysfunction above and below the pelvis. For all of these reasons the pelvis must be evaluated and treated. For assessment and treatment techniques turn to Chapter 15.

Foot examination. We began inspecting the general structure of the feet during gait, while the patient arose from sitting, and while he performed a miniature squat. In addition to this we must examine the foot with the patient prone so we can look for asymmetries including forefoot varus, rearfoot varus, rearfoot valgus, and so on. Manual examination is performed after this to determine the general mobility (or lack thereof) of the foot, with special attention paid to the amount of dorsiflexion at the first MTP and talocrural joints. Remember that restrictions in these two joints in the sagittal plane often force compensations throughout the entire system.

Besides creating mechanical strain throughout the body, foot dysfunction impacts the nervous system. Authors such as Rothbart point out the importance of proper biomechanics so that the nervous system is given the right stimulation to coordinate patterns of muscle contraction and inhibition necessary for normal gait.[44] In applied kinesiology this concept is echoed, as foot dysfunction is often blamed for cases of neurological disorganization. There are even reflex points along the feet (termed gait reflexes) applied kinesiologists treat to stimulate proper upper and lower extremity coordination during gait.

If anyone is still not convinced what a major role the feet play in the health of the entire individual, just consider the field of reflexology. Practitioners using reflexology can affect the entire body just by working on the feet. This is considered an energy-based technique, and it is incredibly useful to the manual therapist. Further discussion of reflexology is presented in Chapter 7, and further information on foot assessment and treatment is presented in Chapter 18.

Stress screen. Determining the involvement of the sympathetic nervous system is integral to an accurate patient assessment. As we have learned, this is because sympathetic dominance negatively impacts the musculoskeletal system and may perpetuate the patient's problem no matter what manual therapy intervention we impart. Consequently, this screen is used to determine how much attention we must focus on treatments to lessen the patient's stress while improving their biochemical/hormonal/emotional status. The components of this screen are as follows:

1. Check pupillary diameter. Stressed individuals tend to have dilated pupils while relaxed individuals have constricted pupils.
2. Check the pupil's ability to hold a constriction. They should be able to hold a constriction for at least one minute before fatiguing. In people with a poorly functioning parasympathetic nervous system, we see the pupils lose their constriction before one minute has elapsed. Oftentimes the pupils undulate in and out, trying to maintain the constriction.
3. Check the temperature of the hands and feet. The sympathetic nervous system shunts blood away from the extremities and causes the hands and feet to become cold. Take this to the extreme and we have Raynaud's phenomenon (a component of FMS).
4. Check the blood pressure as the patient rises from a supine position (Ragland's test). Ideally, the systolic reading should go up 10mmHg. In individuals with adrenal fatigue the systolic pressure does not rise and often drops! These people have stressed their systems for so long that the sympathetic nervous system can no longer act quickly when pressed (as when arising from supine).
5. Palpation of flexor muscles and the 18 points used in diagnosing fibromyalgia syndrome. Tenderness of these muscles gives us a general idea of how stressed the musculoskeletal system is. This can be from sustained contraction, as we see with any facilitated muscle. It can also be due to biochemical issues including excessive lactic acid production and/or deficient waste removal.

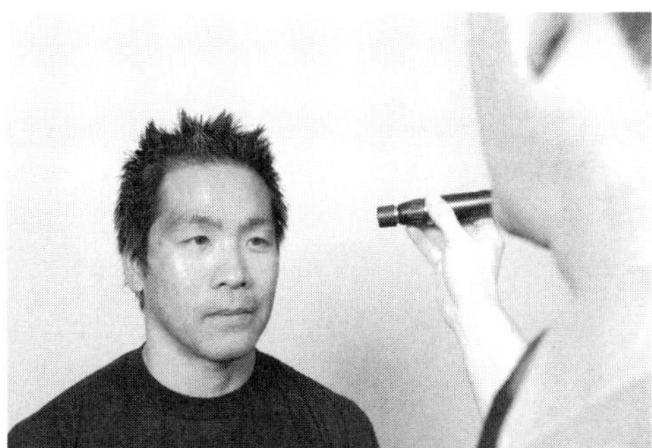

Fig. 3-11 Check the pupil's ability to hold a constriction.

The tender points used in diagnosing fibromyalgia are especially helpful in determining the sensitivity of the musculoskeletal system (Fig. 3-11). Remember that these points do not signify that the person has a dreaded bacterial or viral disease. Instead, these are points which become painful due to changes within the body. Abnormal sympathetic nervous system function and all of its related sequelae are certainly likely causes.

An excellent example of this cause-effect relationship is presented by Buskilia, who studied the onset of fibromyalgia syndrome following cervical spine injury.[45] He found that 21% of subjects who sustained cervical spine injury developed fibromyalgia within 3.2 months of the injury. By contrast, only 1.7% of people who suffered a fractured leg developed fibromyalgia after the same period of time. Without a doubt, this is an amazing piece of research. Just consider its implications. First of all, it reiterates the importance of the cervical spine in comparison to other parts of the body. Secondly, it illustrates how idiopathic conditions such as FMS really do have a causative factor. Moreover, these "conditions" are usually nothing more than physiological adaptations made by the body. Lastly, this study demonstrates how rapidly the body can deteriorate from a state of health and wellness to one of chronic pain. This substantiates the need to treat the patient expeditiously and thoroughly.

Added to the points already made connecting the stress response with musculoskeletal dysfunction is yet one more. It is of the vagus nerve's function in suppressing inflammation. According to Tracey, the vagus nerve inhibits macrophage synthesis and tumor necrosis factor.[46] This is very beneficial to the overall health of the individual, as systemic increases in TNF depress cardiac output,

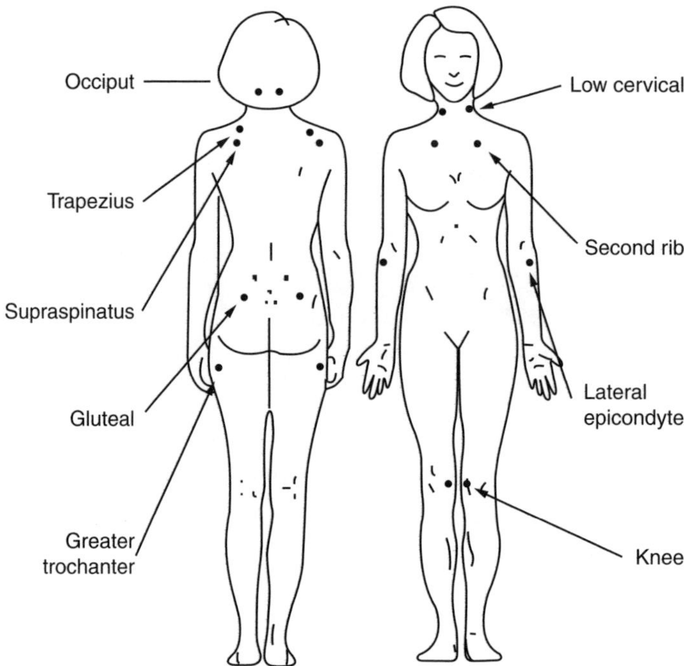

Fig. 3-12 The 18 tender points used in diagnosing fibromyalgia.

amplifies and "prolongs the inflammatory response by activating other cells to release both cytokines such as interleukin-1 and high mobility group B1, and mediators such as eicosanoids, nitric oxide and reactive oxygen species, which promote further inflammation and tissue injury."[46] On a local level, inhibiting the TNF level decreases the cardinal signs of inflammation. Therefore, one can expect that TNF attenuation will result in decreased joint pain and edema. Altogether, this research ties-in the sympathetic nervous system with inflammation once and for all. Thus, one can easily see the value of balancing her patient's autonomic function no matter what musculoskeletal condition is being treated.

As mentioned earlier in the chapter, the components of this screen are "high-yield" ones to the practitioner. That is, for the short period of time it takes the clinician to examine and treat each one, the payoff can be immense. Conversely, ignoring dysfunction involving any one of them can prevent patient improvement.

These components are equally important because they are the best "entry points" into the patient's system. They help streamline the entire process for the clinician, as he does not have to check and treat every possible stressor to the patient's system right away. This gives the therapist insight into the patient's mechanical, neurological, energetic, and movement pattern status in a short period of time. This makes integrating the applied homeostasis approach into one's current practice easy.

4 Mechanical Considerations

MECHANICAL FACTORS PLAY A TREMENDOUS ROLE IN THE ASSESSMENT AND TREATMENT OF THE musculoskeletal system. In fact, it is probably safe to say that this approach dominates the decision-making process of the physical therapist, orthopedist, physiatrist, podiatrist, and ergonomics specialist. This is especially true in this era of evidence-based medicine, where there is an emphasis on treatment we can explain with linear thinking. Moreover, it is easy to compile research reports and data to support a specific treatment regimen that has roots in biomechanics.

The laws of physics dictate the mechanical forces placed upon the locomotor system. Factors such as shear, tension, load, and torque can be determined to help quantify demands placed upon certain muscles and joint structures. To the orthopedic surgeon, these calculations are vital to the success of a particular procedure. The diameter of a screw or perhaps its exact placement may mean the difference between success and failure.

To the manual therapist, knowledge of biomechanics is equally important to success. In fact, the manual therapist's grasp of biomechanics may have to be even more keen. That is because she must know the precise arthrokinematics of each joint, as well as the ways in which one joint affects another, which affects another, and so on. For instance, consider a common mechanical dysfunction such as 1st metatarsophalangeal joint pain. At the local level, we normally find general stiffness with mobility testing. More specifically, we find that the proximal phalanx is not gliding as far dorsally as is required during normal gait. This creates pain with virtually every step and helps set the stage for further irritation and possibly even osteophyte formation at the dorsal aspect of the joint. Local treatment for this problem is directed at restoring normal osteokinematics and arthrokinematics. This therapy is expected to be successful if a traumatic injury was the cause of the patient's problem in the first place. But if there is no incident that precipitated the patient's symptoms, we should look further into the exact cause of the MTP pain. This is necessary because the metatarsalphalangeal pain may only be the proverbial "weak link in the chain." If that is the case, trying to treat the joint locally will only provide temporary relief. Instead, we must look at other joints which have the potential to place extra strain on this region. Among these, restrictions in talocrural dorsiflexion and hip extension will place greater dorsiflexion demands on the 1st MTP joint. Using this reasoning, one can imagine how limitations there place added stress upon all joints in the chain. In this scenario, the 1st MTP joint might become hypermobile initially. Maybe it is able to handle the extra workload for some time without difficulty. However, after repetitive strain on a daily basis, the added motion and stress cause inflammation. This recurrent inflammation causes thickening of the joint capsule and spurring of the dorsal joint. This leaves the joint in a state of degeneration, requiring intensive local treatment and global treatment to treat the causative factor(s).

The example above illustrates how we can use knowledge of biomechanics to guide our treatment—on a local and a global level. On a local level, knowledge of joint mechanics and pathomechanics is of paramount importance. It helps the clinician determine the exact problem within a joint and helps him implement local treatment. It is also on this level the clinician manually assesses joint **mobility**—arguably the major tenet of manual therapy. The diagnosis he makes—whether the joint is normal, hypomobile, or hypermobile—will impact care as much as any other finding.

On a global level, understanding joint mechanics and pathomechanics is just as important. The clinician must know how the patient's **structure**, including postural deviations and asymmetry, can influence the symptomatic area. He must also understand the intricate workings of the **kinetic chain** and be able to link the patient's complaint with any abnormalities in the entire mechanism. Granted, understanding the global influences on a local problem is more difficult than just focusing on the area of chief complaint. Nevertheless, it is absolutely necessary to be able to do this in order to apply a comprehensive therapy regimen.

In the sections that follow, the aforementioned principles are discussed in detail. The reader is urged to utilize these principles with every patient—on a local as well as a global level. Chances are that the mechanical system is involved with every patient to at least some extent. Even when no direct correlation can be made between the patient's presenting complaint and this system, the practitioner can use his expertise to optimize mechanical function and lessen strain to facilitate healing. Where indicated, specific details regarding treatment are also presented here. For the most part, this is when a theory or technique is (a) applicable to the entire body or (b) has the capacity to influence the entire body. Otherwise, specific mechanically-oriented therapies are presented in the regional chapters.

MOBILITY

Joint mobility is the basis of many manual therapy approaches. Too little motion is termed hypomobility. This is where manual therapy plays its most valuable role. Too much motion is called hypermobility. It can be as equally destructive as hypomobility, although the pathomechanics are much different. It can also be treated with manual therapy, just with much different means than we use for hypomobility.

JOINT HYPOMOBILITY

Joint hypomobility is generally considered the primary focus of manual therapy. Numerous approaches from the fields of chiropractic medicine, osteopathy, and physical therapy revolve around the identification and treatment of the hypomobile joint. Many of these approaches view hypomobility primarily as a mechanical problem with a mechanical solution. That is why this topic is presented here (although joint dysfunction is far from being void of influence from the nervous system). In any case, restoring normal motion is certainly a priority for most manual therapy approaches.

There are many reasons why manual therapists focus on eliminating hypomobility. Simply put, hypomobility is usually linked to patients' complaints of pain and/or loss of function. This can be by creating a patient's problem. At other times it is the result of the patient's problem.

Hypomobility is also infamous for creating asymmetry. The concept of asymmetry is well-understood by patients for causing pain and disability. That is because it is a visible, tangible extension of an articular or myofascial restriction. Many of these people consult a chiropractor to put them "back into alignment." They do not realize that the chiropractor is actually "restoring lost motion in order to facilitate proper alignment." Nevertheless, when their motion and symmetry are restored, they are usually delighted to also notice a reduction or elimination of pain.

The effects of hypomobility are not limited solely to the exact area of restriction. In the spine, this is best seen in segments cephalad to a hypomobile vertebra. This may be by way of the kinetic chain, as the body will typically compensate for lost motion in one joint by increasing motion in another. The resultant hypermobility then becomes symptomatic due to increased wear and tear. Further discussion of hypermobility is reserved for a later section.

Degeneration

A major reason for addressing hypomobility is its role in creating spinal degeneration. According to Kirkaldy-Willis, the process of spinal degeneration is often initiated by motion segment dysfunction resulting from altered segmental tone and function.[47] Hypomobility results from this, causing altered segmental biomechanics. This creates repetitive abnormal loading, leading to fatigue of the articular soft tissues.[47] Joint instability then develops as a result of capsular laxity and internal disruption of the intervertebral disc.[48,49,50] If the mechanical derangement is substantial, the body then begins trying to stabilize itself by creating fibrosis and bony exostosis.[49] These changes are now radiographically visible and this added growth may begin to compromise neighboring structures including the spinal cord and exiting nerve roots.[9,50]

Types of Hypomobility

There are several different types of hypomobility. Meadows classifies them as: (1) myofascial, (2) pericapsular, and (3) pathomechanical or subluxation hypomobility.[51] The first category, myofascial hypomobility, refers to the shortening of muscle and fascia. This can be the result of hypertonicity, scarring/adhesions, or adaptive shortening. It results in a non-capsular pattern of physiological motion loss, but arthrokinematic motion is unaffected. Muscle hypertonicity is discussed in Chapter 5, Neurological Considerations.

The second classification, pericapsular hypomobility, is caused by shortening of the joint capsule or ligaments. As with myofascial hypomobility, this dysfunction can be due to scars/adhesions and adaptive shortening. It can also be caused by more severe joint pathology including arthritis, arthrosis, and fibrosis. A capsular pattern of motion restriction is seen in addition to diminished physiological and arthrokinematic movements.

The third classification is pathomechanical or subluxation hypomobility. Quite different from the previous two categories, this form of motion loss occurs when the joint is jammed at one end of the range and motion into the opposite direction is blocked. This occurs due to traumatic injury or repetitive microtrauma. Clinically this manifests as normal range of motion with a normal end-feel into the direction of subluxation. Physiologic and arthrokinematic motion away from the subluxation is limited and comes to an abrupt stop.

Several authors also point to interarticular derangement as a source of hypomobility. Two examples of this form of derangement include the interarticular block and the interdiscal block. Two popular models attempt to explain the interarticular block. The first, suggested by Bogduk and Jull, entails meniscoid *extrapment*. This is said to occur when the meniscoid is pulled out of its normal position by the inferior articular process of a zygapophyseal joint as it moves superiorly during flexion.[47] The meniscoid then occupies space when this process glides downward during extension. This creates pain and limited extension.

The second model is exactly the opposite. Maigne and others believe that meniscoid *entrapment* creates joint dysfunction.[67] This occurs when the meniscoid migrates too far into the joint during poorly coordinated spinal movements or sustained stressful postures.[47] When the patient assumes his/her normal posture, the meniscoid is trapped or the articular capsule is tractioned. This results in pain and muscle spasm.

Interdiscal blocking describes joint dysfunction created by disc derangement. In this model, it is proposed that the nucleus pulposus migrates into a radial fissure of the annulus. It is also believed that fragments of the nucleus can become lodged in the posterior annulus.[47] This creates pain, muscle guarding, and joint locking.

Added to this list of traditional causal factors is Mulligan's structural fault. The structural fault (or malposition) is basically a subtle joint misalignment causing restricted motion. This restriction may be perceived as a soft or hard end-feel, as with other dysfunctions. However, when the joints are aligned properly (with manual pressure), immediate restoration of normal mobility occurs. Thus, the previous hypothesis of muscular or capsular contracture is deemed inaccurate.

Understanding the causes behind hypomobility is unquestionably important in order to formulate an effective treatment plan. Equally important is understanding the implications of hypomobility upon the motion segment. This helps the clinician gain an appreciation for the pathomechanics occurring in the presence of a specific dysfunction, which in turn facilitates the treatment process. But first and foremost, the clinician must have a working knowledge of biomechanics in order to understand pathomechanics. A brief discussion of biomechanics and its relationship to joint dysfunction is presented below.

Hypomobility of the Spine

In order to effectively diagnose and treat hypomobility, one must first understand basic biomechanics. The field of osteopathy has contributed a tremendous amount of work to the field of spinal biomechanics, so its model of joint mobility is presented here. First of all, let us consider the biomechanics of the spine from C2 to L5. When the spine flexes forward, the inferior facet joints of the superior vertebra glide superiorly and forward on the superior facet joints of the inferior vertebra. This motion is termed flexing, and as inferred it entails the *opening* of the facet joints. On the contrary, extension of the spine involves the inferior facet joints of the superior vertebra gliding inferior and posterior on the superior facet joints of the inferior vertebra. This effectively *closes* the facet joints.

The concepts outlined above help explain vertebral dysfunction while also adding more complexity to the entire process. That is, the vertebrae do not move in only one plane of motion, they move in all three. Moreover, motion is not limited to a single joint; rather, it occurs on at least two facet joints under normal circumstances. Again, these possibilities only help expand the number of ways in which the vertebra can become "stuck." Terms such as Flexed, Rotated, and Sidebent (FRS) and Extended, Rotated, and Sidebent (ERS) describe the positional fault of a dysfunctional vertebra. FRS refers to a vertebra which is simply stuck in flexion. One of its inferior facet joints is unable to glide inferior and posterior on the vertebra below it. This leaves the facet joint on the involved side superior and anterior to the facet joint on the uninvolved side. Therefore, the affected vertebra is rotated and sidebent to the opposite side of its extension limitation.

The ERS dysfunction is different. It occurs secondary to the facet joint being stuck in extension, unable to flex on the facet below. In effect, this restriction causes rotation and sidebending towards the side of involvement, as the opposite facet joint is superior and anterior relative to the ipsilateral facet.

Examination techniques are used to differentiate the presence of an FRS from an ERS, and vice versa. This differentiation is important because it allows for the accurate implementation of treatment. For example, let us assume that a vertebra is rotated and sidebent to the right. It that because it is unable to extend on the left, thereby leaving the left facet anterior and superior to the right facet? Or, is it because the right facet is unable to open, again appearing inferior and posterior to the left facet? Proper testing to determine the side of involvement uses a mixture of static and dynamic testing, thus changing osteopathy's viewpoint of a vertebra being simply "out of alignment" to being "out of alignment secondary to an inability to move into a specific direction."

One advantage of this approach is that it does not limit its scope to solely structural asymmetry. While terms such as ERS and FRS are used to describe positional faults, greater emphasis is placed on the motion restriction occurring along with asymmetry. That is why the spine is palpated during motion and at different end-ranges of motion. Osteopathic treatment, therefore, combines restoration of structural symmetry with restoration of function and normal mobility.

The osteopathic model is not the only discipline to describe spinal biomechanics. Both chiropractic medicine and physical therapy offer similar theories and treatment techniques to restore lost spinal motion. Some of the more common approaches and techniques are shared in the chapters dealing with treatment of spinal dysfunction.

Hypomobility of the Extremities

The function of the extremity joints can be visualized as long as the practitioner has a clear understanding of 2 things: the anatomy of each joint and the kinesiology of each joint. It is assumed the reader already has a good foundation in anatomy so joint structure will not be described here. However, the concept that is shared with the reader is that of Kaltenborn's model of arthrokinematics. Basically, this model of arthrokinematics helps describe the specific motion occurring at a given joint. The basic motions available at a given joint are traction, compression, spinning, rolling, and gliding. Traction, compression, and spinning are just as they sound. Traction involves a degree of joint separation, compression involves the approximation of joint surfaces, and spinning is the rotation of a bone about its long axis.

Rolling and gliding motions are possibly a little more complex, as they are dependent upon the shape of the involved joints. Rolling is described just as one would expect. It involves the concave joint surface moving in the same direction as its osteokinematic motion. On the other hand, gliding involves a convex joint surface moving on a concave surface. This results in the osteokinematic and arthrokinematic movements going in opposite directions of one another.

Mobility testing. There are almost as many techniques to evaluate for mobility as there are approaches in manual therapy. However, despite the differences in style, the goals of almost all of these approaches are the same. That is, they attempt to find out: (1) the quantity of movement as well as the (2) quality of movement.

As stated, it is important for the clinician to pinpoint the exact tissues responsible for creating and perpetuating a hypomobility dysfunction. While many approaches have tests to accomplish this task, there are two popular approaches probably used more than any others. The first approach is described by Cyriax. His method is well-regarded by many for its simplicity and ease of application. Simply put, it applies selective tissue testing in order to differentiate offending structures. The second approach is slightly more subtle than the first. It uses the concept of end-feel to determine which tissue is involved. Each of these approaches is discussed below.

Selective tissue testing. When testing the joints, Cyriax made great distinction between contractile and inert structures. Contractile structures include muscles, tendons, and attachments to bone. They are stressed with resisted movements, not passive ones. Resisted motion testing is used to determine both their integrity and degree of involvement. The results of resisted movement testing are interpreted as follows:[52]

1. Strong and painless: nothing is wrong with the contractile structure.
2. Strong and painful: this signifies a minor lesion of contractile tissue.
3. Weak and painless: this suggests either a ruptured muscle/tendon but is more frequently due to nervous system malfunction.
4. Weak and painful: this occurs when serious trouble is present.
5. Painful on repetition: this may indicate intermittent claudication.
6. All resisted movements hurt: this may be due to a proximal lesion or a capsular restriction.

Inert structures include the joint capsule, ligaments, bursae, fascia, displacements, dura mater, and nerve roots.[52] They are tested with passive movements instead of with resisted ones. Cyriax points out that this type of testing also helps the clinician determine an important piece of information. That is, does the lesion involve the entire capsule or another inert structure? A capsular lesion is one which affects the entire joint capsule and its motion will be limited in a particular pattern specific to that joint. To clarify, while the amount of motion loss may vary, the proportion of loss between planes of motion is an important diagnostic point. One of the best-known examples of capsular limitation is in adhesive capsulitis. The glenohumeral joint is most limited in external rotation, followed by abduction, followed by internal rotation. Patients may present with motion limitations of varying intensities, but the proportion of loss between planes of motion will be identical.

When passive motion loss is not in a capsular pattern, the most common causes are internal derangement, ligamentous sprain, and bursitis. These non-capsular lesions often affect only one or two planes of motion instead of more numerous planes as seen with capsular lesions. An example of a non-capsular pattern would be limited shoulder flexion with all other motions free to move normally. This is in contradiction to the established capsular pattern for the shoulder. Therefore, the clinician has to consider the possibility of internal derangement, ligamentous sprain, or bursitis as being responsible for the limitation.

End-Feel. The resistance a joint gives to passive motion at the end of its range is its end-feel. Because each joint has its own normal end-feel, the significance of end-feel testing is in comparing the patient's presentation to that of the established norm. By contrasting the two, the clinician has another means to differentiate what tissue is responsible for creating hypomobility.

The common end-feels are: capsular, bony, ligamentous, soft-tissue approximation, muscular, muscle spasm, interarticular, and empty. A brief description of these end-feels along with a normal example is given in Table 4-1:[47,51]

The implications for this form of testing can be significant. In the case of a pathomechanical end-feel, the clinician may be forewarned to consult a

TABLE 4-1

End-Feel	Sensation	Normal Example
Capsular	Firm but giving; feels like stretching a piece of leather	External rotation of the shoulder
Ligamentous	Like capsular but more Firm	Knee extension
Bony	Hard, non-giving abrupt Stop	Elbow extension
Muscular	Firm but giving; not as stiff as capsular	Hip flexion
Muscle Spasm	Guarded; resisted by muscle contraction	Protective muscle splinting in the presence of acute pain/injury
Pathomechanical	Very hard or springy	Meniscal tear
Empty	No end-feel is reached	N/A

specialist if the patient's problem requires a surgical consult. In other cases, the presence of an empty end-feel alerts the clinician to the seriousness of the patient's condition. However, in most cases, the assessment of end-feel helps the clinician decide what structure is preventing normal joint motion. This allows him or her to plan treatment accordingly.

Treatment concepts. As mentioned above, most approaches in manual therapy center around the treatment of hypomobility. While many of these approaches are similar to one another, there also exists many differences both in their theories and techniques. Let's take a look at some of the more popular approaches to see how they address limited movement:

- *McKenzie.* In his model of dysfunction (not derangement), he approaches a limitation by repetitively moving into the restriction.
- *Faye.* Manipulation is in the direction of segmental motion limitation.
- *Greenman.* Muscle energy techniques and manipulation are performed into the direction of limitation.
- *Maitland.* Mobilizes and manipulates into the pain-free direction early-on; he approaches the painful side only when it is clear that soft tissue restrictions are causing the patient's pain and need to be addressed directly.
- *Maigne.* Mobilizes and manipulates into the pain-free direction so that the patient's condition is not aggravated.
- *Diversified and Gonstead techniques.* Both approaches adjust to correct movement or structural asymmetry directly.
- *Thompson Technique.* The unilateral cervical syndrome is adjusted on the side of the tender facet with the head turned to the opposite side (usually the pain-free side).
- *Jones' Strain-Counterstrain.* This puts the spine or bodypart into the direction of ease, thereby putting the tender soft tissues on a slack. For tender points on the posterior cervical spine, for instance, this involves rotation in the opposite direction.

As illustrated above, many successful approaches in manual therapy use techniques that appear to be 180 degrees apart from one another. *But how can that be? How can two approaches following such opposing principles possibly be effective?* The answer lies in the nature of the limitation.

As outlined previously, there are several different causes for hypomobility. These differences must be taken into account to understand why a specific treatment works. They also explain why a specific treatment does not always work. The rationale is as follows:

- *Capsular tightness.* This is consistent with McKenzie, Faye, and others who use a direct approach to increase mobility. Especially in the absence of a neurological component or structural fault, capsular tightness must be addressed directly in order to stretch shortened tissue or break adhesions. McKenzie advocates frequent stretching in order to remodel collagen.
- *Muscle/tissue shortening.* This is consistent with several approaches. Directly stretching, mobilizing and manipulating into the direction of restriction are ways to address this type of limitation.
- *Muscle hypertonicity.* This is consistent with Jones' strain-counterstrain, Thompson's unilateral cervical syndrome and other indirect techniques that reduce the neural input to the muscle. The author believes this category also encompasses Maigne and Maitland, both of whom propose mobilization/manipulation away from the side of pain.
- *Meniscoid entrapment or other loose body.* Paris proposes that some cases of neck or low back pain are caused by meniscoid entrapment. He suggests an exercise which recruits the multifidi, which subsequently pull the meniscoid out from the joint space.[53]
- *Structural fault.* The presence of a structural fault is simultaneously proven and corrected by the application of a Mulligan technique. However, because it frequently needs to be re-applied by the patient, there is obviously concomitant tissue shortening or hypertonicity perpetuating it.

Accurate differential diagnosis is vital for effective treatment. In some cases, choosing the wrong approach only serves to only irritate the patient's condition. This occurs when approaching a structural fault, entrapment, or facilitated muscle with aggressive stretching into the restriction. This is probably why Maitland and Maigne suggest manipulating away from the pain, especially in acute and subacute conditions. On the other hand, by addressing a capsular restriction indirectly, it is unlikely to break adhesions or lengthen shortened tissues. Maitland addresses this problem as well. His suggested treatment progression illustrates both of these points. Treatment begins by going away from pain, and as the patient improves more direct treatment is implemented. This progression is used in the spine and extremities.

As our discussion of hypomobility was focused on mechanical considerations, our discussion of proposed treatment is also limited to those methods grounded in mechanical theory. The reader must be aware that the influence of the neurological system is not to be understated. Even in treatment which theoretically affects only the mechanical system, the nervous system is collecting data and responding in ways we may or may not be aware of. See Chapter 5 for further discussion.

JOINT HYPERMOBILITY

While hypomobility is the primary focus of manual therapy, hypermobility is a concept widely neglected by manual therapists. Perhaps this is because hypermobility is more difficult to identify than its counterpart. Or, maybe it is because hypermobility is more difficult to manage than hypomobility. Certainly, cases of hypermobility do not respond in the same way to manual therapy as hypomobility does. There are no quick fixes with hypermobility, either. But that is not to say the manual therapist does not have any treatment options to benefit these patients. In actuality, he is in an excellent position to treat this condition. He just has to alter his typical mentality and adopt a philosophy built on stabilization instead of mobilization. This begins with understanding the different forms of hypermobility. These are presented below.

Instability

The term instability refers to the loss of the passive restraints to joint motion—namely the ligaments. This typically occurs secondary to trauma, where the ligaments are torn and joint integrity is lost. This allows the joint to move past its normal end-range during movement. It usually also results in slight separation of the joint surfaces, leading to aberrant motion of one articular surface on the other. Together, these abnormalities promote joint destruction. This case of hypermobility is best treated by the orthopedic surgeon.

On the other hand, there are two other causes of instability well-within the scope of manual therapy treatment. They are microtrauma and joint degeneration. With microtrauma, poor postural patterns and structural asymmetries overstretch ligaments, leading to a loss in joint integrity. With degeneration, loss of disc height and articular cartilage thickness lead to a loss in tension in the surrounding ligaments, creating a degree of instability as well. This is the second stage Kirkaldy-Willis describes. It results from hypomobility, which created the degeneration in the first place.

Localized Hypermobility

The term 'localized hypermobility' refers to a joint (or a limited number of joints) with an excessive amount of motion. This is distinguished from systemic hypermobility in that it involves an isolated region instead of the entire body. It is distinguished from instability in that instability involves a pathological increase in motion whereas hypermobility indicates a joint has an increased amount of motion—but it is still within normal anatomical restraints. Nonetheless, hypermobility still increases stress on the joint surfaces while also forcing supporting musculature to work harder than normal.

Isolated hypermobility can be due to several different factors. The most common one is a neighboring hypomobility, which creates the hypermobility just to compensate for lost motion. In chiropractic this concept is well-accepted. Chiropractors recognize the importance of finding and adjusting the hypomobile segment regardless of where the patient experiences symptoms. This is fortunate, as the hypermobile area is frequently more symptomatic than the hypomobile one. This is usually due to increased stress on the area as well as compensatory muscle spasm attempting to splint the area. Taken to a greater degree, one sees the long-term results of spinal fusion in the segments adjacent to the surgical stabilization. These levels become hypermobile and degenerate very quickly.

Another common cause of localized hypermobility is altered function of the active subsystem (muscles) and the control subsystem (mechanoreceptors and the neural control centers). This compromises the ability of these two subsystems to prevent movement exceeding the normal neutral zones when internal or external perturbations are introduced.[54] This results in delayed response of the active subsystem, and stability is effectively lost. Wear and tear of the joint ensues.

Treatment for this disorder starts by addressing joint dysfunction, as it is the decrease in afferentation from joint mechanoreceptors which begins this chain reaction in the first place. In addition to this, weakened/atrophied muscles must be strengthened so they can perform their normal duties. Last but not least, the patient should undergo a thorough program of sensorimotor training to integrate these changes into improved overall function. Please see Chapter 6 for further details on this regimen.

Systemic Hypermobility

As the name implies, systemic hypermobility refers to hypermobility throughout the entire body. While this can be due to pathological conditions such as

Erlos-Danlos Syndrome, systemic lupus erythematosus, Marfan Syndrome, or rheumatoid arthritis, the focus in this text is on its most common form, Hypermobility Syndrome. Hypermobility syndrome (HMS) is basically a systemic collagen abnormality affecting the musculoskeletal system, cardiac tissue, and the smooth muscles in the gastrointestinal system and female genital system.[55] Most notable is its effects on the musculoskeletal system, however, as criteria for HMS is actually based on articular hypermobility. One of the first such methods to diagnose hypermobility was presented by Beighton et al.[56] To qualify, the patient must have a score of at least 5 out of nine (See Table 4-2) on a standardized scale.

TABLE 4-2 Beighton scale for hypermobility. Score one point per extremity for the first four tests. Score maximum of 1 point for the last test.

1.	Apposition of the thumb to the forearm. Do bilaterally.
2.	Hyperextension of the 5th MCP joints to 90 degrees. Do bilaterally.
3.	Hyperextension of the elbow, >10 degrees. Do bilaterally.
4.	Hyperextension of the knee, >10 degrees. Do bilaterally.
5.	Trunk flexion whereby the palms lie flat on the floor.

In addition to the Beighton scale, there are certain areas of the body the practitioner can quickly examine to aid in the diagnosis of hypermobility. Keer and Grahame list several areas as 'potentially fruitful' ones in which to observe hypermobility.[57] They include:

- Extension of the hands and fingers while actively outstretched
- Excessive wrist flexion and extension
- Lateral rotation of the shoulder (>90 degrees)
- Cervical spine rotation greater than 90 degrees, lateral flexion greater than 60 degrees.
- Ability to insert four fingers vertically placed into open mouth
- Thoracic spine rotation of 90 degrees
- Internal + external hip rotation of 150 degrees
- Ankle dorsiflexion and plantarflexion of 90 degrees
- Passive hyperextension of the 1st MTP greater than 90 degrees

As one would expect, HMS predisposes the patient to excessive wear-and-tear on joint surfaces and soft tissue structures. This is in good part due to abnormal joint mechanics on a local level, as the ligamentous laxity allows aberrant joint motion (loss of passive stability). On a global level, hypermobility also leads to an exaggeration of the common pattern—which is readily evidenced by the patient's posture. Expect these patients to suffer from many of the sequelae of this pattern.

To make matters worse, the nature of hypermobility syndrome makes the patient more susceptible to the effects of trauma while also making it more difficult for them to heal. This combination undoubtedly confounds manual therapists, and it earns many of these patients the stigma of being "difficult to work with." This unresponsiveness to conventional treatment is not their fault, of course. It just underscores the importance of recognizing and treating this syndrome appropriately. For the most part, treatment must stabilize rather than mobilize. The clinician should prescribe supports, where appropriate, to protect vulnerable structures. Activities at work and home must be altered to reduce stress and strain on the system as much as possible. Really, every secondary factor must be evaluated and addressed. Therapeutic exercise plays an important role with these patients as well. Strengthening exercises as opposed to stretching exercises are highly indicated—although the clinician must take care to be sure the patient is not doing more harm than good.

More important than traditional strengthening is sensorimotor training. Studies show that patients with HMS often have impaired joint proprioceptive acuity.[57] In effect, this allows excessive motion in the joint's neutral zone, which will stress the joint further. Sensorimotor training exercises help re-train the active and neural control systems, thereby optimizing dynamic stability. This is exactly what these patients need to lessen stress on joint and soft tissue structures. Please see Chapter 6 for further details on this regimen.

STRUCTURE

Many approaches/professions in manual therapy focus on structure as an important piece of the puzzle. One way they do this is by observing the patient's posture. Now, while posture was mentioned as a secondary factor, it is also a primary factor. That is because many practitioners use methods to physically change the client's posture—making this a dynamic entity instead of a static, unchanging one.

A second important way therapists integrate structural ideas into practice is by looking for patterns of asymmetry. These are seen almost everywhere we look. Some of these can be corrected with manual therapy. Other times, the therapist can only provide the patient with supports to compensate for the asymmetry. In both cases, it is necessary the therapist know how to recognize and treat structural asymmetry. A manual therapy approach to posture and structural asymmetry is presented below.

POSTURE

Examination of the patient's posture can lend invaluable insight to his or her condition. By analyzing the person's structure in all three planes—sagittal, coronal, and transverse—the clinician can detect asymmetry or abnormality. Then, by using the laws of physics, he or she can predict specific areas of the body that are prone to excessive stress and strain. With this knowledge, the clinician can begin forming an idea why the patient's problem occurred and then formulate a treatment plan.

Postural analysis consists of observing the body from all sides. Analysis from the side is frequently done with the help of a plumb line. This is used to help the practitioner make a more accurate, objective postural assessment. Ideally, the plumb line should pass through the following structures (Fig. 4-1):[58]

1. the external auditory meatus
2. the bodies of the cervical vertebrae
3. the glenohumeral joint
4. slightly anterior to the bodies of the thoracic vertebrae
5. transect the vertebrae at the thoracolumbar junction
6. the bodies of the lumbar vertebrae
7. the sacral promontory
8. slightly posterior to the coronal axis of the hip joint
9. slightly anterior to the coronal axis of the knee joint
10. slightly anterior to the talocrural joint
11. across the naviculocalcaneo-cuboid joint

From the posterior perspective, the plumb line should pass:[47]

1. through the midline of the skull
2. through the spinous processes

3. through the gluteal crease

4. midway between the knees

5. midway between the ankles

Specific landmarks should also be inspected for unleveling or asymmetry, including:[47]

1. gluteal folds

2. gluteal contours

3. iliac crests

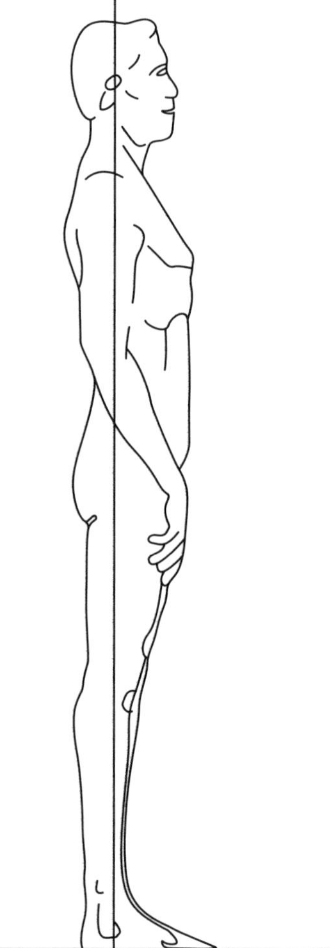

Fig. 4-1

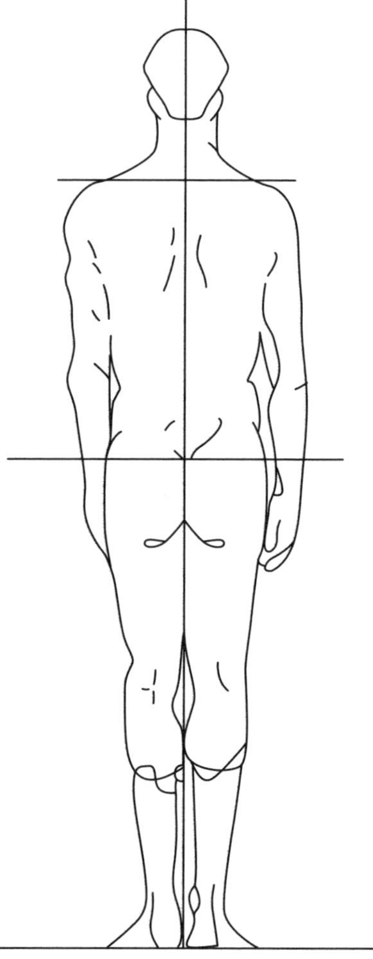

Fig. 4-2

4. PSISs
5. rib cage
6. inferior angles of the scapula
7. vertebral borders of the scapula
8. acromioclavicular joints
9. ear lobes

On the local level, information should be collected regarding specific details. Among other things, this includes the position of the affected bodypart and any difference in landmark height to its counterpart. In the shoulder, for instance, we should examine the position of the scapula. Any asymmetry in height compared to the opposite scapula is significant. We should also note the relative position of the scapula in all planes. It is tilted forward in the sagittal plane? Is it rotated downward in the coronal plane? Is it protracted in the transverse plane? All of this information is important because it will affect the shoulder's function. In fact, a specific finding may tell the clinician why the patient's "insidious onset" shoulder pain developed. This connection may then be used in the patient's treatment. In the case of shoulder pain, the clinician may take measures to change the scapula's position in order to reduce stress on the symptomatic glenohumeral joint.

We can also use the posture of the entire body to help in our assessment and treatment planning. Mechanically, we can use the laws of physics to help us predict increased areas of stress due to distant postural faults. This is especially helpful when it comes to problems such as forward head posture, which has widespread effects throughout the entire body. Further discussion of this destructive, common postural fault is presented below. Please note that this postural fault is presented in this chapter because it is traditionally considered as a mechanical dysfunction, but in actuality it also greatly affects the nervous system.

Forward Head Posture

As its name implies, forward head posture (FHP) is identified as the anterior displacement of the head relative to the body. The results of this common postural fault involve more than just the head and neck. Instead, the forces of gravity are altered all the way down to the feet. This makes sense from a mechanical perspective, which is why FHP is included in this chapter. However, there are many theories to explain this common pattern that are much different than the mechanical model. Each of them has logical reasoning on its side, and each will be discussed in its respective chapter. For the purposes of this section we will discuss the mechanical causes and subsequent changes that accompany forward head posture. These changes not only alter joint function locally but they also affect distant joints. In essence, we are looking at a very complex chain reaction when the head is displaced forward.

Mechanically, or traditionally speaking, forward head posture is the result of several factors. Habitually, we put the head in a forward position quite frequently. A good example of this is when we read or write. We tend to not only translate the head forward, but we also end up looking downwards to see the text. Forward head posture can also be due to prolonged sitting, which we are all guilty of. When we sit we usually fall forward and rest ourselves on the ligaments in the posterior spine. Once again, of course, the head is thrust forward. It is easy to see how certain structures become shortened and others become lengthened, thus causing this posture to become permanent. Less benign than these examples is the case of osteoporosis. Osteoporosis and subsequent loss of vertebral height set the stage for a flexed posture as well. Now let's examine the physics of forward head posture.

Starting at the top, the occiput glides anteriorly on the atlas to maintain the head in a level position. This is also known as capital extension. Compression results in the suboccipital area and the hypertonic suboccipitals shorten. Besides possibly causing an OA flexion restriction, this pulls the mandible posteriorly. Thus, increased TMJ compression results.

At shoulder level, the posterior musculature must now contract violently to prevent further anterior migration of the skull. The shoulder girdle is pulled into elevation and protraction. The pectorals have also tightened, and the glenohumeral joints become internally rotated. All of these factors are bringing the weight of the body forward. In order to prevent further flexion, the body must compensate. This may be with increased lumbar lordosis, or a sway-back posture. This brings the weight of the upper thorax backwards and lessens the flexion moment.

Along with the excessive lumbar lordosis is the anterior pelvic tilt. This internally rotates the hips as well. Moreover, because the line of gravity is anterior to the knee and ankle, the person stands with the knees hyperextended and is adding too much weight to the balls of his feet. Altogether, one can see the potential stress and strain on the entire structure due to FHP.

Coronal and Transverse Plane Deviations

Besides deviations in the sagittal plane, the clinician must also look for asymmetries in the coronal and transverse planes. These can be due to multiple factors including idiopathic scoliosis, asymmetrical muscle activation patterns, altered movement patterns, certain occupation and lifestyle-related activities, and vertebral or pelvic subluxations. Hruska theorizes that many deviations in these planes are due to internal asymmetry, especially that of the diaphragmatic domes.[59] This is certainly a valid point. Yet another likely cause is structural inadequacy. Please see the following section for common structural asymmetries as well as an in-depth discussion regarding the effects of coronal and transverse plane postural deviations.

STRUCTURAL INADEQUACIES

Travell and Simons use the term structural inadequacy (SI) to describe a set of mechanical factors whose presence tends to perpetuate myofascial trigger points. This group includes skeletal shortcomings, unilateral or bilateral, that deviate from normal. Generally speaking, these inadequacies create factors such as excessive compression, excessive tension, suboptimal circulation/neural supply, altered proprioception, and poor mechanical leverage. Over time, the results of these problems may rise to a clinical level and present themselves. Or, they may stay at a subclinical level and play a less evident role. In either case, their presence will undoubtedly have a negative consequence for the musculoskeletal system. This influence can take two forms. First, it can act to produce symptoms. In other words, the inadequacy may be directly responsible for causing the patient's symptoms. In this situation, the patient will typically present with symptoms of insidious onset. Consequently, as is often the case, the practitioner must become part-sleuth to determine the exact cause of the patient's problem. Treatment in this case will address the inadequacy and very likely lead to the resolution of symptoms.

As stated, a structural inadequacy can also play an important role in perpetuating symptoms. Take a patient presenting with acute-onset low back pain secondary to a fall. Considering that this person was pain-free prior to her fall, we must assume that a structural inadequacy did not directly cause her back pain. However, now that she is trying to recover from an injury, the asymmetry may become clinically relevant. The increased demands placed on the system while trying to repair itself are challenging in their own rite. To battle these and at the same time battle factors related to an added stressor may be too great a demand on the system. Thus, in this case of indirect involvement, action must be taken in order to facilitate recovery. Again, the clinician has to play part-sleuth in order to find this important perpetuating factor. In many ways, the clinician's job in this situation is more difficult than in the previously-described situation. That is, we as practitioners are accustomed to searching for causal factors in cases of insidious onset. On the other hand, in a traumatic injury, the guesswork is seemingly eliminated. The patient knows exactly what happened, and in all likelihood he or she does not undergo the same trauma on a daily basis. Therefore, it is easy for the practitioner to resign him/herself to treating the injured tissue in isolation without checking for factors that make healing more difficult or even impossible. This omission can mean the difference between symptom improvement and stagnation; therefore, the reader is urged to always examine for SI regardless of the mechanism of injury (or lack thereof).

Leg-Length Inequality

Leg-length inequality (LLI) refers to the asymmetrical length of the lower extremities. Although functional LLI is more common than structural (anatomical) LLI, our discussion in this section centers on the latter version. This is due to its inclusion in numerous research studies and the ease with which mechanical inferences may be made when discussing its clinical implications. However, many of the findings seen in structural LLI are equal to those seen with functional LLI. Most consistent are changes above the sacral base, as in either case the body's goal is to attain upright posture. Specific pathology and compensatory patterns are outlined below.

Pathology. Leg-length inequality is known to cause widespread damage to the locomotor system. Among those bodyparts directly affected are the knees, hips, pelvis, and lumbar spine. Beginning from the bottom, the knee of the long lower extremity has been shown by Dixon and Campbell-Smith[60] to develop valgus deformity, destruction of the lateral tibiofemoral compartment, and osteoarthrosis. Assuming a valgus posture is often a way to shorten a long lower extremity.

The hip on the high side is also prone to damage, typically in the form of degenerative osteoarthritis.[61] This etiology comes as no surprise when the biomechanics of the hip are studied. Looking at the hip on the long leg side, the joint is relatively adducted due to the inferior tilt of the contralateral hemipelvis. This relationship causes increased weight-bearing on the lateral portion of the acetabulum. Unfortunately, this area of the acetabulum is smaller than the normal area available for weight bearing. Consequently, the joint surface must encounter increased pressure per surface area. This change ultimately promotes premature chondral damage.

Perhaps most often associated with LLI is low back pain. Numerous studies have used it as a barometer to determine the amount of LLI that is clinically significant. Travell and Simons believe differences of ½ inch (1.3 cm) are clinically significant and should be corrected.[31] On the other hand, Rush and Steiner report that an LLI as small as 3⁄16 inch (0.5 cm) can lead to low back pain.[62] Other studies have reported the onset of symptoms by adding height to one shoe. One experiment created pain within only three days by adding ¾ inch (1.9 cm). After three weeks of increasing pain, the lift was removed. The subject's low back pain disappeared after 2 weeks.[63]

As with the knee and hip, the majority of problems in the lumbar spine due to LLI are on the side of the long leg. As the spine side-bends towards the long side, there is increased compression on the ipsilateral half of the lumbar vertebrae. Giles and Taylor showed that this causes a wedging effect on the vertebrae, possibly creating a structural scoliosis from a functional one.[64] The development of osteophytes has also been found on the side of the concavity.

Other Findings. Structural LLI can also create other problems for the body. It forces the foot and ankle to compensate in order to achieve symmetry. On the long-leg side, increased pronation helps reduce overall length.[65] On the short-leg side, increased supination helps increase overall length.

The pelvis also changes its structure in order to help reduce an asymmetry. This can occur via anterior innominate rotation on the short-leg side and posterior innominate rotation on the long-leg side. The net effect of this rotation is a gain of 1–2 mm.[43]

Other iliosacral compensatory mechanisms include an inferior translation of the sacrum on the ilium of the long-leg side. This may be accompanied by superior translation of the ilium on the short-leg side.[43] Tilting of the sacrum in the coronal plane is another measure taken to level the base. This involves "intrinsic adaptive mechanisms" attempting to tip the sacrum into the position normally assumed during side-bending.[43]

In any event, this phenomenon acts as proof that a thorough assessment of leg length is necessary. Otherwise, the practitioner may be satisfied that the pelvis is symmetrical if he/she only examines the malleoli. Or, he may expend energy trying to correct an apparent pelvic asymmetry that is endlessly perpetuated by an LLI.

Leg-length discrepancy also creates scoliotic curves in the spine. Travell and Simons describe these curvatures as either "C" or "S" curves. As an example, take a patient with a long right leg. In this instance, a "C" curve involves lumbar sidebending towards the right. This is accomplished by the quadratus lumborum and torso muscles on the right side pulling inferiorly on the trunk. Higher up in the spine, this curve is compensated for by contraction of the left neck muscles to bring the head to the neutral position.[31] The S-curve occurs in a similar fashion to the C-curve. The quadratus lumborum contracts to bring the lower rib cage inferiorly. Then, the lateral chest muscles on the short-leg side contract to bring the upper trunk to the left. This leaves the cervical spine sidebent to the left. As expected, the lateral neck muscles on the right side must then contract in order to bring the head into an upright position.

Not every author describes this same pattern of compensation. Schamberger notes that the curves associated with functional and anatomical leg-length inequalities are often unpredictable. Moreover, he reports observing a more frequent pattern of lumbar convexity towards the long-leg side.

Clinical Implications. The effects of LLI on the lower extremity, hip, pelvis, and lumbar spine were previously discussed. However, they do not end there. As long as the curvature of the spine has been altered there will be ramifications for the rest of the spine and the upper extremities. Many of these distant effects have been detailed by Schamberger. Beginning with the cervical and thoracic spines, the compensatory curves automatically cause decreased mobility in certain directions. Normally, this limitation is in the same direction as the curvature. To clarify, assume the thoracic spine is sidebent to the left and rotated to the right. This position then limits the range of motion available into right sidebending and left rotation. The result of this limitation is a potential strain due to lack of available motion as dictated by structure. Another byproduct of compensatory curvature is increased stress at the transitional vertebrae. Where the compensatory curves of the spine come together, there is increased potential for injury and subsequent damage. This is because two vertebrae in very opposing positions are actually joined to one another. To make matters worse, this transition frequently occurs at the points of transition for the natural curves of the spine. Thus, the curves in the coronal plane (mostly compensatory) meet with the curves in the sagittal plane (natural). The exact point of transition for either curve may fall a few segments away from the anatomical transition points, leading to localized symptoms in this area. A good example of this is in the upper thoracic spine, where an inferiorly shifted curve reversal may help create the all-too-common pain in the scapular region. Hruska also believes this syndrome is due to excessive vertebral and costal rotation.[59] Often, it is reported in the right upper thoracic spine due to counterclockwise rotation of the vertebrae with subsequent forward torsion of the connecting rib. This gives the scapula less surface area to articulate with, thereby irritating adjoining structures.

The position and function of the upper extremities is also altered by the malposition of the rest of the spine. Schamberger lists some of the common findings secondary to a pelvic asymmetry with a subsequent thoracic curve, convex left.[66] They are as follows:

1. the right shoulder girdle is retracted, depressed, and inferiorly tilted.
2. the left shoulder girdle is protracted, elevated, and superiorly tilted.
3. right shoulder internal rotation is limited, whereas left shoulder external rotation is limited.
4. right elbow supination is limited, whereas left elbow pronation is limited.

While these findings are intended for discussion regarding pelvic rotation, many of the same principles apply. Spinal curvature creates asymmetrical placement of the thoracic spine, cervical spine and upper extremities. Together with altered muscle tension, this leads to altered function. Please note that this list is not conclusive. There are other common asymmetries stemming from pelvic asymmetry. Some of these are mentioned throughout this text, but the reader is urged to consult Schamberger's work for a more comprehensive list of these findings.

Lift Therapy. Lift therapy is a very common and effective approach to treating LLI. Travell and Simons advocate full correction of LLI with a heel lift, but encourage use of a full-sole lift for any lift over 13 mm (½ in).[43] The exact amount of lift to use is normally obtained by performing standing radiographs. However, it is also believed that the patient's perception of symmetry and muscle strain is valuable.[43] This second technique is basically a trial-and-error approach, where sheets of paper are added under the short-leg until the patient reports greatest improvement.

Although it is effective, lift therapy should not be used indiscriminately with every patient. Instead, factors including the spine's adaptability need to be considered first and foremost. In a patient with a stiff spine, the addition of a lift will most likely create other problems. The scoliotic curves will not diminish, and symptoms may increase or appear in new areas. In this case, the use of mobilization instead of lift therapy will be more effective.[43] Even when using lift therapy, it is wise to have a "break-in" period to allow the body time to adapt. Maigne advocates starting with half of the correction and progressing to the full lift after one month.[67]

Hemipelvic Asymmetry

Another important structural asymmetry is the small hemipelvis. It is often a part of a defined pattern, accompanied by a smaller face, shorter upper limb, and short lower extremity on the same side. Unlike a leg-length inequality, hemipelvic asymmetry is made worse with sitting instead of standing. This is because weight bearing is placed on the ischial tuberosities, which are not in a symmetrical position in this patient population.

The compensation for a small hemipelvis is similar to that with an LLI.[68] The approach to treatment is also similar, although in this case the patient is fitted with a lift under the small-side ischial tuberosity when seated. As with a patient with an LLI, the correct reduction of this asymmetry should yield positive results from the start. Likewise, a lift placed on the opposite side should cause increased pain.

Although this asymmetry is normally considered as solely a superior-inferior discrepancy, it can also explain a difference in anterior-posterior hemipelvic size. In this case, symptoms are made worse by lying.[68] This is because the pelvis is tilted downwards on the small side, causing strain. Treatment involves placing adequate support under the small hemipelvis side while the patient is supine, thereby eliminating compensatory strain.

Short Upper Arms

Shortness of the upper arms is a SI wherein the length of the humerus is too short relative to the length of the torso. As described by Travell and Simons, it is a relatively frequent clinical finding and is a common perpetuating factor for myofascial trigger points. It is best observed in the standing patient. Normally, the patient's elbows come down to the level of the iliac crests. In the case of short upper arms, the elbows do not come down quite this far. This is clinically relevant because it makes sitting uncomfortable for the patient. Instead of being able to rest his/her elbows on the armrests, the patient often leans forward or to one side in order to bring the elbows down to the level of the armrests. Prolonged forward flexion in this manner creates increased stress on the back extensors. Prolonged sidebending is equally stressful, as it places increased strain on the quadratus lumborum and scalenii.[68]

Short upper arms are addressed by altering the height of the armrests. This can be done by building up the height of the armrests to the height of the elbows. The use of a chair with sloping armrests is also helpful, as it contains armrest heights of all varieties inherent in its design.[68]

Morton's Foot

Morton's foot is the fourth and final structural inadequacy listed by Travell and Simons. Briefly, it is described as a short first and long second metatarsal. Great importance is placed on this foot structure for several reasons. First, it is quite prevalent. Studies show it is present in up to 40% of the population.[69] Second, it has rather far-reaching effects. Besides creating trigger points in the peroneus longus, it also frequently affects the vastus medialis, gluteus medius, and gluteus minimus. The vastus medialis TrP causes medial knee pain, the gluteus medius trigger points refer pain to the low back, and the gluteus minimus trigger points typically cause posterior thigh and calf pain.

The wide-ranging effects of the Morton's foot configuration do not end here. Trigger points in the lower extremities can also have a negative effect on the muscles of the head and neck. This interaction creates limited mobility in the cervical spine and craniomandibular joint. In fact, increased interincisal opening has been observed following inactivation of TrPs in involved lower extremities.[31] This phenomenon occurred when opening was previously restricted by the presence of TrPs.

The theory and rationale for most of this influence is grounded in biomechanical principles. As expected, it starts with the structural inadequacy of the first metatarsal. The first metatarsal is normally expected to bear more weight than the second metatarsal. However, when it is shorter than its neighbor, the weight of the body begins to "rock" itself on the second metatarsal. To bring the body's weight onto the first metatarsal, the patient walks with an altered gait. This involves a lateral heel strike followed by excessive pronation. The stance phase finishes with eversion of the forefoot and increased weight bearing on its medial aspect. Consequently, the peroneus longus becomes strained and develops TrPs. The excessive pronation creates internal rotation of the femur, which overloads the medial knee and the lateral rotators of the hip.[31] This demand explains trigger point formation in the vastus medialis, gluteus minimus and medius from a mechanical perspective.

Examination. Examination for Morton's foot is fairly straightforward. According to Simons and Travell, there are two popular methods used to identify a Morton's foot. First, start by flexing the toe joints while supporting the metatarsals. The dorsal crease formed at the metatarsophalangeal joint becomes apparent. Next, mark the prominence of each metatarsal head and then have the patient stand. In weight bearing, the presence of a Morton's foot is confirmed if the second metatarsal is longer than the first metatarsal.

The second examination method is even easier. Extend the phalanges of the first and second toes and compare the length of the metatarsals. By eliminating the phalanges from the exam, the clinician is given a clear picture of which metatarsal is longer. This is important, as a patient with a longer second metatarsal may also possess short phalanges.[31]

Treatment. Treatment of Morton's foot centers around one important concept: support the first metatarsal. By "bringing the ground up" to the first ray, the body is free to bear weight on the first metatarsal, which is what it is designed for. Consequently, the foot and ankle no longer have to compensate in order to bring the first metatarsal down to the ground. The elimination of this compensation then has a chain reaction effect on the rest of the body. The knees and hips no longer have to forcibly contract in an attempt to prevent further genu valgus and hip internal rotation.

As described by Travell and Simons, supporting the first ray is very simple. An insert is cut-out to extend past the first metatarsal head, but just short of the interphalangeal joint. The rest of the insert should not extend underneath the other metatarsal heads. Rather, it should end just posterior to them.[31]

THE FASCIAL SYSTEM

The fascial system is another important way by which the body's structure affects the musculoskeletal system. In short, the reason for this influence is because of two factors. First, the fascial system envelops every structure of the body—down to the level of the cell. Second, fascia is known to have a very strong tensile strength. Put these two factors together and it is easily understood why practitioners of techniques such as myofascial release believe that working on restrictions in one part of the body can benefit distant areas.

A visual used by the myofascial release approach is that of a shirt with a hook pulling on one corner. This causes distortion throughout the shirt, depicted by a change in the shape of the shirt and the asymmetric pattern of the threads. This is an excellent way to look at the effects of fascial restriction, but it is not the only way fascia influences the entire person. There is also the concept of tensegrity. This is more of a three-dimensional model of fascial influence. It helps explain how fascia is connected in different planes and even how it supports the person's structure. This provides one more perspective how manual therapy applied in one part of the body, addressing local restrictions, can affect a distant area.

So, what are some of the ways fascia is involved? Well, fascia is involved anytime there is inflammation in an area. It is also affected by muscular holding patterns. More severe fascial injuries occur with lacerations or surgery, as scar tissue binds up numerous fascial layers. Upledger, for instance, remarks on the widespread effects of scars in his text, Craniosacral Therapy. He points to several different cases where his patients' long-standing headaches were caused by scar tissue, and direct scar release eliminated these headaches. In one of these cases, he found that mobilizing an appendectomy scar of 24 years duration eliminated headaches a woman had experienced for over 20 years. Other bizarre cases he describes includes headaches resolving after scar mobilization in patients after medial meniscal surgery, right kidney suspension, coccygectomy, and ganglionectomy of the left wrist.[70]

These examples illustrate how important the fascial system is in treatment and justifies treatment in one part of the body in order to affect a distant area. This may be a situation where the location of the person's symptoms is just the weak link in the chain. Only a thorough evaluation of the entire body will yield the practitioner with the information as to where the true problem lies.

Later in this text several myofascial release techniques are presented, including the suboccipital release, the lower extremity pull, and the diaphragmatic release. These are just a few of the many techniques taught under myofascial release. They are known to be especially beneficial to the bodypart they are working on. However, keep in mind that myofascial release technique's benefit is not limited to the bodypart on which it is applied. It has the potential to benefit the entire body.

THE KINETIC CHAIN

Many fields in manual therapy use the kinetic chain concept as an aid in mechanical diagnosis and treatment. Most often, it is used to aid the practitioner in gait analysis and correction—certainly a valuable use of the concept—but not the only one. We must not forget the kinetic chain also works from the top-down and from the inside-out. For this reason, the core concept is included under this heading as well. The reader is encouraged to learn both applications in problem assessment and treatment.

GAIT

It is important for the clinician to understand even minute details when it comes to the biomechanics of gait. This is because he or she needs to be able to recognize potential faults in the kinetic chain that may lead to overuse syndromes. Likewise, this knowledge may then be used to treat a particular problem by creating positive change at the site of symptoms or elsewhere along the kinetic chain. For the purpose of this section, we will only discuss biomechanics from the ground on up through the lumbar spine. In the section titled "Functional Hallux Limitus," an extension of the kinetic chain concept is discussed that explains how problems as high as the cervical spine can have their roots in the foot.

The foot and lower extremity

Discussion of lower extremity biomechanics begins with a description of the mechanics of the foot. With regards to these biomechanics, the two terms most frequently used to describe motion are pronation and supination. Pronation is a popular term clinicians are very familiar with. In short, it is defined as the tri-planar "unlocking" of the foot as contact is made with the ground. During initial contact and weight acceptance, this helps dissipate force while also promoting surface adaptation. This chain reaction begins with initial contact of the posterolateral heel with the ground. Directly following this contact, the ankle plantarflexes and the subtalar joint pronates. More specifically, the talus adducts and plantarflexes while the calcaneus everts. This lowers the ankle mortise, thereby dissipating energy. The forefoot unlocks, dorsiflexing, abducting, and inverting (the opposite motions of what is occurring at the rearfoot.) Simultaneously, the internal rotation of the tibia creates an unlocking of the extended knee.[71] This flexion moment reduces shock as well. Movement in these planes traverses superiorly, medially rotating the tibia and femur. Femoral internal rotation causes anterior rotation of the innominate and increased lordosis of the lumbar spine. In the coronal plane, weight moves medially when the calcaneus everts. This brings the knee medially, forcing the joint into valgus and the hip into increased adduction.

The midstance period marks the next phase of gait. This phase begins at full forefoot load and ends at heel lift. Within this portion of the gait cycle the foot goes from a state of pronation to a state of supination. This transformation is set into motion when the pelvis passes over the foot. In doing so, the head of the femur passes anterior to the greater trochanter, thereby externally rotating the femur and tibia. This has the effect of abducting and dorsiflexing the talus. The calcaneus then inverts and the rearfoot is expected to be in its subtalar neutral position by the end of the midstance period. In order to do so, it must rely on eversion of the forefoot in order to become locked. This eversion includes plantarflexion of the first ray and dorsiflexion of the lateral forefoot.[71] Again, the motions of the forefoot and rearfoot oppose one another. This combination transforms the foot from a loose "bag of bones" to a rigid lever as the propulsive period is entered.

The propulsive period lasts from heel lift to toe-off. It is in this phase that normal supination is absolutely necessary. This is because the body will soon utilize the foot as a lever from which to propel itself through space. To achieve supination, several factors come into play. First of all, the forward migration of the body helps aid in rearfoot supination, as discussed in the previous paragraph. Secondly, the windlass mechanism is activated when the toes are passively dorsiflexed. This occurs as the plantar fascia is stretched around the metatarsal heads, thus pulling the anterior and posterior pillars of the longitudinal arch together.[71] Further assistance is given by the muscular system. This includes the foot intrinsics, soleus, and peroneus longus. Of these muscles, the peroneus longus plays an especially important role. Its first job is to aid ground reaction forces by pushing the cuboid dorsally into the calcaneus. This osseous locking is necessary to lock the forefoot on the rearfoot. Secondly, it must plantarflex the first ray. Along with its effects on the lateral column, this eversion of the forefoot helps direct body weight medially instead of laterally. This is important for the sake of efficiency, as the medial column is longer than the lateral column. Besides this, the first metatarsal is much larger than the other metatarsals, thereby making it more structurally suited to bear the weight of the body.

The pelvis and lumbar spine

The relationship between the pelvis and lumbar spine during gait has been described by Greenman.[72] Beginning with right heel strike, the right innominate rotates posteriorly and the left anteriorly. Both the sacrum and the lumbar spine are rotated to the left. The sacrum is specifically described as being rotated left on its left oblique axis. As the right lower extremity reaches midstance, the innominates begin moving in the opposite direction. At midstance, the sacrum is rotated right, side-bent left, and L5 is rotated left and side-bent right. Following midstance, the right lower extremity progresses into the toe-off phase. At this point, the right innominate is in anterior rotation and the left innominate is in posterior rotation. The lumbar spine is now rotated right and the sacrum is rotated right on its right oblique axis.

Specific maladies due to faulty biomechanics are discussed in their respective chapters later in the text. Instead of describing each of them in this chapter, it is the author's goal to acquaint the reader with what is normal. Only by knowing what is normal can the clinician can recognize what is abnormal. Moreover, by understanding the exact mechanical relationships between the joints of the locomotor system, the reader can predict sites of stress and strain. In the context of this section, this may include the foot's influence on the other joints involved in normal gait. Along with improved clinical assessment comes more effective treatment planning. In the case where a patient has symptoms secondary to a distant cause, this ability to recognize and treat the *source* is invaluable.

A thorough examination is necessary when evaluating the role of faulty mechanics. Static structural examination must include inspection of the feet, knees, and hips. The structure of the feet is especially important. Common faults include forefoot varus and rearfoot varus, which both contribute to over-pronation. In weight-bearing, the height of the medial longitudinal arch should be examined. The attitude of the knees including the Q-angle should be observed. The position of the hips in the coronal and transverse planes is especially important and often goes hand-in-hand with the Q-angle. Dynamic evaluation includes gait analysis as well as the performance of several functional tasks. Gait analysis is aided with the use of a video camera. This allows the clinician time to slow the person's movements down and more thoroughly study his or her motion patterns. In the over-pronator, this allows the clinician the opportunity to view the breakdown of the midfoot and resultant rotational genu valgus. Conversely, it may prove excessive hip adduction is causing over-pronation due to medial deviation of the person's bodyweight. The combination of these factors is a common pattern seen in rehabilitation clinics. It is termed miserable malalignment.[73] Of course, the patient's structure may be the exact opposite of the pattern just described. He or she may have a rigid foot prone to supination and have a genu varus deformity. In either case, the clinician can use knowledge of biomechanics to make an assessment and plan treatment accordingly. In the next section the topic of orthotic therapy is introduced. This is the most popular method of treating biomechanical dysfunction with origins in the feet. Subsequently, it is used by several professions to treat symptoms in the feet, knees, and hips. Treatment of the lower extremity kinetic chain (LEKC) via treatment of the superior/proximal components is covered in later sections.

TREATMENT

Biomechanical orthotics are the most popular means to address faulty mechanics of the lower extremities. Whether custom-made or pre-fabricated, orthotics have been proven effective at reducing foot, ankle, and knee pain when indicated. In the patient with excessive pronation, the orthotics' role is to provide increased support, thus reducing the amount of pronation. This is frequently achieved with the use of a rearfoot or forefoot post. The rearfoot post (varus post) is used to alter mechanics occurring from heelstrike to footflat.[73] It is placed medially in the rear of the orthotic to support the calcaneus in varus. This reduces the amount of calcaneal eversion, as reported by several authors.[73] The use of a forefoot post helps support the forefoot and midfoot during propulsion. It is frequently used medially in order to address a forefoot varus structure. In essence, its purpose is to bring the ground up to the medial forefoot. Otherwise, the medial forefoot has to drop farther than normal in order to reach the ground. This is not damaging on its own accord, but it forces the subtalar joint to compensate by pronating excessively.

With these approaches or with other techniques, the goal is to reduce breakdown of the offending structure. In doing so, the foot is better able to perform the important functions needed during the start of stance phase. In addition, reduction of excessive pronation may be of great benefit at the end of stance phase. This is applicable in the instance the foot stays pronated for too long. As discussed, this compromises the foot's function as a rigid lever.

The goal of orthotics for the patient with excessive supination is quite different. First and foremost, the purpose is to provide enhanced shock absorption. This is often accomplished with the qualities inherent to a soft orthotic, as it provides extra material between the foot and the walking surface. However, this is not the only way orthotics benefit an excessively supinated foot. In a custom-fabricated orthotic, the patient's foot is cast in subtalar neutral, as it is with a pronated foot. This process is sometimes enough to bring a supinated foot into slightly more pronation. Thus, the patient's foot is already predisposed to pronation from the moment of initial contact.

FUNCTIONAL HALLUX LIMITUS

Examination and treatment of functional hallux limitus (FHL) is specialized. The reason for this is that FHL is not present during non-weight bearing. In other words, the patient will demonstrate normal first metatarsal-phalangeal dorsiflexion during physical examination. Only upon weight bearing is the restriction present, as when pushing dorsally upon the metatarsal head. This brings the dorsiflexion restriction into view so the clinician can make the diagnosis.

This functional dorsiflexion restriction creates important problems during the gait cycle, as it prevents normal sagittal-plane motion. This creates problems up the kinetic chain. Among other things, Dananberg notes that forward head posture often results from this condition, as the body is trying to vault itself over the restriction.[74] The best way to do this, he postulates, is by trying to bring the head, neck, and upper body over the joint in question.

Treatment for FHL is specialized as well. It requires a specific orthotic to change the mechanics of the first ray. This allows for normal MTP dorsiflexion and restore normal mechanics. The manual therapist is encouraged to scan for this problem and refer to a podiatrist when indicated.

THE CORE CONCEPT

The sections above detail the effects from the bottom to the top of the kinetic chain. While this connection is a powerful one, it is not the only one. The pelvic girdle also has a great influence downwards towards the feet. Much has been written recently on the importance of "core" strength to the stability of the rest of the body. This concept and others center around strengthening the stabilizing muscles of the pelvis and lumbar spine, the pelvic floor muscles, abdominal obliques, and transversus abdominis. Mechanically speaking, this influence is believed to be the result of increased stability. With this comes less aberrant motion of the spine, pelvic girdle, hip complex, etcetera. This in turn leads to less stress and strain on all structures of the lower extremities.

The advent of the Protonics knee brace probably serves as the best evidence that the lower extremities are influenced from above. This brace was developed primarily to treat patellofemoral dysfunction. Simply put, it applies an extension force to the user's knee. This forces the user to constantly contract his hamstrings in order to avoid hyperextension. While the brace is on, the patient can oftentimes perform a normally painful movement—such as squatting—without pain. Originally, this instantaneous improvement was thought to be due to reciprocal inhibition of the quadriceps. However, later deliberations attributed much of the device's success to a mechanical explanation. That reasoning is as follows: contraction of the hamstrings creates an inferior pull on the ischial tuberosity. Because the ischial tuberosity is posterior to the innominate's axis of rotation, this creates posterior innominate rotation. This posterior rotation automatically externally rotates the femurs. This brings the lateral epicondyle of the femur away from the patella, thereby reducing or eliminating any pain generated by abnormal compression of these two structures.

This is not the first time a connection has been made between pelvic/hip stability and patellofemoral syndrome. Practitioners have known for a long time that the position, function, and overall strength of the pelvis and hip influence knee function. In fact, the chain reaction stemming from pelvic dysfunction does not stop at the knee. This is because as the femurs externally rotate, the tibia and fibula externally rotate. This externally rotates the talus and inverts the calcaneus. Therefore, motion of the pelvic girdle effectively changes the alignment of the feet. Take note that this connection is made possible on a myofascial level as well, notes Myers.[162] He reports that this change in pelvic tilt will also pull the Spiral Line superiorly, thereby lifting the medial longitudinal arch. This is just one more connection between the pelvis and feet.

A solid foundation undoubtedly benefits the shoulder girdles as well. Like the lower extremities, they need a firm platform from which to operate. If the core musculature is not providing this stability then aberrant scapular motion will result. This leads to local problems including rotator cuff dysfunction and scapulothoracic pain. It also places added stress on the suspensory muscles of the scapula and tractions the brachial plexus. This is just one more example how important the mechanical system is to the manual therapist. Be sure to utilize everything discussed so far in order to ensure successful clinical outcomes.

5 Neurological Considerations

LIKE THE MECHANICAL SYSTEM, THE NERVOUS SYSTEM PLAYS AN IMPORTANT ROLE IN THE development of musculoskeletal disorders. It also plays an important role in the treatment of musculoskeletal disorders. In fact, it is safe to say that the majority of manual therapy interventions influence the nervous system even if that is not their primary intention. A good example of this is the use of spinal manipulation. While manipulation has been used successfully for many years, its effects are not limited to structural "repositioning" of a spinal segment. This notion may be partially true, but the majority of immediate improvement following manipulation is not due to the vertebra falling into its proper place. Instead, this immediate reduction in pain is due to neurological factors, such as the stimulation of mechanoreceptors, the inhibition of nociceptors, and the restoration of normal muscle tone. Altogether, these neurological changes often let the vertebra glide back into its neutral position. This example is just one small way the nervous system is influenced in treatment. It plays a role in almost everything we clinicians do for our patients; many of these mechanisms are discussed later.

Because the nervous system is so complex and is such a broad topic, it is impossible to cover it thoroughly in this text or any other. With that being said, the goal here is not to cover the topic of neurophysiology. Nor is an attempt made to explain complicated neural pathways. Instead, the goal in this chapter is to focus on the more practical aspects of the nervous system and its role in manual therapy. To do this, we will attempt to simplify this incredibly complex system by classifying the *ways* the nervous system influences the musculoskeletal system. From there, we delve into subcategories where we see not only differences in the extent of this influence but also the wide-ranging ways *how* this influence occurs. This will help the clinician assess and treat the patient on different levels according to what he/she needs. It will also help him/her to become cognizant of the many neurological phenomena which can interfere with a patient's capacity to succeed with therapy. Where indicated, specific treatment techniques are explained in this chapter. This is done for two reasons. The first reason is that a given theory or technique is applicable to all areas of the body, not just a single region. The second reason is that a given theory or technique has the capability to influence the entire body—not just a single region. In both instances, the reader is expected to utilize these techniques no matter what bodypart is symptomatic; assuming of course that her examination indicates a need for them. For information on other specific treatment techniques please consult later chapters of this text corresponding with individual bodyparts.

INTERFERENCE WITH NERVE CONDUCTION

The first (and most simple) way neurological dysfunction influences the musculoskeletal system is by interfering with nerve conduction. This refers to the mechanical action of neural structure compression or tension, leading to diminished signal transmission to an intended target. This will cause reduced motor output if the nerve is an efferent fiber. Likewise, it will cause decreased sensation, proprioception, etc., if this nerve is an afferent fiber. In many instances, this stress irritates the nerve and causes hyperalgesia.

Problems due to altered signal transmission are frequently seen in the manual therapist's office. They include common compression syndromes like lumbar and cervical radiculopathy, carpal tunnel syndrome, thoracic outlet syndrome, cubital tunnel syndrome, and radial tunnel syndrome, among others. They also include less common (or at least less frequently recognized) dysfunctions including double and triple crush syndromes, where more than one area of the body is impinging a nerve along its path.

Recognition of most entrapment neuropathies is achieved with orthopedic testing. This makes the diagnosis easy in many instances. In other cases, their recognition is more difficult; they may not produce a characteristic pattern of altered sensation, pain, or weakness. Instead, they may produce a subtle alteration in function which leads to slow changes over time, thereby causing another structure to work harder and break down as a result. Again, the manual therapist must be aware of all potential entrapment syndromes, obvious and subtle, so that he/she is treating the source of the patient's problem and not just the end result.

The principles guiding treatment of the entrapment syndromes are actually quite simple. For the most part, they involve treating the tissues surrounding the nerve in order to either reduce excessive compression or tension upon it. In the spine, for instance, treatment is geared at increasing the diameter of the intervertebral foramen so that the spinal nerves are allowed to pass without interruption. Traction, mobilization, and manipulation are popular ways to accomplish this.

In the extremities, this usually involves soft tissue work applied to the structure directly impinging the nerve, such as the flexor retinaculum or pronator teres for the median nerve. It also involves any treatment known to benefit the nerve either proximally or distally. This includes releasing other tissues along the nerve's path so that it is allowed to glide as optimally as possible.

Nerve gliding (or nerve flossing) is an option advocated by Butler and Elvey. This involves gliding the nerve back and forth using a modified tension-testing position. This is done in order to improve the nerve's mobility in relation to surrounding structures. However, please note that it is not advocated to directly stretch the nerve, as nervous tissue: (1) does not lengthen with repetitive stretching and (2) is quite sensitive.

Additional considerations are the patient's postural status (static and dynamic), as well as occupational factors which may either directly stress the nerve or cause hypertrophy of structures surrounding it. These are issues recognized as causing carpal and cubital tunnel syndromes, and they are probably responsible for many others. Addressing these stressors is *vitally important* to the success of manual therapy. If they are allowed to exist unchecked they will lead to an unsuccessful outcome. Please see later chapters for further discussion of specific entrapment syndromes and their appropriate treatment.

FACILITATION AND INHIBITION

While there are many ways the nervous system influences the musculoskeletal system, probably the best way to describe this influence is by looking at the methods of facilitation and inhibition. After all, just consider what goes on within the nervous system at all levels. Certain neurotransmitters are excitatory and others are inhibitory. Some neurons are excitatory and others are inhibitory. Even when we palpate for muscle tone or perform a deep tendon reflex we are primarily testing facilitation and inhibition within the nervous system.

Given that the nervous system utilizes patterns of facilitation and inhibition for normal function, it is no surprise that these same means are responsible for creating most cases of neuropathology. We see this in disorders like epilepsy and Parkinson's due to inadequate amounts of certain neurotransmitters. We also see this on a larger scale when injury to the cortex destroys its inhibitory effect on powerful reflexes: the result is the assumption of characteristic neurological patterns which leave the patient with permanent disability.

Of course, not all patterns of facilitation and inhibition are this harmful. Nevertheless, they often play an important role in the creation and perpetuation of musculoskeletal dysfunction. For this reason they must be treated—on all levels—by the manual therapist. Below we describe some of the ways facilitation and inhibition affects the body, and discuss some of the methods manual therapists utilize to manage it. To start with, let's break this subject down into several subcategories according to the scope of influence: local, segmental, and global.

LOCAL

Local facilitation/inhibition refers to the isolated facilitation and inhibition of a given muscle or soft tissue structure. This may result from any one of many stressors. Conventionally, we think of different types of trauma as being the culprit. A macrotrauma, such as a quadriceps strain could do it. Or, it may be due to a microtrauma, such as assembly-line work or slouching in front of a computer all day. In any event, the result is the same: muscles become either facilitated or inhibited.

Unfortunately, the body often has a difficult time trying to balance these dysfunctional states. A strained, overworked muscle causes its antagonist to become inhibited even further due to reciprocal inhibition. At the same time, the facilitated muscle becomes even more facilitated due to the lack of opposition as well as factors within its own intrafusal fibers (muscle spindles). Myofascial trigger points and tender points (referenced in regard to strain-counterstrain) often develop, adding into this cycle. This creates widespread patterns of muscle guarding to oppose further strain.

Treatment for these cases is usually confined to the affected area. Popular approaches such as positional release therapy or strain-counterstrain are excellent at reducing tone in specific muscles (Fig. 5-1). So is the hold-relax technique of muscle stretching used in many muscle energy techniques, which utilizes the principle of post-isometric relaxation to help reduce muscle facilitation (Fig. 5-2).

Other approaches take a different view of this dysfunction. Namely, applied kinesiology and muscle activation technique focus on restoring normal tone to

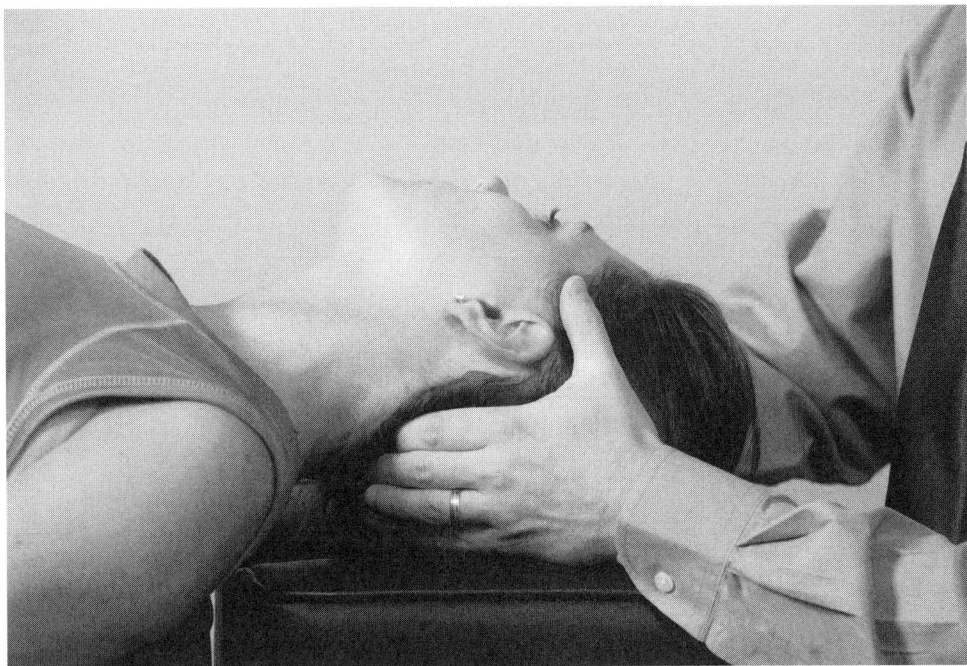

Fig. 5-1 Strain-counterstrain of the suboccipitals.

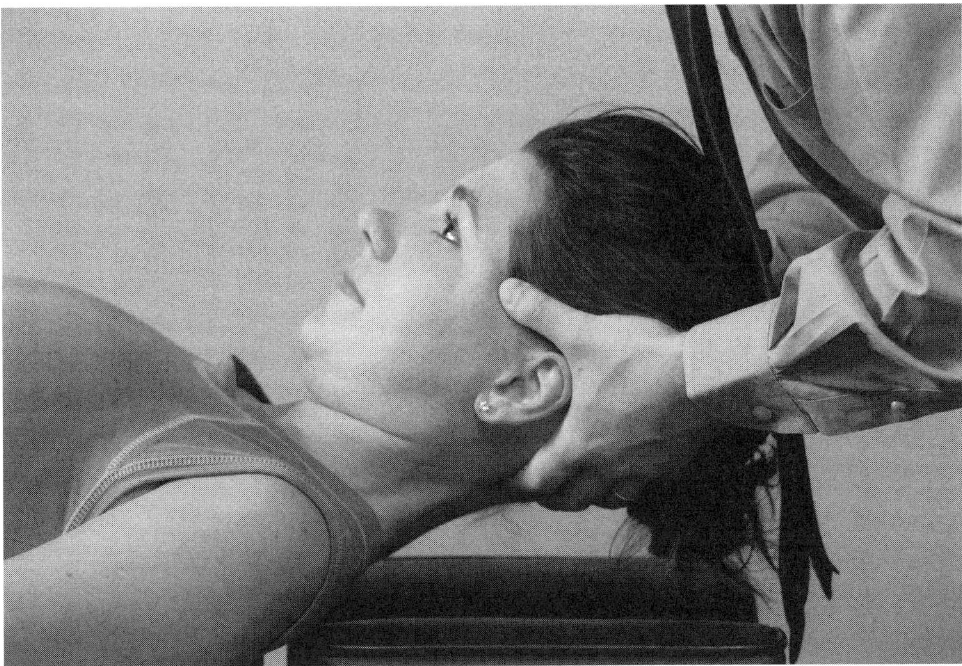

Fig. 5-2 Muscle energy technique applied to the suboccipitals.

inhibited muscles instead of trying to down-regulate tone of facilitated muscles. This can be through a variety of techniques, including different reflex techniques, spinal adjusting, acupressure, and origin-insertion techniques (Fig. 5-3). These methods are based on research showing that there are many stressors which can cause muscle inhibition, ranging from meridian imbalances to cranial imbalances to altered gait reflexes, among others. To say the least, it is beyond the scope of this text to describe all of these stressors and their corresponding treatment. For further information please read David Walther's *Applied Kinesiology: Synopsis.*

Treatment of myofascial trigger points is a little different from these techniques and deserves special attention. That is because authorities agree it needs to be more aggressive to be effective. The most popular treatment method is the use of ischemic compression. This is a simple technique involving little more than applying continuous pressure to the trigger point for 90 seconds (Fig 5-4). This method is thought to create ischemia to the area followed by a rapid influx of fresh blood. One must assume it has a powerful neurological and mechanical effect as well.

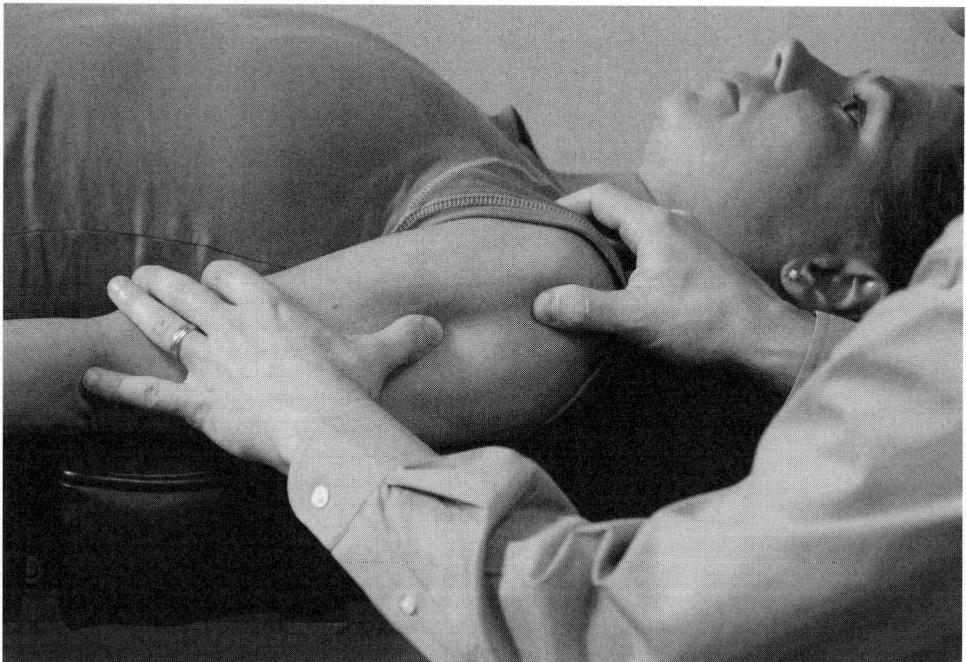

Fig. 5-3 Origin-insertion technique to facilitate muscle strength.

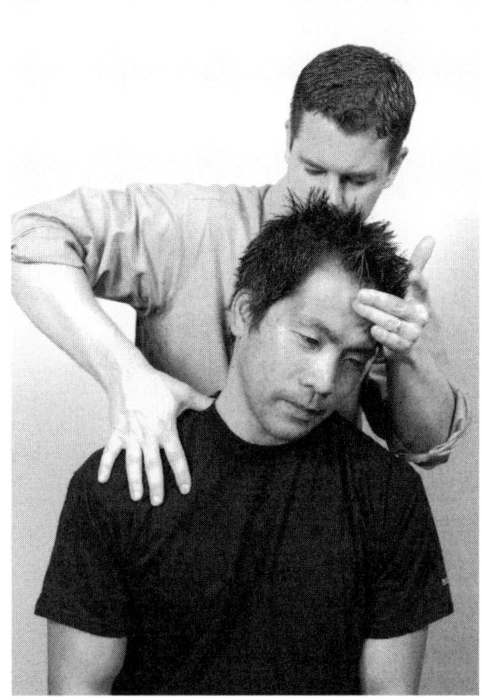

Fig. 5-4 Ischemic compression applied to the upper trapezius.

SEGMENTAL

Segmental facilitation and inhibition refers to a more widespread method of influence than we saw with local facilitation and inhibition. Instead of involving just a single agonist and antagonist, this pattern involves tissues along an entire spinal segment. Because of this widespread influence, the segmental pattern of facilitation and inhibition is responsible for creating many of the problems manual therapists treat every day. This can be by increasing tone in a muscle, leading to fatigue and pain (and the development of tender/trigger points). Or, it can be by altering the function of muscles surrounding a joint, thereby causing joint dysfunction and postural distortion. It both cases, it is necessary for the therapist to be able to recognize this connection so that the true cause of the patient's symptoms is addressed.

So, what causes this problem in the first place, one might ask? Generally speaking, most chiropractors and osteopaths consider vertebral dysfunction as the primary causative factor. This does not have to include frank nerve root impingement. Instead, it can include any type of local irritation or alteration in vertebral motion, with the result being local and peripheral facilitation/

inhibition (as well as other phenomena including sympathetic vasoconstriction, lowered nociception thresholds resulting in increased nociceptive input, central sensitization, and decreased mechanoreception under chiropractic's Vertebral Subluxation Complex model). Because the peripheral involvement affects tissues in a myotomal and sclerotomal distribution, the therapist can predict which tissues are involved by locating the level of vertebral involvement. This greatly aids the assessment and treatment process. See Fig. 5-5 for a list of some of the more common vertebral segment—muscular trigger point connections.[75]

Dysfunctional joint	Muscle involved
Occipital-atlantal	Suboccipitals
C0/1 and C2/3	Sternocleidomastoid
C3/4, C4-5	Levator scapula
TMJ	Muscles of mastication
L3/4 (hip)	Rectus femoris
L4/5 (coccyx)	Piriformis[75]
L5/S1 (coccyx)	Iliacus

Fig. 5-5 Segmental dysfunction and its corresponding muscular involvement.

In addition to these connections are those described by Maigne, who connects segmental dysfunction to common musculoskeletal ailments and specific symptoms. This is very helpful to the manual therapist, as the conditions he addresses are often mistaken for localized dysfunction. Thus, knowing about these connections aids the practitioner in finding the root of the problem and then implementing appropriate treatment. See Figure 5-6 for a list of these connections.[67]

Dysfunctional joint	Symptom/Syndrome
C5/6, C6/7	Shoulder pain
C5/6, C6/7	Lateral epicondylar pain
C7/T1	Medial epicondylar pain
C5/6,C6/7,C7/T1	Mid-thoracic pain*
T12/L1	Low back pain, false hip pain, pubic tenderness, irritable bowel symptomatology, lower abdominal pain**
L2/3, L3/4	Knee pain
L2/3	Meralgia paresthetica
L4/5	Gluteus medius/hip pain

*Maigne's 'cervical point of the back.' Characterized by a tender point 2cm lateral from midline at the level of T5 or T6. Maigne reports that when this syndrome is present there will be ipsilateral tenderness at a lower cervical segment. Treating this segment will eliminate the thoracic symptoms.

**Maigne's thoracolumbar junction syndrome. May also include T11/12 and L1/2.

Fig. 5-6 Dysfunctional joints and their corresponding symptoms/syndromes.

In addition to creating trigger points and contributing to *specific* pain syndromes, segmental dysfunction is also responsible for inhibiting muscle function. This is considered an especially important factor in applied kinesiology. It is evaluated by having the patient therapy localize (touch) the area of the spine responsible for the primary nerve supply to an inhibited muscle. For instance, if one were testing the tensor fascia lata, he or she would therapy localize over L4, L5, and S1. If the vertebra(e) in question is responsible for the muscle's inhibition, the muscle will now test strong. The practitioner then uses additional tests to determine the vector of manipulation most suitable for the patient's disorder. See Figures 5-7 and 5-8.

Besides the central-to-peripheral relationship just described, the manual therapist must also be cognizant that the reverse relationship can occur. That is, it is possible for peripheral joint dysfunction to create central/proximal dysfunction. This was illustrated in a research study by Bullock-Saxton, who found that patients with ankle sprain demonstrate weakened gluteal muscle function.[76]

In chiropractic this concept is reinforced by several examination techniques. For instance, the gluteus medius, quadriceps, and psoas are strength tested in order to identify problems with the cuboid, metatarsals, and navicular, respectively.

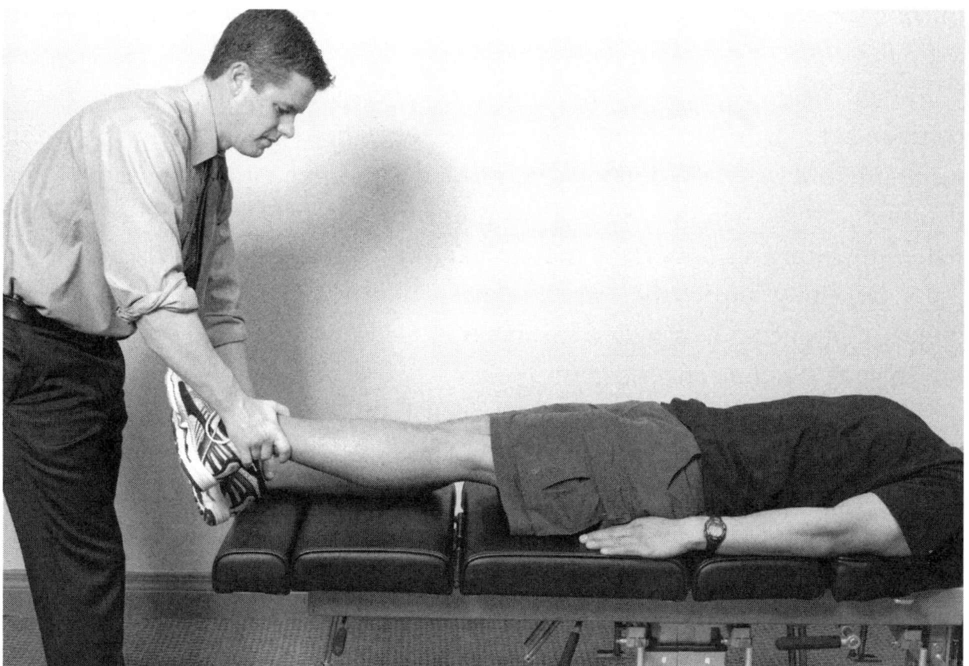

Fig. 5-7 Manual muscle testing of the tensor fascia lata demonstrating muscle inhibition.

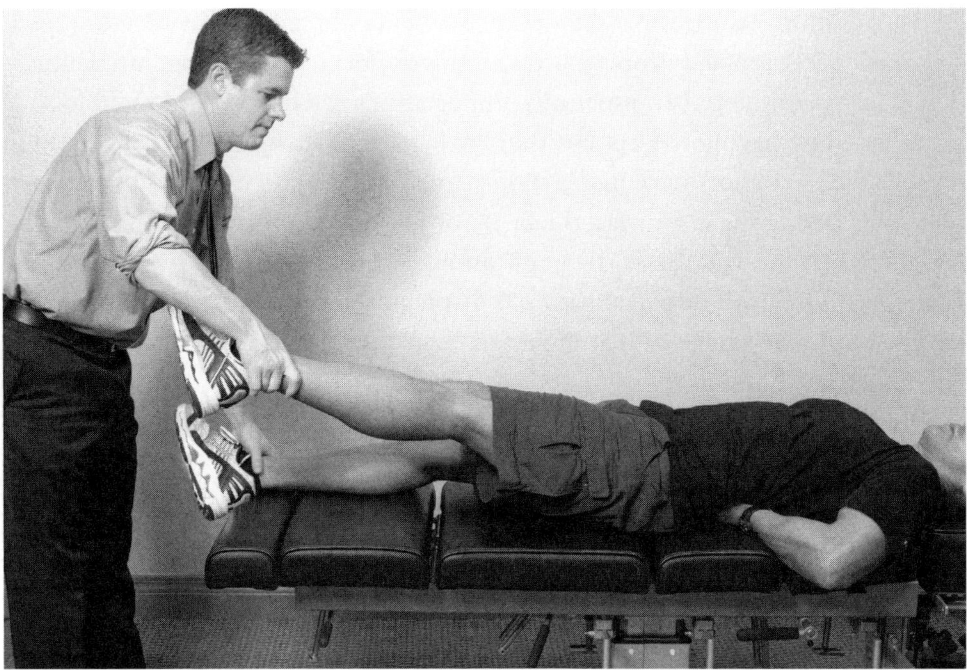

Fig. 5-8 Manual muscle testing of the TFL while the patient therapy localizes the L4 vertebrae. Muscle strengthening indicates involvement of L4 in the TFL's inhibition.

Effective treatment directed to the foot leads to immediate strengthening of these muscles.

These are just a few examples how the periphery can influence central components. There are many other ways; some have been documented but many others have not. With that being said, we must remember to examine the periphery even when the patient's symptoms are centrally located. A segmental reflex inhibiting an important muscle like the gluteus medius, quadriceps, or psoas can easily impact the spine, as one would imagine. Besides this, altered proprioception and heightened nociception feeds into the central nervous system, having systemic effects.

Treatment for cases involving segmental facilitation and inhibition is relatively the same as it is for the local pattern. This includes manipulation, mobilization, strain-counterstrain, muscle energy techniques, massage, myofascial release, Mulligan techniques, and ischemic compression. The important distinction in this case is that the clinician must be sure to treat the *cause* of the problem as well as the symptomatic area. This ensures that the issue driving the problem is resolved. Additionally, by removing the effects of segmental dysfunction (tender points, trigger points, altered joint mechanics), one is ensuring that these issues do not feed back into the system.

GLOBAL

Global patterns of facilitation and inhibition are the third group. As expected, this group encompasses an even greater area than the other two groups. It is also more "holistic," meaning that the input and output driving these reflexes involves the entire nervous system instead of being relegated to a single nerve or spinal segment. Consequently, we see that these patterns are activated by almost anything affecting the system as a whole. We can also see why the global patterns have the capacity to affect the entire body when they are (over) activated.

So, what exactly does the global pattern of facilitation and inhibition include? From a purely neuromusculoskeletal point-of-view, the answer is simple. It is the common pattern described in Chapters 2 and 9. In short, the common pattern is a synergy the body "defaults" to secondary to stressors including pain, abnormal neurological function (especially due to abnormal/inadequate mechanoreceptor input), emotional stress, brain damage (TBI, CVA), and virtually anything else which disrupts homeostasis (components of this pattern are mentioned by Janda, Hanna, Alexander, and Greenman).

Besides being extremely common (it is present to some degree in most individuals), the common pattern is also extremely influential. This is because it has the capacity to change the entire structure and neurological function of the body, thereby challenging the musculoskeletal system. Because of this powerful influence, any potential causative factors must be addressed in addition to the different components of the pattern itself.

With this being said, one could argue that virtually any treatment which restores homeostasis will reduce or eliminate the presence of the global pattern of influence. This is undoubtedly true (especially when we address the "high-yield" regions introduced in Chapter 3). In fact, there are several approaches which embody this philosophy more than any others; they are based entirely on treating one area of the body no matter where the patient's complaints are located. Thus, it is through their respective successes which we see the true power of the nervous system—in both its ability to create pathology when it is disrupted and in its ability to heal when it is working normally.

UPPER CERVICAL COMPLEX

The upper cervical spine has an enormous influence over the entire body. It is no wonder why so many professions and approaches attempt to treat it. In chiropractic it was B.J. Palmer who turned his focus on the upper cervical spine in the late 1920's.[77] He referred to his technique as the HIO (Hole In One) technique, and used it to treat thousands of chronically ill patients with excellent results at his research clinic in Davenport, Iowa.

Of course, to some practitioners it seems absurd to limit one's treatment to a single part of the body. However, if we consider the tremendous influence the upper cervical spine has on the CNS, this approach makes more sense. Summarized below are several reasons why the upper cervical spine is so vital to the general health and musculoskeletal well-being of the individual:

1. A large number of spinoreticular fibers originate in the upper cervical spine. These synapse on many areas of the pontomedullary reticular formation.[29] The pontomedullary reticular formation inhibits flexor muscle tone and intermediolateral column activity (thereby opposing sympathetic nervous system activity).
2. The superior and inferior obliquus capitis muscles have the most dense concentration of muscle spindles in the entire body.[78] This means that these muscles, as well as some of the other muscles of the upper cervical spine, play a huge role in providing the body's proprioceptive sensation. Consequently, when they are not functioning normally they influence the *entire* body in a negative fashion.
3. Primitive reflexes, including the tonic neck reflex, influence muscle activation patterns even in adults. Dysfunction in this part of the spine can cause hyperactivity of these reflexes, which then create abnormal patterns of spinal and extremity hypertonicity/inhibition.
4. Hack et al. discovered a myodural bridge running between the rectus capitis posterior minor and the dura mater.[79] This creates a connection (literally) between the soft tissues of the cervical spine and the highly-innervated dura mater of the spinal cord.
5. Several of the dura mater's few connections to the vertebral column are at the occiput, C2 and C3 (the others are at the sacrum and coccyx). Misalignment in the upper cervical spine leads to undue torque and tension on the dura mater.
6. The dentate (also called denticulate) ligaments connecting the pia and dura mater are yet another explanation for the upper cervical spine's importance.

Experts including Grostic[80] and Harrison[81] mention these ligaments in their writings as viable reasons why correction of vertebral subluxations and restoration of normal spinal alignment/curvature in this area is so important—because the surface of the spinal cord is actually tractioned when the dura is torqued.

Mounting research from upper cervical practitioners illustrates the extent of the upper cervical spine's influence better than anything else. Listed below is just a small sample of some of the incredible results seen with upper cervical care. Consistent with the theme of this text, these studies reinforce the potential for a specific therapy to influence the musculoskeletal system on a local and global scale while also normalizing autonomic function and improving the patient's systemic health (typically by activating the parasympathetic nervous system). The reader is asked to ponder each abstract individually to best appreciate the widespread benefit of correcting upper cervical dysfunction.

- A recent study published in the Journal of Human Hypertension demonstrated the effect of upper cervical technique on reducing high blood pressure. Researchers in this double-blinded, placebo-controlled study found that NUCCA-style adjustments led to a significant reduction in systolic and diastolic blood pressure, while the amount of atlas laterality diminished as well.[82]
- Selano et al. researched the effects of upper cervical manipulation on the T-helper (T4) cell levels in HIV positive patients.[83] In this study, they found that the group receiving manipulative treatment had a 48% increase in T4 levels while those in the control group (receiving a sham adjustment) had a 7.96% decrease in T4 levels over the duration of the study. Granted, this study was small (only 5 experimental subjects and 5 controls), but the results are impressive nevertheless.
- Upper cervical chiropractor Erin Elster has published several articles describing her success in treating patients with multiple sclerosis and Parkinson disease.[84] Although her studies are not performed with the strict standards of a randomized-controlled trial format we must concede that any amount of improvement for these patients is tremendous. Not only that, but it is eye-opening for these successes to occur with manual therapy.
- Pollard and Ward found subjects receiving upper cervical manipulation demonstrated a greater increase in passive hip flexion (SLR) than those receiving sacroiliac manipulation.[85]

- Pollard and Ward also compared the effects of suboccipital and hamstring stretching on subjects' hip flexion range of motion.[86] They found that repetitive suboccipital contraction led to a greater improvement in ROM than hamstring contraction performed at the end-range of hip flexion.
- Karel Lewit discovered a strong connection between atlanto-occipital blockage and the presence of pelvic distortion in young children.[75] He found that while studying 75 children aged 3-6 years, there was pelvic distortion in 24 of them. Twenty-three of these children had restricted atlanto-occipital movement. To further demonstrate the link between these findings, he found that manipulation of the OA joint led to the elimination of the distortion.[75]
- Robinson et al. found that upper cervical treatment was effective as a stand-alone treatment for low back pain.[87]
- Kessigner and Boneva found that upper cervical adjustment (knee-chest) led to an increase in subjects' lumbar range of motion (flexion, extension, lateral flexion) whereas the control group experienced no change.[88]
- Rochester performed a retrospective case series to assess the effect of upper cervical adjustments on neck pain and disability outcomes. He found this treatment significantly decreased neck pain and disability (NDI) after an average of just 13.6 days involving just 5.7 office visits and only 2.7 adjustments. No adverse effects of care were noted in any of the sixty-six cases studied.[89]
- Wiles studied the effects of atlas adjustment on stomach function. It was found that the manipulation led to an increase in the basic gastric tone and the "normalization" of the wave pattern.[90]
- Amalu studied the effect of upper cervical care on 23 successive patients with primary fibromyalgia and chronic fatigue syndrome.[91] The results indicate that every patient was able to resume normal activities at the conclusion of care. Additionally, all patients reported maintaining these improvements at 1 to 1.5 years later.
- In the Trigeminal Neuralgia Association's patient handbook, Weigel and Casey report that upper cervical care is proven to be especially beneficial in treating this condition.[92] They point to a survey of upper cervical chiropractors who have found that 73.5% of patients with trigeminal neuralgia experience complete relief, 21% experience some relief, while only 6% are not helped at all.
- Whittingham et al. tested the effect of upper cervical toggle manipulation on headaches.[93] They found these adjustments led to improvements in headache frequency, duration and severity in all but two of 24 participants.

So, what does all this mean to the manual therapist, one might ask? It means that the upper cervical spine must be addressed; it is just too important to bypass. But do not worry. Treatment does not have to include manipulation if that is out of one's scope of practice. Instead, there are many techniques from many approaches available to the manual therapist. Specific treatment is described in Chapter 11, The Cervical Spine.

CRANIOSACRAL AND SACRO-OCCIPITAL TECHNIQUE

These techniques come from osteopathic and chiropractic physicians, respectively. Both offer further insight into the complexity of the nervous system. That is because each of these approaches deals with the vital flow of cerebrospinal fluid and the delicate relationship between the cranial and sacral respiratory mechanisms. Thus, by correcting dysfunction in this system, clinicians are able to correct a wide variety of patient complaints. The reader is urged to attend seminars in either technique in order to fully understand the concepts of the craniosacral rhythm and to gain hands-on experience performing these techniques. It is beyond the scope of this text to cover either approach thoroughly.

As mentioned at the top of this section, treatment of the global pattern involves anything which brings the patient back to homeostasis. This might be by using a neurologically-based technique, but it could also be achieved with treatment along any one of the other three primary factors. Likewise, it could even be done by addressing the secondary factors. All in all, a treatment most likely to work is one which addresses the stressors creating the pattern in the first place.

NEUROLOGICAL DISORGANIZATION

Neurological disorganization is the third important way that neurological dysfunction can affect the body. For the most part, this is a concept recognized solely by Applied Kinesiologists because it is detected with muscle testing. In short, it is described as a "functional problem in the neuromuscular system that results in specific patterns of abnormal muscle function."[94] This means that the nervous system is not activating/inhibiting muscles in a typical, predictable manner. A classic example of this occurrence is when a patient displays an obvious postural fault—such as an elevated shoulder—but does not demonstrate a weak latissimus and strong upper trapezius on the same side. Another example is an alteration in muscle recruitment patterns during the gait cycle. For instance, instead of an inhibited shoulder flexor and facilitated shoulder extensor on the side of lower extremity advancement, the opposite pattern is found. Of course, there are many other manifestations of neurological disorganization, as well as many clinical implications of this condition. As Maffetone points out, this condition can "predispose a person to injury, prevent an injury from being corrected even when the proper therapy is applied, and may cause a continual recurrence of another injury or imbalance."[94]

Optimal assessment of this condition is carried out by applied kinesiology examination. In the absence of this, the clinician would be wise to consider this disorder as a possibility when the patient's body is not behaving as it should, or even when the patient seems a little "mixed-up" at times. This may be a person who lies on his back when told to go face down, or vice versa. These individuals just seem to be neurologically "switched," as prior terminology described them.

Treatment for neurological disorganization is to correct the problem causing the disorganization in the first place. With AK, the clinician can quickly find this disorder, correct it, and retest the patient to see if the condition is resolved. Without AK this process is slower and several causative factors cannot be found. Fortunately, the most common causes of neurological disorganization are problems the manual therapist *can* find and fix. Among these are the cranials, the pelvis, the feet (subluxations and gait reflexes), and the TMJ. Therefore, by treating these areas, the clinician without AK experience can address the common causes of this disorder.

After reading this chapter, it should be fairly obvious why assessing and treating the nervous system—on all levels—is imperative to a successful outcome. To this point, the preceding sections provide an excellent framework for the clinician attempting to do as much. Not only do they categorize the ways in which the nervous system acts upon the body, but they also detail many successful ways the clinician can implement treatment. Among these means of influence and treatment were theories the reader was likely familiar with, and therefore can identify with. But also included is a more abstract theory—that of the nervous system as an open-ended system. It is under this theory that we can rationalize how any disturbance of the system can have widespread, far-reaching effects. This realm has always been the "X-factor" for chiropractors and osteopaths alike, whose treatments sometimes cure seemingly unrelated somatovisceral or viscerosomatic problems—and at other times do not.

With the help of authors such as Orbach[95] and Chestnut this phenomenon has been "demystified" in recent years. Both authors outline the neural circuitry explaining how minor alterations in function (often of afferent activity) lead to disruptions in all systemic functions of the body (especially by synapsing in the hypothalamus and increasing activity of the sympathetic nervous system). Indeed, they have taken out part of the "magic" of manual therapy with their logical explanations (hah)!

In later chapters of this text many of these techniques—both logical and "mystical"—are described in detail. For the most part, they are included in the chapter corresponding to the area in which treatment is applied. However, at other times they are placed in a chapter corresponding to the area in which pathology resides. Regardless of their placement the reader is urged to keep in mind that placing these techniques and pathologies into nice, neat categories is done for convenience only. Remember, virtually any technique affecting the body will affect the nervous system, and vice versa.

6 Movement Pattern Considerations

FOR THE PURPOSE OF THIS TEXT, THE TERM "MOVEMENT PATTERN" REFERS TO THE *WAY* THE BODY moves. While this subject is a combination of mechanical and neurological factors, it is presented here as a separate consideration worthy of independent discussion. In general orthopedic terms, the term movement pattern is defined as the quality and symmetry with which a joint or bodypart moves. These factors are very important and are separate from the objective range-of-motion data we normally focus on. While range-of-motion is primarily a mechanical concern, the movement pattern is primarily a neurological one. It is the result of firing patterns and the brain's ability to recruit specific muscles in a specific sequence.

Learning to identify and correct faulty movement patterns should be a top priority to the manual therapist. The first reason for this is that the faulty movement pattern is often responsible for *causing* the patient's joint-related pain. This may be due to altered osteokinematics or arthrokinematics causing abnormal stress to the joint and adjoining soft-tissues. In fact, Lewit believes that "disturbance of function appears much earlier in the locomotor system than do degenerative morphological changes."[75] An example of this relationship is seen in the hip, where weakness of the gluteus medius has been shown to precede degenerative changes. A similar situation is seen in the spine, where inhibition and atrophy of the intrinsic muscles leads to instability and degeneration. Other disorders, including rotator cuff impingement, patellofemoral dysfunction, lateral epicondylitis and many others are also frequently caused by faulty movement patterns.

The second reason movement pattern correction is so important is that faulty movement patterns *perpetuate* existing conditions. In other words, they make a bad condition worse. This is by altering osteokinematics and arthrokinematic relationships as previously discussed. It is also through protective muscle spasm in the case of localized injury and pain. Helpful in the short term, the inability to "shut off" increased muscle tone leads to a new pain—one of muscular origin. Prolonged hypertonicity does not allow the muscle time to heal or for blood to circulate. This plays into the "pain-spasm-pain" cycle. In this vicious cycle, joint pain is responsible for causing muscle spasm. Prolonged muscle spasm causes more pain. More pain causes more muscle spasm, and so on.

Abnormal movement patterns often follow the common pattern in that the body tends to use or initiate movement with a facilitated muscle while further neglecting inhibited muscles. This is the neurological influence of our hard-wiring, and awareness of this tendency certainly helps streamline the identification and treatment of faulty patterns for the therapist. Treatment should focus on methods to reduce the influence of the common pattern—segmentally and suprasegmentally—as presented throughout this book. It should also include the use of sensorimotor training exercises. These were designed by Vladimir Janda as a way to treat the upper and lower crossed syndromes, which are basically the same as the common pattern. These exercises are presented later in this chapter.

The different movement-based therapy approaches provide useful ways to treat the common pattern as well. For instance, the fields of yoga, Pilates, Alexander technique and Somatic technique all have ways to address the anterior pelvic tilt—hyperlordosis pattern. They all do so with methods requiring strict concentration and muscle recruitment on the part of the patient while he/she performs other motions. This helps integrate the lost motion into the person's skill set for greater carry-over into the real world.

If treating the common pattern is not the "common ground" for these approaches, it is only second to another important concept: awareness. Yes, it is awareness—or lack thereof—which the movement therapies hold most important. The masters behind the techniques—Alexander, Hanna, and Feldenkrais—each emphasized the importance of static and dynamic awareness in their teachings. They recognized long ago that most individuals were unaware of their place in space, they were unaware of the way they breathed, they were unaware of the way they moved. These men designed treatment techniques to help the person become aware of these things and to use his body properly. A big part of this is in teaching the person to activate muscles he is not using and inactivate muscles unconsciously activated. Alexander's Primary Control is one example of this and Hanna's techniques to contract and relax muscles with "sensory-motor amnesia" are another.

Once again, it is fortunate that the primary teachings of these men fall in with the common pattern. This eliminates the need to learn yet another concept. At the same time they provide valuable ways to help retrain weak, forgotten muscles and take stress off vulnerable joints. Moreover, the methods these techniques utilize are easily integrated with normal function, thus maximizing their efficacy. Later in this text two of these movement patterns are described in detail: respiration and Alexander's Primary Control. Each of these is chosen for its important influence on the entire system.

Besides the neurological influences on the patient's movement patterns, we must also remember the mechanical system plays an important role here as well. This is really what traditional physical therapists are trained in. It is what we do when we study a patient's work environment or teach a back care class. We look at the mechanical influences of his surroundings. Similarly, when we observe a person's gait or the way he swings a golf club we use the same methodology by looking at factors such as velocity, acceleration, mass, and lever arm length to calculate the effects on the person's body. Yes, this is the basis behind gait analysis, golf swing analysis, throwing analysis, and so on. Because it is based more in physics than it is in neurology (as presented in this text), this form of movement pattern dysfunction is less predictable. This makes it more difficult for the therapist to evaluate, as he is not able to simply fall back on the common pattern as the mechanism driving it.

We begin our discussion below by exploring the neurologically-based concepts of movement therapy including sensorimotor training, awareness, respiration, and the Primary Control. Following this, we turn our focus towards mechanically-based ideals. This includes an overview of the kinetic chain and also provides the reader with an approach to make decisions on mechanically-based movement therapy.

SENSORIMOTOR TRAINING

Per Greenman,[5] sensorimotor training "restores symmetrical muscle firing patterns for control of motor function." It achieves this by bombarding the central nervous system with afferent impulses. This aids the CNS in forming the proper movement patterns which are "harmonious and coordinated and that provide stability to the locomotor system."[54]

In essence, besides addressing the common pattern, sensorimotor training greatly benefits the patient's dynamic stability by training the active and neural control subsystems. Referenced in Chapter 4, these components are vastly important for keeping joints in neutral during internal or external perturbation. In a sense, these exercises are the bridge between just strengthening a muscle and really integrating the strength increase into the patient's movement pattern.

The indications for sensorimotor training are numerous. Listed below are a few of the more common ones:

- Presence of the upper/lower crossed syndrome or common pattern.
- Balance deficit in any form.
- Abnormal shoulder elevation recruitment pattern.
- Abnormal hip extension recruitment pattern.
- Abnormal hip abduction recruitment pattern.
- Conditions suggestive of joint instability including localized or systemic hypermobility.
- Pain syndromes in any part of the spine.

From this list, the reader can see that these exercises are useful in treating the entire body. This is because they help normalize function of the CNS. This makes them important in treating almost every condition involving the spine or extremities. Presented below is a version of sensorimotor training adapted from Murphy, who presents a comprehensive retraining regimen in his text.[54]

Preparation

As these exercises are designed to bombard the CNS with afferent input, it is important to make sure this input is ideal. For this reason, it is necessary to have the patient do three things during each exercise. They are:

1. Maintain a short foot. This consists of contracting muscles on the sole of the foot in order to bring the forefoot and rearfoot together, thereby lifting the medial longitudinal arch. Take care to avoid toe flexion.
2. Place the tongue in the proper resting position. Ideally, this is just behind the incisors on the hard palate. It helps to have the patient make a clucking sound, as this will accomplish the task at hand. This position helps assure input from the TMJ, mouth, and throat is optimal.

3. Assume an Alexandrian posture. This refers to asserting one's primary control, which is mentioned in the next section. This involves allowing the posterior-superior portion of the head to raise, freeing the suboccipitals and lengthening the spine. Additionally, the patient is asked to expand the shoulders and visualize the legs extending towards the floor, moving away from the body.

Rocker Board Exercises

A rocker board allows movement in two directions. Begin by standing on the board with both feet, assuming the three prerequisites mentioned above. Once quiet standing is achieved, turn the board 90 degrees to the side. Once quiet standing is achieved in this plane, turn the board 45 degrees to one side. This forces motion in an oblique angle to the patient. Then turn it 90 degrees from here to create motion through the other oblique plane. Once the patient can stand in each position without difficulty, increase the level of difficulty by having him cross his arms. Then, have him close his eyes with his arms by his side. Next, have him stand with the eyes closed and arms crossed. Once this is achieved, start all over on just one leg (Fig. 6-1). Progress in the same fashion.

Wobble Board Exercises

After the patient masters the rocker board, progress him to the wobble board. This allows motion in 360 degrees and is more difficult than the rocker board. Progress him in the same way as done with the rocker board: eyes open, arms down to eyes open, arms crossed to eyes closed, arms down to eyes closed, arms crossed. Then have him stand on one leg instead of two and progress through the same stages (Fig. 6-2).

From this point, add perturbations to the patient. External perturbations are given by the clinician and internal perturbations are created by active patient movement. Murphy details several useful external perturbations, as they specifically activate weak, inhibited muscles. The first is pushing the patient's upper thoracic spine. This creates chin protrusion, which activates the deep cervical flexors to stop it. The second is a perturbation to the lumbosacral area. This forces abdominal contraction in order to halt excessive lumbosacral extension. The third perturbation is applied to the anterior pelvic girdle. This creates a hip flexor moment, thereby activating the gluteus maximus muscle to prevent it.

Internal perturbations are accomplished by having the patient do anything that compromises stability. This includes actions like swinging the arm or free

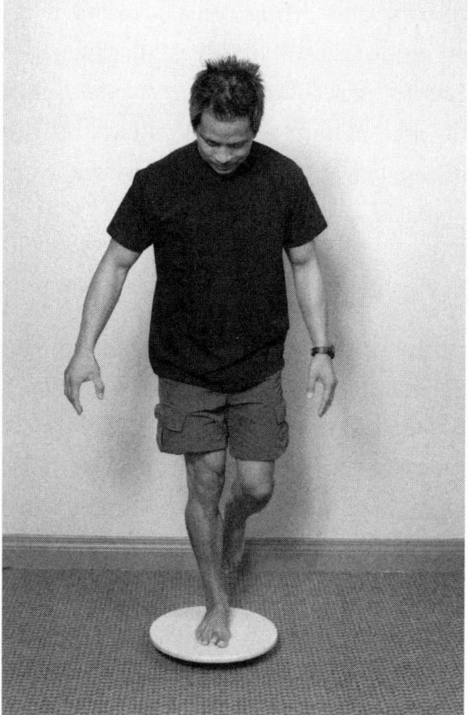

Fig. 6-1 Single leg standing on the rocker board.

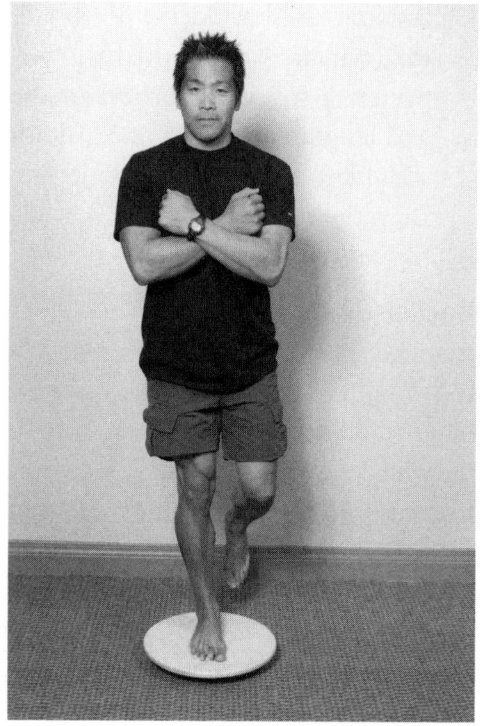

Fig. 6-2 Eyes open, arms crossed on wobble board.

leg in space, throwing and catching a ball, and even performing postural exercises (a valuable use of time). All of these challenge the body's stability and thus result in enhanced stability through repetition.

Head, Neck and Eye Coordination

Murphy describes several exercises to improve head, neck, and eye coordination. Ideally, he writes, these exercises are performed by the patient who is able to stand on the wobble board on one leg. If this is not possible, standing on both legs is allowable. The first exercise he describes is fairly simple. Have the patient focus their gaze on an object, such as a pen in the clinician's hand. Next, bring the pen to one side and have the patient track it with the eyes while also moving the head. Continue moving the pen to the patient's maximal range. After this, go to the opposite side, followed by going up and down and at oblique angles to the patient.

Another valuable exercise is to have the patient focus on an object in the clinician's hand while moving the head and neck in one direction and then the other—all the while maintaining a fixed gaze. This is progressed to neck motions in other planes, still maintaining a stable gaze. Additional drills involve having the patient follow a slow moving ball with his eyes to activate smooth pursuit or having him read a magazine aloud, thereby stimulating saccadic function.

It is the author's opinion that eye function is more important than most practitioners realize—so much so that it should be examined in all patients. For instance, just consider the fact that there are entire approaches based on eye exercises. One of them, Eye Movement Desensitization and Reprocessing technique is a progressive approach in psychology used to treat numerous psychological disorders. In chiropractic, the Conjugative Gaze Adjustive Technique simply has the patient turn his eyes away from the side of involvement and presto—spasm on the involved side diminishes while tone on the opposite side increases.

It is no wonder why these techniques are so far-reaching. The eyes have a tremendous influence on the nervous system. Just consider the fact that there are three cranial nerves dedicated to its movement. Then there is general sensation, riding along yet another nerve. Visual input travels along another cranial nerve, providing a great amount of input to the cerebral cortex. Altogether, it is no surprise some practitioners can focus solely on the eyes and get great results. Consequently, it is a must we consider eye function in the management of our patients.

RESPIRATION

Many practitioners in traditional medicine forget about the importance of proper respiration. We often examine and treat the ribcage, but we neglect the actual process of breathing. By ignoring this important action, we are failing to restore optimal health from two different perspectives. The first of these is from a systemic perspective. We know that proper breathing is necessary to oxygenate the blood. The brain and other organs need adequately oxygenated blood in order to survive. When the process of breathing fails to properly oxygenate blood, these organs and other tissues cannot function properly. Not only are they unable to perform normal maintenance tasks efficiently, but they are unable to repair themselves following injury. Besides this obvious function of respiration, some believe that respiration also plays an important role in aiding circulation. Mitchell points out that the heart is only responsible for pumping one-fourth of the body's total blood volume.[96] The remaining three-fourths is pumped by the action of the diaphragm and striated muscles.[96] Consequently, ineffective respiration leads to not only poor oxygenation of the blood, but also diminished tissue perfusion. One can surmise that this lack of help from the diaphragm makes the heart work that much harder.

The other important perspective concerning respiration involves its demands on the musculoskeletal system. Like any repetitive activity, the act of respiration has the power to negatively impact the musculoskeletal system. To perform normal breathing, numerous muscles must contract in synchrony to achieve inspiration and expiration. At the same time, numerous joints must have adequate mobility to allow proper inspiration and expiration to take place. Any deviation from normal in the recruitment of specific respiratory muscles creates problems in the long run. In addition, lack of adequate muscle strength or joint flexibility adds overwhelming stress to another portion of the functional unit, thus creating symptoms in one form or another. For the patient with symptoms already present, it is easy to understand how dysfunctional breathing will perpetuate these symptoms.

We begin this section with a preliminary description of normal and abnormal respiratory dynamics. Following this, we will cover important treatment strategies. For the most part, this portion is borne out of the work of movement therapists. This is because their approaches were the first to truly change the breathing process. Practitioners of the Alexander and Feldenkrais techniques train people to change the way they breathe. It is this entire breathing process we are interested in for the sake of this chapter.

Normal Breathing

Normal breathing is more complicated than the simple act of breathing in and breathing out. By the time we are adults there are many factors which can alter our respiratory pattern and hinder its function. For this reason, it is helpful to look for certain characteristics indicative of normal breathing in our patients. According to Gray,[97] several of these components are as follows:

- Lateral movement of the ribcage (especially the lower ribcage) without excessive upward and downward movement of the sternum.
- The shoulders should not rise with breathing, and the muscles of the neck should be quiet.
- The exhalation phase should be two to three times longer than the inspiration phase.
- Diaphragmatic contraction creates a vacuum effect which pulls air into the lungs; there is no need to "suck" air in.

- The abdominal muscles should not be overly tight and contracted during breathing. A slight contraction at the end of exhalation is acceptable as long as this contraction is immediately released to allow full inspiration.
- The abdomen should not pooch out excessively.

For the most part, adults do not breathe properly and the clinician will have to examine many patients before finding one with a healthy breathing pattern. However, if one wants to see an example of proper breathing it is not hard. Just watch a healthy child breathe. They do not have faulty movement patterns, emotional stress, or fascial and articular restrictions limiting this natural motion (in most cases). They breathe free and without effort—just as we are supposed to. This is consistent with the concept that the body functions in a perfect way under normal circumstances. It is only with the accumulation of life's stressors that the body's innate function is altered.

Abnormal Breathing

The most common abnormal breathing pattern is consistent with the common pattern (startle response, Hanna's Red Light Reflex). It involves shallow chest breathing instead of deep, diaphragmatic breathing. In essence, this leads to all of the problems described above ranging from poor oxygenation to the overuse of the muscles raising the chest (scalenii, sternocleidomastoids, pectorals). This pattern also plays into a harmful cycle echoed throughout this text in that it promotes systemic acidification[98] and sympathetic nervous system dominance. It is for this reason that authors including Young[98] suggest proper diaphragmatic breathing as a way to optimal health. Likewise, it is for this reason that exercises which emphasize deep, rhythmical breathing such as Yoga are proven to benefit the participant across the health spectrum.[99]

To observe this faulty pattern, simply observe the chest during inspiration. One will see the entire thorax lift concurrent with a breath in (Fig. 6-3).[75] Palpation will substantiate this visual finding. As noted above, this motion is created by the contraction of the cervical muscles, including the sternocleidomastoid and scalenii. These muscles will often be prominent when this pattern is present for a long time. In the lower ribcage of these patients, the clinician will note that there is an overall lack of widening. This may be due to the lack of abdominal muscle contraction to counteract the diaphragm. Or, it may be due to the patient's inability to breathe into the posterior thorax.[75] The end result is that the

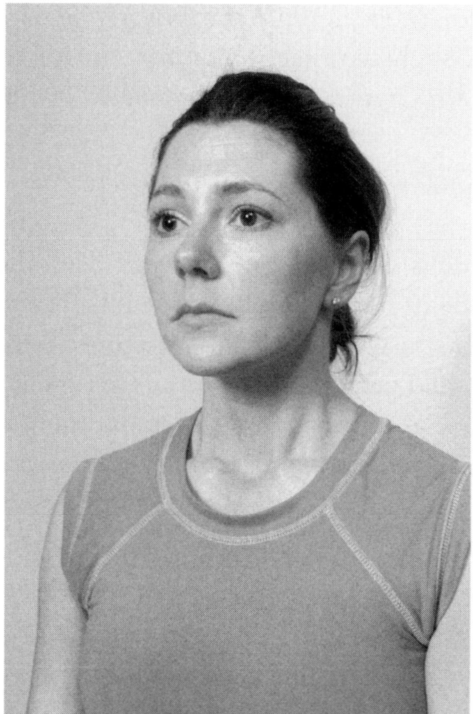

Fig. 6-3 Excessive chest elevation during breathing. Also note the contraction of the SCM.

thoracic spine does not go through its normal range of flexion and extension. This helps maintain movement restrictions in the thoracic spine.[75]

Treatment Strategies

As mentioned previously, most of the work to improve the quality of respiration has been done by movement therapists. In the teachings of Alexander and Feldenkrais, proper breathing is an important topic. In fact, it is said that F.M. Alexander was called "the breathing man" during his early days of teaching.[100] The thought of spending more than a few seconds to teach proper breathing is a new concept to most of us. But, given the ramifications of abnormal breathing, this is something we must add to our repertoire.

As stated, teachers of Alexander Technique and the Feldenkrais Method spend a great deal of time helping their clients regain normal respiratory function. While a discussion of this depth is out of the scope of this text, suffice it say that therapy begins with making the patient aware of his improper breathing pattern. Then, after he is aware of this, he should be taught how to breathe properly, adhering to the principles of normal breathing described above. The manual therapist can aid this process by implementing the primary control concept (described below) with the patient in order to optimize alignment and neurological recruitment. Additionally, manual techniques to improve soft tissue and articular mobility (especially of the thoracic spine and ribcage) will allow the body to be more free in performing motions it is not accustomed to. For further information on proper breathing, please consult a book devoted to one of these approaches.

Research has substantiated the efficacy of the Alexander Technique in improving respiratory function. In a study published in *Chest*, subjects who were taught the Alexander Technique improved in peak expiratory flow, maximal voluntary ventilation, maximal inspiratory mouth pressure, and maximal expiratory mouth pressure.[101] The authors of this report gave four possible causes for such improvements:

1. *Increased length of the muscles of the torso.* This refers to the inhibition of slumping patterns including a reduction in cervical lordosis and a lengthening of the rectus abdominis. The reduction in excessive cervical lordosis allows for a greater passage of air to the lungs.
2. *Increased strength and/or endurance of muscles of the abdominal wall.*
3. *Decreased resting tension of chest wall muscles.* This reduction in muscle tone allows for more freedom of motion of the ribs.
4. *Enhanced coordination of the respiratory muscles.* By increasing the length and decreasing the resting tension of various chest and abdominal muscles, the breathing mechanism faces less interference. Therefore, it is able to work more efficiently.

ALEXANDER'S PRIMARY CONTROL

F.M. Alexander is mentioned extensively throughout this text. While he is known for many contributions to the field of movement therapy, certainly one of the most functionally relevant to the manual therapist is his concept of the Primary Control. Briefly stated, the Primary Control is a conscious effort on the part of the patient to raise the posterior-superior part of the skull, thereby freeing the head to move upwards and slightly forwards. This frees the skull and cervical spine (and rest of the body) from the effects of what Alexander calls the Downward Pull—an involuntary contraction of the suboccipital muscles resulting in occipital extension upon the cervical spine and exaggerated lordosis of the lumbar spine.

Training patients to activate the Primary Control is beneficial in many ways. It helps lengthen the spine and allows the scapulae to drop down and back (Fig. 6-4). Neurologically, the suboccipitals and sternocleidomastoids are inhibited with this action, so the patient is effectively breaking up a pathological synergistic pattern. This undoubtedly benefits recruitment patterns in the entire body as well—making this a valuable concept to share with all patients.

One of the most commonly used ways of integrating Hanna's Primary Control concept into practice is by guiding the patient as she arises from sitting. This involves placing the clinician's hands on the patient's mastoid processes and lightly lifting the posterior skull up and forward as she stands (Fig. 6-5). This helps train the patient to use the muscles which perform this same motion voluntarily. In effect, this prevents occipital extension upon standing, which is a common faulty pattern. Coupled with this, the patient is asked to lengthen the entire spine including the lumbar spine. This prevents excessive lumbar lordosis

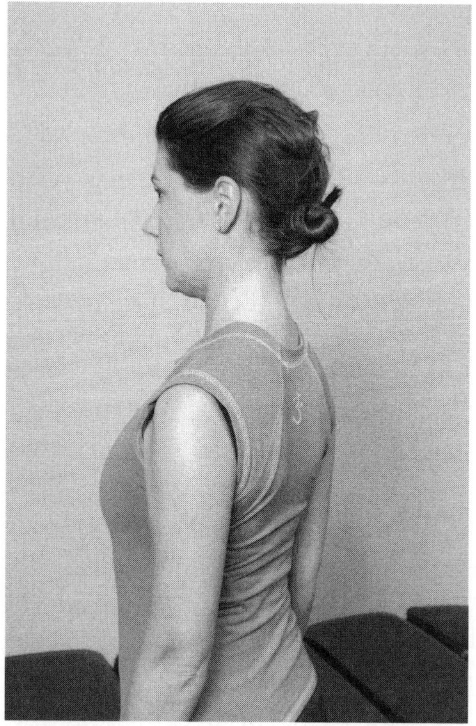

Fig. 6-4 Asserting the Primary Control lengthens the spine and allows the scapulae to drop down and back.

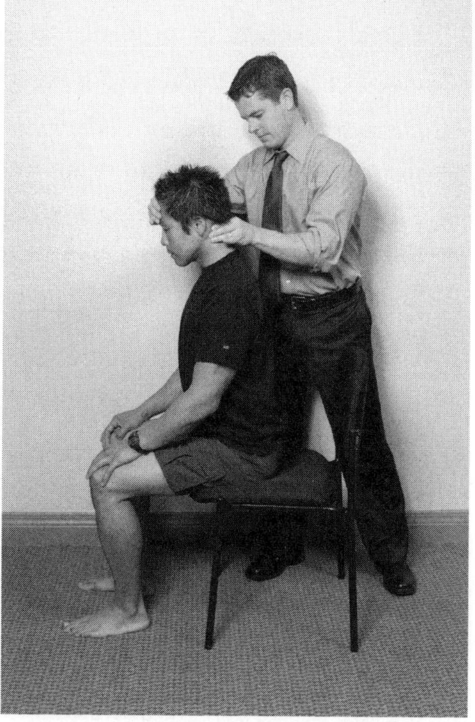

Fig. 6-5 Training the patient to use the Primary Control while arising from sitting. Gently lift the posterior occiput anteriorly and superiorly as the patient stands, asking him to flex the upper cervical spine at the same time.

when arising from sitting—a common aggravating factor for many patients with low back pain. In fact, as published in the September 1997 issue of the Journal of Orthopedic and Sports Physical Therapy, Cottingham and Maitland found this technique especially helpful in treating a patient with pain in the low back and buttock.[102] Guided sit-to-stand, stand-to-sit, and squatting exercises not only helped reduce the patient's pain but also helped maintain structural correction of the pelvic girdle.

KINETIC CHAIN REACTION

In school we are trained to examine the movement of each bodypart as though it exists completely independent of the rest of the body. This of course is hardly the case, but it is probably the most practical approach in the classroom and the clinic. After all, examining a single joint for movement quality and quantity is fairly easy to master. Likewise, formulating a treatment plan based on these findings is rather straightforward. Unfortunately, this approach does not take into consideration the "dynamic dependence" of the kinetic chain.

The kinetic chain concept was discussed in the section Mechanical Considerations. It is highlighted in this chapter due to its importance in understanding the body's dynamic relationships. By understanding and then applying the principles of this theory the clinician has one more tool to use in the diagnosis and treatment of musculoskeletal disorders.

In the context of diagnosis, the kinetic chain concept helps the clinician predict areas of undue stress. The author has taken the liberty of creating a classification scheme to describe the numerous sources of stress and strain during a multi-joint movement. These categories are as follows:

1. Inherent Stress
2. Compensatory/Intrinsic Stress
3. Compensatory/Extrinsic Stress

The first category, Inherent Stress, refers to the direct stress the joint endures during a specific motion. This includes the joint's end-range motion, position, velocity, and resultant torque during an activity. We can predict these factors via clinical observation and then use this information to focus on a particular motion known to be especially stressful on a given joint. Take the effects of the baseball throw on the shoulder joint. During cocking, the shoulder has been observed to go into 175 degrees of external rotation.[103] This is obviously very stressful on the anterior structures of the shoulder joint. Not only are the active restraints to external rotation placed under extreme load, but the anterior ligaments are stretched as well. Following ball release, the shoulder undergoes extreme stress once again. The external rotators are maximally contracted to decelerate the humerus. The passive elements in the posterior shoulder are also stretched to a maximal degree. By taking this knowledge and combining it with other aspects of the examination, the clinician is better able to formulate a cause-and-effect hypothesis of the patient's problem.

The second classification, Compensatory/Intrinsic Stress, refers to the added stress a joint undergoes when it is not functioning at an optimal level. This may be due to joint pathology, hypermobility, hypomobility, weakness, etc. Any limitation that does not allow the joint to function normally only serves to cause further strain. To succeed in performing the desired movement without causing increased strain, the body must compensate. Again, let's use the baseball pitch as an example. In the cocking phase, the pitcher is trained to bring the baseball behind his head to the same point in space every time. To do this, a certain amount of motion must occur in all three physical planes. In the transverse plane, the shoulder must horizontally abduct a specific amount. In the sagittal plane, the shoulder undergoes flexion. In the coronal plane, the shoulder abducts. The contribution of each plane to the end-goal is specific. When a restriction prevents optimal motion in one plane, the body can compensate by increasing motion in another. In the example of the right-handed pitcher, imagine that his latissimus dorsi is tight. This restricts flexion, a sagittal plane motion. To compensate for this, he may now have to abduct his arm more than normal. While this compensation may be successful temporarily, it is likely to cause joint damage in the long run. Considering the velocity and torque generated when throwing, it is likely that the athlete will now develop a secondary problem such as impingement.

The final category is called Compensatory/Extrinsic Stress. This term signifies the added stress a joint endures due to dysfunction in a neighboring or distant joint along the kinetic chain. Once again, we are considering compensation as a means to an end. It is used to allow the body to successfully perform a task. Or, it may even be a way of protecting itself while maintaining the same level of function. In the context of the Extrinsic Stress category, we must realize the body has the capacity to go far beyond the restricted/painful joint to achieve its goal. It can use all of the laws of physics in order to bypass a bodypart that is not co-operating. To illustrate this concept in action, let's again turn to the cocking phase of the baseball pitch. First and foremost, remember that the brain's goal is to place the ball at a specific point behind the pitcher's head at the end of the cocking phase. To do this, countless three-dimensional movements occur all the way from the ground up to the hand. With that being said, imagine that the pitcher's trunk rotation to the right is restricted. Somehow, the body now must achieve more clockwise motion in the transverse plane or the ball will not reach its desired placement. This may take the form of increased right hip internal rotation. Or, the shoulder may now go into further horizontal abduction.

The compensations may not be completely limited to the same plane. They may be a combination of other available planes. Using the case of restricted right thoracic rotation, the ramifications could be widespread. The humerus may externally rotate excessively, the scapula may tilt posteriorly, or the shoulder may flex more than normal. The combination of possible compensations is limitless.

These categories of compensation are not limited to competitive athletics. They are used by all of us consciously and subconsciously on a daily basis. We elevate our shoulder girdle to aid us in putting a dish away. We extend our low back to enhance hip extension. We rotate our thoracic spine when it is painful to turn the cervical spine. Unfortunately, our patient's bodies may be so skilled at compensating that we sometimes only treat the symptomatic bodypart, believing that it is the root of the problem. This occurs when symptoms are the result of dysfunction elsewhere. This trickery is undoubtedly responsible for countless cases of "failed therapy" every year.

Implications for Treatment

Once the clinician has identified the motion(s) responsible for stressing the problematic joint, it is time to teach the patient how to lessen these stresses. This should involve local as well as global modifications to his movement patterns. Locally, teach him ways to protect the symptomatic bodypart during a given motion if that action causes excessive movement or strain to the bodypart. For instance, a patient with low back pain can brace himself by assuming a neutral pelvic tilt with the navel pulled posteriorly while performing stressful activities. This minimizes local stress and strain and protects the back.

Outside this region, the therapist can teach the patient to use other bodyparts to assume more of the workload to further take stress off the low back. Oftentimes in cases of low back pain we find the hips are not used as much as they should be. Therefore, teaching the patient to use his/her hips with forward flexion or rotation is extremely helpful in protecting an acute or subacute back condition.

This is just one example how this treatment strategy can benefit the patient. There are many, many others. Therapists are urged to always look outside the symptomatic bodypart when performing movement analysis. It is there that one often finds the cause of the patient's problem. Consequently, it is there that the best treatment resides.

GAIT

The biomechanics of normal gait were discussed in Chapter 4, Mechanical Considerations. In that chapter, human gait was broken down into a series of individual movements that occurred in a strictly mechanical, chain-reaction format. Accordingly, treatment under the mechanical model involves the use of mechanical tools—such as orthotics—to correct improper motion. In this chapter, the mode of treatment is different. Instead of just supporting a structural fault, the clinician is encouraged to retrain the client's faulty movement pattern. To do this, begin by assessing the gait pattern in the same fashion as was performed previously. Remark on any deviations from normal. Include notations about gait speed, cadence, step length, and stride length. Look for toe in/out posturing, as well as deviation from initial contact to toe off. Look at the position of the knee during swing and stance phases. Does it buckle? Does it fully extend? Does the person actually walk on the forefoot instead of passing from the hindfoot to the forefoot? What do their shoes look like, for that matter? Is there unequal wear and tear? Does the opposite hip drop during single leg stance? Are the hips rotated or are they straight?

As the reader is well aware, gait analysis is not easy to master. Actually, in some respects, it is a lot like reading an x-ray. One must have a system instead of just looking all around for a while, hoping she won't miss anything. Gait analysis is no different. Whether the practitioner wants to start at the bottom and work her way up or start at the top and work her way down does not matter. However, a good system must be in place so that she looks at the same things every time and does not miss anything.

After gait analysis comes gait correction. Work with the patient by first informing them of any deviation. In many cases they are unaware of their asymmetry and can correct it right away. Other times it will take repetition to make proper gait a habit. In other instances, the person's gait abnormality is due to an orthopedic problem requiring attention—in this case it is the clinician's duty to perform the needed correction and then re-train gait.

7 Energetic Considerations

ENERGY MEDICINE IS THE FOURTH AND FINAL PRIMARY FACTOR. IT IS BY FAR THE LEAST UNDERSTOOD of the primary factors and the most controversial. Speaking from personal experience, I can recall laughing the first time I saw the word "ch'i" in an acupuncture text. As a traditionally-trained physical therapist, I thought the idea of subtle energy flow through one's body was ridiculous. I do not know what a recent physical therapy graduate thinks of energy medicine at this point in time, but I can assume his thoughts are similar to my initial ones on the subject. Compounded with this, in a time of evidence-based medicine, practitioners want to see the research behind a therapy. To address these issues, this topic is presented by letting the research do the talking.

In the first section of this chapter the age-old question is addressed: how do these techniques work? After all, do acupuncture and other techniques really influence energy flow or do they just influence neurology? Well, truthfully, the verdict is still out on this issue. But what is not a mystery is that these techniques really do alter physiology, and there are many studies to prove it.

The second section answers a more important question than the "how" behind energy medicine. It answers the question "does energy medicine work?" Once again, the reader is presented with numerous research studies proving that energy-based therapies are effective in treating various problems.

Finally, after the barrage of research on this topic, several of the more popular "energy-based" techniques are presented. For the purposes of this text, a mere introduction to these techniques is given. It is hoped that this gives the reader a general idea of what these methods do and spurs a greater interest in them.

THE HOW

Below are the summaries of numerous studies trying to explain the precise effects of "energy medicine":

- Volf studied the somatosensory evoked potentials created by auricular acupuncture stimulation.[104] She found that stimulating the point on the ear corresponding with the wrist activated the same cortical area as did direct median nerve stimulation at the wrist.
- Uchida and Hotta studied the effects of acupuncture on blood flow in the cerebral cortex and the uterus in anesthetized rats.[105] They found stimulation to the face, forepaw and hindpaw increased cortical blood flow and stimulation to the hindpaw and perineal area increased uterine blood flow.
- Yim et al. studied the effect of electroacupuncture on acupoint ST36 in collagen-induced arthritic mice.[106] They found electroacupuncture on this point reduced the incidence of collagen-induced arthritis and levels of IL-6, TNF-α, INF-γ, collagen II antibody, IgG and IgM levels while preventing knee joint destruction. Needle retention without electrical stimulation was effective as well, though not as effective as electroacupuncture.
- Felhendler and Lisander designed a randomized-controlled trial to study the effect of acupressure on the cardiovascular system.[107] They found that acupuncture, as compared with stroking the meridians, led to significant decreases in systolic arterial pressure, diastolic arterial pressure, mean arterial pressure, heart rate and skin blood flow.
- Mori et al. studied the effects of acupuncture on pupillary diameter, heart rate, and pulse wave amplitude.[108] They found acupuncture led to a decrease in all three parameters. This is consistent with claims that acupuncture affects the autonomic nervous system.
- Liu et al. studied the effect of auricular pellet acupressure on antioxidative system function in patients with diabetes mellitus.[109] They found that patients receiving treatment for 20 days had significantly higher concentrations of superoxide dismutase and catalase compared with a control group receiving no treatment.
- Ohnishi et al. studied the effects of Kozo Nishino, a Japanese Ki expert, sending ki-energy into cultured osteoblastic MC3T3-E1 cells.[110] They found the number of cells in the dish with Ki-exposure was significantly greater than that in the control group. Further testing revealed increased

levels of mRNA expressions related to bone mineralization as well as elevated alkaline phosphatase and osteocalcin. In another study testing the effects on bone resorption, they found the number of osteoclast-like cells in dishes with Ki exposure were fewer than those in control dishes.

- Ohnishi and Ohnishi studied the effects of Kozo Nishino, a Japanese Ki expert, sending ki-energy into cell samples.[111] They found his ki-energy inhibited cell division of cancer cells, protected isolated mitochondria from heat deterioration and reduced lipid peroxidation in heat-treated mitochondria. They also reported that they found his energy (at least one form of it) to be infrared radiation between the wavelength range of .8 and 2.7 micrometers.
- Yamaguchi et al. studied the effect of acupuncture on leukocyte subpopulations in peripheral blood.[112] They found acupuncture promoted humoral and cellular immunity. Among the changes observed were increases in the number of CD2+, CD4+, CD8+, CD11b+, CD16+, CD19+, CD56+ cells and IL-4, IL-1β and IFN-γ levels in the cells.
- Napadow et al. studied the effects of acupuncture on somatosensory cortical plasticity in patients with carpal tunnel syndrome.[113] They found acupuncture reduced the size of fMRI activity in contralateral Brodmann Areas 1 and 4 when the third digit was stimulated. These were originally increased in size compared with control subjects' activation patterns. Also noted was lateral shifting of the cortical activation when the second digit was stimulated in post-treatment testing. Collectively, these findings were consistent with the patient's reports of decreased paresthesias and improved ability to distinguish sensation in the second and third digits. The authors conclude that acupuncture shows promise in inducing "beneficial cortical plasticity manifested by more focused digital representations."
- Inoue et al. found that acupuncture applied to the lumbar musculature, the pudendal nerve, and sciatic nerve led to an increase in sciatic nerve blood flow.[114] Of these, sciatic nerve stimulation sustained the increase longer than the pudendal nerve stimulation. The authors speculate that there was likely a change in the circulation of the cauda equina and nerve roots as well.
- Gaponjuk and Sherkovina describe the neurophysiological basis for using auricular acupuncture to lower blood pressure.[115] They point out that branches of the trigeminal, facial, glossopharyngeal, vagus and cervical nerves are all present on the ear surface. Therefore, by stimulating the ear at different locations, the practitioner can treat patients with different forms of hypertension

(hyperkinetic, hypokinetic, and eukinetic) in a specific fashion. The authors outline specific details behind treatment of each form of hypertension, including the mechanism by which acupuncture helps.

- Karavis summarizes the many ways acupuncture affects neurophysiology.[116] Among these are local, regional, and general effects. Locally, there are immune responses, the generation of an electric injury potential, and the release of opioid peptides, bradykinin, serotonin and proteolytic enzymes at the site of entry. Regionally, acupuncture creates changes covering several dermatomes due to activation of several reflexes, including cutaneo-visceral, cutaneo-muscular and viscera-muscular reflexes. Karavis lists the general effects of acupuncture as being mediated by opioid, non-opioid and central sympathetic inhibitory mechanisms.

As the reader can tell from these studies, there is no doubt that energy-based techniques influence physiology. But do they really have anything to do with "energy?" After reading this research it appears we can explain the majority of these techniques' efficacy just by observing their influence on the nervous system. However, before we entirely write-off the existence of "energy" in the healing arts, it is only fair to mention texts by Becker, Gerber and Oschman. These authors provide copious details on the role of energy in both health and disease, and make an excellent case for energy medicine. Gerber does an especially good job at summarizing numerous studies describing how certain energy-based practitioners use their energy to do different things, ranging from helping plants grow to preventing goiters from enlarging. Granted, much of this data does not fall under the "evidence-based medicine" umbrella, but it is definitely worth a second look.

Yet another compelling case for energy medicine is presented by authors including Oschman,[117,118,119] Cheralier,[119] and Mori.[119] These researchers propose that free electrons from the earth can be used to help heal the body. These electrons, which are transmitted to us when we physically touch the ground (as when walking barefoot), are believed to act as antioxidants in the body. Supporting this theory are several research studies showing that sleeping on "earthing beds" (beds electrically connected to the ground) results in changes in cortisol levels, sleeping habits, trapezius muscle tone (chosen specifically as a marker of stress), cortical activation and pain levels. This is definitely an exciting piece of research as it links energy flow with inflammation and free radical damage, each regarded as the agents responsible for almost every degenerative disease humans face. In fact, this research is even consistent with other authors' claims that systemic acidity (a heightened positive charge) is responsible for the same chronic degenerative conditions.

DOES IT WORK?

Many high-quality studies point to the efficacy of energy-based therapies. Several of these are listed below.

- Quinn et al. performed a randomized controlled trial to determine the effect of reflexology on low back pain.[120] They found that true reflexology led to a significant decrease in low back pain as compared with a control group receiving sham reflexology.
- Jensen et al. designed a randomized-controlled trial to study the effects of acupuncture on patients with patellofemoral pain syndrome.[121] They found that one month of treatment led to improvements in the Cincinnati Knee Rating System by a significant margin at follow-up 12 months later.
- Haslam designed a randomized-controlled trial to compare the effects of acupuncture with exercises and advice on patients with hip osteoarthritis.[122] He found the group receiving acupuncture once per week for six weeks experienced significant improvement immediately after the course of treatment and at eight-week follow-up.
- Ebneshahidi et al. studied the effects of low energy laser acupuncture on chronic tension headache.[123] They found the group receiving low energy laser acupuncture experienced significant improvements over the placebo group in headache intensity, median duration of attacks, and median number of days with headache per month.
- Johansson et al. performed a randomized controlled trial comparing the effects of acupuncture and home exercises with those of ultrasound and home exercises on patients with shoulder impingement.[124] They found that both groups improved, but the acupuncture and exercise group had a larger improvement in the combined score.
- Guerra de Hoyos et al. performed a randomized controlled trial comparing the effects of acupuncture on patients with shoulder pain.[125] They found that the group receiving electro-acupuncture demonstrated consistent improvements over the control group (placebo acupuncture) in pain level, functional ability, quality of life, range of motion, global satisfaction, and NSAID intake.

- Vas et al. performed a randomized-controlled trial to determine the effects of the addition of single-point acupuncture to a physical therapy regimen for patients with shoulder pain.[126] They found the addition of acupuncture to the physical therapy regimen led to significantly greater improvements in pain level than physical therapy alone.
- Barker et al. studied the effects of auricular acupressure in patients with hip fracture.[127] In a randomized double-blinded trial, they found auricular acupressure applied to points corresponding to hip pain resulted in patients having less pain, anxiety and a lower heart rate compared with those receiving sham auricular acupressure.
- Usichenko et al. performed a randomized controlled trial to study the effect of auricular acupuncture on pain levels after total hip arthroplasty.[128] They found auricular acupuncture was successful in reducing pain levels.

Besides being valuable in the treatment of musculoskeletal disorders, there is also a substantial amount of evidence showing that energy-based techniques can be used to treat certain non-musculoskeletal conditions. A few of these studies are presented below.

- Zhang et al. performed a randomized controlled trial studying the effects of acupuncture on diabetic nephropathies.[129] They found acupuncture had a protective effect on the kidney and led to therapeutic improvement in terms of blood sugar, blood lipids, urinary albumin excretion rate, urinary monocyte chemotactic protein-1, glomerular filtration rate, and renal blood flow.
- Zhang et al. studied the effects of acupuncture on diabetic retinopathy.[130] It was found that acupuncture to regulate the spleen and stomach improved eye fundus condition and led to improved levels of vascular active substances nitric oxide and endothelin.
- Wang et al. conducted a meta-analysis of eight randomized controlled trials studying the effect of acupuncture on depression.[131] The authors found these eight studies including 477 subjects confirmed that acupuncture significantly reduced the severity of depression using the Hamilton rating scale for depression and the Beck Depression Inventory.
- Stener-Victorin and Humaidan reviewed the efficacy of acupuncture as an adjuvant to conventional treatment in assisted reproductive technology.[132] In short, the authors reviewed four published randomized controlled trials.

Of these four studies, three revealed significantly higher pregnancy rates in the acupuncture groups compared with the control groups.

- Chen et al. performed a double-blinded clinical trial to determine if acupressure or meridian massage had an effect on increasing body weight in premature infants.[133] Compared with the control group, the infants receiving acupressure and meridian massage gained significantly more weight than the control group receiving routine care.
- Oleson and Flocco studied the effect of ear, hand and foot reflexology on premenstrual symptoms in a randomized controlled trial.[134] They found reflexology reduced symptoms of premenstrual syndrome.

Altogether, this research says it all. Acupuncture, auriculotherapy, acupressure and reflexology *are* effective at treating a wide variety of musculoskeletal problems—the exact same problems manual therapists deal with every day. By way of many different mechanisms they bring the patient closer to a state of balance. In the patient with musculoskeletal complaints this entails a reduction in pain and a restoration in joint mobility. In patients with non-musculoskeletal complaints this trend almost invariably goes toward a state of parasympathetic activation. Whether the end result be increased protection against oxidative stress, improved reproductive function, enhanced bone formation, decreased bone resorption, weight gain in a premature infant, normalization of blood glucose and lipid levels in a diabetic, or improvement in immune function, relatively the same thing happens: activation of the body's rest and digest system and the blunting of our fight-or-flight mechanism. By now the reader should recognize this trend: dampening the stress response results in improved outcomes. Period.

Given the efficacy of the "energy-based" techniques in treating musculoskeletal problems it is obvious they must be integrated into the manual therapist's repertoire. For this reason the reader is urged to learn one of the techniques mentioned so that it can be added to his or her current treatment regimen. Ideally, if he or she is able to learn and then practice acupuncture this is strongly encouraged based on the research at hand. If, on the other hand, this is impossible then one of the less invasive techniques is suggested. There are many good seminars and texts to teach the reader the theory and practice behind these techniques.

To begin the reader's indoctrination into "energy-medicine," an abbreviated version of auriculotherapy and reflexology has been added to each chapter on regional treatment. Please remember that this is merely an introduction to these fascinating techniques and is not comprehensive by any means (comprehensive treatment with these methods involves much more than just one or two reflex points). However, it is a good starting point for the reader to begin learning where some of these points are and how they are utilized. It will also serve as an example of how the four primary factors are addressed with a *complete* manual therapy approach.

8 Secondary Factors

THE SECONDARY FACTORS ARE THE SECOND CATEGORY OF STRESSORS WHICH INFLUENCE THE BODY. Simply put, this category includes all potential stressors not included as primary factors. Of course, these stressors still work via the same physical mechanisms as the primary factors. They also have the power to create or perpetuate physical problems, just as the primary factors do. The main difference between these stressors and the primary factors is that the secondary factors do not present themselves physically as do their primary counterparts. Therefore, they are often neglected by the clinician and deemed less important than the more apparent stressors. This is unfortunate because the problems they create are very real.

Sometimes a single secondary factor can create dysfunction on its own. Most often, though, the secondary factors work on a summative basis. This means the presence of multiple factors tends to push the body further into a dysfunctional state than would occur if just one factor was involved. This can occur by directly stressing a particular bodypart. Or, it may work indirectly by stressing the entire body. This latter mechanism involves the concept of musculoskeletal homeostasis presented in Chapter 2.

This leads to a breach of the symptomatic threshold in an otherwise healthy bodypart(s). Most often, this breach occurs in a joint already under abnormal strain compared with the rest of the system. This may be in a pitcher's shoulder or a basketball player's knee, for instance. Or, it may involve the low back of a sedentary individual. In any case, the secondary factors often go unnoticed and are left untreated when practitioners do not look at the entire system.

The primary goal of this chapter is to better acquaint the reader with the secondary factors so they no longer go overlooked. To achieve this, each stressor and its clinical implications are described in detail. (Please note that some of these factors were discussed in detail in Chapter 3 and are only briefly mentioned here.) When applicable, treatment to address each stressor is outlined as well. Again, please bear in mind the importance of addressing all potential stressors, even if the connection between the person's symptoms and the stressor is unclear. As long as no harm is done to the patient, unloading strain from the person's system will only benefit him.

The stressors below are organized according to how they affect the system. The first group, the Internal Stressors, involves stressors acting on the inside of the body. This includes matters ranging from diet to illness to emotional considerations. Briefly put, these stressors influence the body's internal physiology and biochemistry. That means they also affect the body's healing power. Consequently, addressing these factors will greatly facilitate the patient's healing response and lead to a much faster, efficient recovery.

The second group of stressors is the External Stressors. These are stressors manual therapists are used to dealing with, including the typical physical stressors resulting from our everyday routines. For the most part, this involves all static and dynamic activities capable of straining the body. This group of stressors is large and has the greatest potential to be helped by treatment.

INTERNAL STRESSORS

As mentioned above, the internal stressors are rarely addressed by manual therapists. This is a shame. As we discussed in Chapters 2 and 3, the internal environment and musculoskeletal system are intimately related. Actually, not only are they related, but oftentimes problems of the musculoskeletal system are due to problems of the internal system. With this being said, it stands to reason that we must treat factors which stress the internal systems of the body.

As we will see below, many of these interventions are easy to implement into anyone's practice. At other times, adequate intervention may be out of the therapist's scope of practice. In this case, it is still helpful to know of these connections because it will facilitate appropriate referral to qualified practitioners.

Diet

Dietary stress can be a major burden upon the patient's musculoskeletal system. For this reason, this issue must be addressed with all patients. Now, while there are countless factors comprising one's nutritional status, going into great depth on the subject is out of the scope of this text. Additionally, nutritional counseling is also out of the scope of practice of many manual therapists. To counter this, a brief synopsis of foods people should avoid and foods they should enjoy is presented below (Fig. 8-1). This is a brief, simple approach to nutritional counseling which any practitioner can utilize in practice. Please note that while this list may seem very basic, the foods included on it are very important. That is, overindulgence in any of the bad foods may contribute to the patient's problem. On the other hand, adequate amounts of the good foods can be just the boost the person's system needs in order to repair a problem. This list is as follows:

Foods to Avoid:

1. Refined sugars.
2. Saturated fats.
3. Trans fats.
4. Artificial sweeteners.
5. Alcohol.
6. Caffeine.
7. Processed foods.
8. Foods high in sodium.
9. Limited intake of starchy foods like white rice, white potatoes, pasta, breads (esp. white bread), and cereals.
10. Red meat.
11. Shellfish (due to cholesterol and pollutant content).
12. Pork products.
13. Dairy products (at least limit consumption of these foods).

Foods to Enjoy:

1. Vegetables. Remember that the greater the variety in color, the greater the variety of antioxidants.
2. Fruits. Again, variety is the key.
3. Certain raw nuts, including almonds and walnuts.

Fig. 8-1 Foods to avoid and foods to enjoy.

(Continued to next page)

4. Whole grains.
5. Foods high in fiber.
6. Foods rich in Omega-3 fatty acids like flaxseed oil and wild salmon. Please note that farm-raised, warm-water salmon does not contain the desired balance of Omega-3's, and often contains high amounts of pollutants including mercury and PCB's.
7. Lean meats including chicken and turkey.

Fig. 8-1 *Continued*—Foods to avoid and foods to enjoy.

Interestingly, these dietary do's and don'ts fall into a common pattern of their own. It seems that almost all well-researched dietary solutions include these do's and don'ts on their lists despite supposedly addressing different topics. This includes conditions ranging from systemic inflammation to excessive acidity to free-radical damage. Indeed, in each case, we see that the same diet is used as a therapy.

Hydration

Hydration is a similar issue in that it can be addressed by the manual therapist. Again, this would be by reinforcing what is common knowledge: drink more water. Most of us have heard we need to drink at least eight-8 ounce glasses of water per day. Despite this, not many people do it. What's more, they substitute the recommended pure water with beverages containing caffeine and alcohol which compromise the body's hydration even further. Because of this poor compliance to such an important tenet of good health, it is only appropriate we not only inquire about a person's drinking habits but also do our best to make them drink, drink, drink! Please see Chapters 2 and 3 for further information on how dehydration affects homeostasis and how it relates to the wellness continuum.

Obesity

Obesity creates many added problems for the musculoskeletal system. The most obvious of these is the added compressive force on the spine and lower extremities. This damages joint surfaces and speeds the degenerative process. The added weight also places opposing muscles and ligaments under greater strain, leading to premature breakdown of these structures as well.

In addition to this added compressive force, obesity also accentuates many postural faults. This is especially true in people with enlarged abdominal areas. This change brings the person's center of gravity forward, causing an increased anterior pelvic tilt, increased lumbar lordosis, and exaggerated forward head carriage.

Besides this added mechanical stress, obesity also produces a systemic inflammatory state. That is because adipocytes sequester arachnidonic acid, which then produces pro-inflammatory eicosanoids. These eicosanoids "generate the production of more pro-inflammatory cytokines in the fat cells, such as interleukin-6 and TNF. Both of these enter the bloodstream, causing a cascade of additional inflammatory responses" throughout the body.[10] Therefore, by losing bodyfat, a person can dramatically alter his biochemical status. This makes it all-the-more important we counsel our patients to lose weight when indicated.

Sleep Quantity

Besides the physical position a person sleeps in, it is also very important to consider the quantity of sleep he or she gets. Sleep, of course, is vital for the body to properly repair itself. It is also absolutely necessary for the CNS. Besides this, sleep is necessary for keeping many important hormones in balance. One of the most powerful of these is cortisol, which increases when the body is in a sleep-deprived state. Interestingly, according to some authors, the reason cortisol is secreted in this instance is because sleep deprivation activates the body's stress response.

Sleep deprivation is known to have many other negative effects on the body. It is shown to reduce emotional and physical well-being.[135] It is also linked to coronary heart disease in women (sleep deprivation as well as too much sleep).[136] Sleep deprivation is even known to increase sensitivity to pain[137] and boost levels of high-sensitivity C–reactive protein[138] and IL-6.[139]

For these reasons it is important to ask the patient how much sleep he/she gets. If it is less than 7–8 hours per night educate them in the importance of sleep. Remember that most people of this day-and-age are sleep deprived—so pursue this issue with all patients. Also remember that all patients will have reasons why they can't sleep longer. Tell them there are no excuses!

Mental/Emotional Stressors

Mental and emotional stress will cause or perpetuate symptoms in the same fashion as the other secondary factors. In fact, some approaches believe the mind has as great an influence on the musculoskeletal system as other physical factors such as structure and internal chemistry (in fact, emotions affect structure and internal chemistry). Because of the scope of its potential importance as well as the complexity of the mind-body connection, a separate chapter has been set aside to cover this topic. Please see Chapter 22, The Mind-Body Connection for an in-depth discussion on the role of the mind in the development and treatment of musculoskeletal problems. Please see Chapter 2 and 3 for an overview of its role in maintaining/disrupting homeostasis.

Lack of Exercise

An adequate amount of exercise is vitally important to the body's well-being. It reduces stress, heightens mood, benefits almost every system of the body, and drives the central nervous system. Needless to say, it also has an incredible impact on the well-being of the musculoskeletal system. Please see Chapter 3 for further discussion on this topic.

Illness/Disease

Acute and chronic illness affects the musculoskeletal system in several ways. In holistic terms, the body must expend valuable energy trying to fight an illness, infection, or disease. This diminishes its capacity to repair the musculoskeletal system, both as a matter of priority as well as an issue of finite resources. In addition to this mechanism, the illness itself can have a direct effect upon the musculoskeletal system. It usually initiates a stress response, as in a fight-or-flight reaction. This creates a state of chronic inflammation, further irritating symptomatic tissues. Depending on the disease process, it can even create widespread hyper- or hypomobility. There are also many correlations between certain diseases and specific musculoskeletal problems. A good example of this is the much higher risk a diabetic person has of developing adhesive capsulitis. While we may not directly treat illness or disease, it is certainly helpful to understand how they may act as causative factors and/or influence a patient's progress with therapy.

Injury

The term injury in this context refers to traumatic injury as opposed to repetitive motion injury. Traumatic injuries occur in many different forms, but for the sake of this text we will categorize them according to their effects upon the body. The first category is the localized pain and inflammation created by an injury. This is a primary focus of traditional medicine. As a result it is usually well-managed by manual therapists. These cases are normally straight-forward. In other words, there is usually no mystery as to what caused the person's symptoms. The second category is the global effects of trauma. These are the effects trauma has upon the entire body. This includes the initiation of the stress response, the subsequent release of cortisol, the initiation of the inflammatory cascade, and the reflexive muscular contraction due to pain. These factors will irritate a distant, concomitant problem. Additionally, as with battling illness, a traumatic injury limits energy available to repair a more chronic problem. The third category is the long-term effects of injury. Many manual therapy approaches agree that trauma is absorbed by the body and permanently changes it. This causes many of the effects mentioned above, but it also affects motor control, binds down layers of fascia, and creates muscle shortening. These dysfunctions may lie dormant for a long time before they finally surface in the form of local or distant symptoms.

A thorough patient history is the best way to catch all traumatic injuries. In the first category, the traumatic injury is often the reason the patient sought medical attention. Therefore, he or she will likely bring up the injury and furnish details. However, the latter two categories will require the practitioner to delve into the patient's past in order to obtain an accurate background. That is because he is unlikely to associate a past injury with his or her current problem. The same goes for a recent or long-ago injury to a distant bodypart. Again, the patient will not willingly mention it because no possible relationship is perceived. To catch these injuries specific questions such as, "Have you ever hurt your ____ before? are often necessary to jog the patient's memory. For instance, many patients with low back pain do not mention an old coccyx injury until they are specifically asked, "Have you ever fallen on your tailbone?" Inevitably, the person who just denied any history of trauma will recall falling onto their coccyx thirty years ago and even be able to give very specific details about the incident.

EXTERNAL STRESSORS

The group of external/habitual stressors has a very powerful influence on the musculoskeletal system. Because of this, they deserve our close attention. Moreover, these are the group of stressors we can exert the most influence over.

As mentioned in the chapter introduction, these stressors are the result of the countless things we do in our everyday lives. However, please note that a special effort has been made to omit actions which fall in the category of "movement patterns." This is its own primary factor. While movement patterns deal with the precise *way* we move, the external/habitual stressors do not. Instead, this category is limited to stressors such as static postures and occupational habits without regard to muscle recruitment, firing patterns, etc.

Most therapists already try to educate their patients in the proper way to do some of these activities. Unfortunately, this is often hit-or-miss. That is because it is very easy to forget about each one of them. For this reason, the therapist should have patients fill out a thorough questionnaire including each of these stressors. This will ensure the clinician has covered each one of them.

STATIC POSTURES

The group of static postures includes everything we do that involves staying still. This involves the things we normally think of—such as sitting and standing. It also includes other activities such as driving and sleeping. In the case of any activity with which we stay relatively motionless, we must consider the physical effects of that immobility. Joints do not get lubricated. Circulation slows. Certain muscles maintain a continuous isometric contraction. Some soft tissues have the opportunity to shorten while their counterparts lengthen. Afferent input is diminished. These are just a few of the harmful effects; there are many others. Understanding that this is what the body undergoes while maintaining static postures, it is reasonable that all these activities be scrutinized and altered where indicated.

Sitting

Prolonged sitting is already recognized as being very stressful on the low back, particularly the intervertebral discs. It is also stressful for other regions of the body, especially the cervical and thoracic spine. For these reasons, patients must be questioned on the amount of time they spend sitting and the position they adopt while doing so. Questioning should not be limited to the person's work, but should also include their habits at home.

Remember that most people do not have any furniture in their living area which promotes good posture. Instead, they have sofas and recliners which exaggerate postural faults. Most sofas are too deep, so the person posteriorly tilts the pelvis and/or presses the thoracic spine backwards to meet the cushions. Meanwhile, sitting in a recliner with the feet elevated again tilts the pelvis posteriorly, thus exaggerating the lumbar and thoracic kyphosis.

Other things to inquire about are tendencies towards asymmetry in the coronal and transverse planes. Coronal plane asymmetries will occur if the person is forced to lean to one side or the other at work, possibly due to the location of the computer or telephone. At home, many people lean on the armrest of the chair or sofa, creating thoracolumbar sidebending. This is made worse when the feet are tucked underneath. Tucking the feet underneath the buttocks also strains the hips and knees.

Besides frontal plane asymmetry, problems in the transverse plane are also fairly common. At work, this occurs on a repetitive or prolonged basis if the person's workstation is arranged improperly. For instance, having the computer monitor to one side or another forces the person to rotate the neck in one direction while the body is rotated in another. At home, this problem can be just as bad or worse. That is because the television is often off to one side or the other, forcing the person to rotate the head or body the entire time he is watching T.V.

Treatment involves correcting asymmetry/dysfunction in each plane. Starting with the sagittal plane, steps must be taken to restore the normal lumbar lordosis. The traditional way to do this is to place a support behind the lumbar spine, which pushes the middle of the lumbar spine anteriorly. There are many cushions available to do this, and they are usually more effective and practical than a small pillow or rolled-up towel. Another way to restore normal lordosis is by altering the hip-to-knee heights. By raising the hips up higher than the knees, the pelvis automatically goes into an anterior tilt. This places the lumbar spine into a lordotic position without applying any direct pressure to the vertebrae.

Practically speaking, this can be done in several ways. The first is by raising the hips. Placing a towel or cushion under the ischial tuberosities (not the length of the femurs) brings the hips higher than the knees. Extra bulk may be needed to provide extra support if the chair or sofa is especially soft. Dropping the knee height is the other way to change this relationship. This can be done by using a chair with a seat capable of tilting forward, thus dropping the knees lower than the hips. Or, the patient can look into specialized furniture designed with this principle in mind. The kneeling chair is one such piece of furniture. It is designed with a forward-tilted seat that anteriorly tilts the pelvis. Instead of placing the soles of the feet on the floor, the knees and upper shins rest on a cushioned support, thereby bending the knees to 90 degrees. This exaggerates the anterior tilt, thereby pulling the upper half of the body posteriorly.

Along with these suggestions, it is important to advise the patient against activities requiring them to look downwards while they are sitting. Instead, if they must sew or read have them do so with their materials or book supported and upright to lessen strain on cervical and thoracic structures. Also, have them avoid sitting in a recliner or sitting on a sofa so deep it forces the knees into extension. Having the knees extended while sitting pulls the pelvis into a posterior tilt and puts the lumbar spine into kyphosis.

Correcting frontal and transverse plane problems requires a little less effort. The most important thing to do is to correct any structural issue at work or at home which forces prolonged or repetitive rotation or sidebending. As mentioned above, this may be due to the television or computer being in the wrong place. Whatever the case is, it must be corrected.

Standing

As with the stress from prolonged sitting, the simple act of maintaining a standing position for too long is stressful to the body. In addition to this, any asymmetry or deviation from optimal posture magnifies the amount of strain. This can be due to the requirements of the activity itself and/or any postural faults the person already displays. Therefore, it is necessary to assess both of these potential sources of strain. Let's start by assessing the patient's activities.

Everyone performs numerous activities each day requiring static standing. At home, these activities include cooking, folding laundry, ironing clothes, washing dishes, showering, shaving, and applying makeup (among others). In public, we spend time standing in lines at the bank, the supermarket, the coffee shop, and the post office. At work, some people spend their entire day standing doing a variety of different tasks. While these activities may vary, our approach to each of them needs to be the same. First, we need to find out how these activities are performed. From this, we can identify any ergonomic "no-no's." Many of these faults are similar in nature to those described in the previous section on sitting. They include deviations from neutral in any of the three planes: sagittal, coronal, and transverse. For instance, an assembly line worker might be twisted to the right side all day long in order to receive something off a conveyor belt. Or, he may have to bend forward to work on a low workstation. Of course, these same principles apply to the person doing chores at home. Therefore, it is necessary to inquire about any activities which require especially poor body positioning. Added to these principles are a few extra concerns regarding flooring and footwear. Specifically, if the person stands on cement flooring at home or work they will incur added compressive stress and reduced shock absorption throughout their whole body. Along these same lines we must inspect the patient's footwear. The thinner the sole and/or the less supportive the shoe, the greater the stress upon the body.

Treatment to address these added stressors is fairly straight-forward. First, try to make every standing activity more ergonomically favorable. This requires working surfaces to be at a favorable height for the patient. They must also be straight-ahead instead of off to one side. This applies even when there is no table or workbench used. Whatever the person is doing while standing, it should be straight in front of him or her. The end-result is that the person should be standing as erect as possible in a neutral position with weight evenly distributed on both lower extremities. Of course, in some situations the patient must adapt to the surroundings instead of trying to make the surroundings adapt to him. That is why patient education is so important. As long as the patient understands the principles behind proper ergonomics, he/she will be able to go home or to work and make changes as needed.

Added to these stressors are any postural faults the patient already displays. For instance, the person may be swaybacked, flat-backed, have a scoliosis, or have a leg length discrepancy. In each case, this deviation from optimal biomechanics magnifies the strain of a stressful activity. Further information on posture is presented in Chapter 4, Mechanical Considerations.

Driving

Driving is another example of an activity we engage in on a daily basis, often for prolonged periods. Even if it was performed symmetrically, the amount of time we spend driving plus the prevalence of unsupportive seats makes it stressful. But it is *not* performed symmetrically. By sheer design of the pedals it will never be a symmetrical activity. To make matters worse, many people drive with an exaggerated asymmetry placing tremendous strain on most of the body. For instance, take a person with average posture. Imagine he is right-hand dominant in a car with the steering wheel on the left side. His posture will look like this:

- Left hip flexed, abducted, and externally rotated. The knee is likely resting on the door.
- The left foot, in order to lie flat on the floorboard, is then everted excessively. Or, the driver may choose to rest the lateral or dorsal surface of the left foot on the floorboard. This forces the ankle into extreme inversion and the knee into extreme flexion.

- The right knee is typically in a position of extension and the right ankle is plantarflexed.
- The lumbar spine, depending on the car seat, is often in a state of kyphosis. In this case, the pelvis is posteriorly tilted and weight is borne on the sacrum instead of the ischial tuberosities.
- If the person steers with both hands, great. If he uses only his left hand, expect him to bear weight on the console with the right elbow. This puts the thoracolumbar spine into a left sidebent position. The right humerus is pressed upwards into the glenoid fossa.
- If he drives with just the right hand, he likely rests the left elbow on the door, compressing the ulnar nerve.
- A forward head posture is adopted.

Treatment follows the same principles as those for other static postural dysfunctions. Because most cars and their car seats foster an excessively kyphotic position, restoring normal lordosis is a priority. Obviously, for those cars with a built-in lumbar support, this feature must be utilized. For cars without this feature, a lumbar roll or small cushion can be used. Next, the right-left asymmetry must be addressed. Sidebending to either side and placing weight on the door or console should be discouraged. Next, the knees should be facing straight ahead and be at the same height. This reduces discrepancies in hip internal/external rotation as well as pelvic torsions in the sagittal plane. Hand position on the steering wheel should be symmetrical for best results.

Sleeping

Sleeping is another potential stressor. Although we generally spend almost 1/3 of our lives asleep, few clinicians address this important activity. This is unfortunate, as it has the potential to be very damaging if the patient's positioning is less than optimal.

Mechanically, numerous structures may be under excessive stress while a person is asleep. This includes a joint that is placed at its end-range for hours on end. Or, it may be a joint that is bearing the body's weight for the duration of the night. In many ways, the effects of these mechanical stressors are similar to the stressors the body faces during the waking hours.

With these factors in mind, it is important to review the patient's sleeping position in order to scan for potential red flags. While a detailed discussion on this topic is beyond the scope of this book, we will highlight common problems associated with each position. The spine is used as an example in this chapter, but the theories behind abnormal stresses and their correction are relatable to any joint in the body.

Prone

Much has been written of the deleterious effects of prone sleeping. Most affected is the cervical spine, which is forced into extension and end-range rotation. This not only stresses the soft-tissues of the cervical spine, but it is also believed to compress the vertebral arteries. The best solution to prone sleeping is to tell the patient to avoid it altogether. McKenzie proposes fixing a thumb tack to the abdomen so that the patient will receive a sharp pain when prone lying is attempted. This is harsh, but it illustrates how bad prone lying is for the neck. For those individuals impervious to pain or who just refuse to sleep in supine or sidelying, we must provide options to lessen the extent of extension and rotation inherent with this positioning. One method of doing this is to rotate the body on the cervical spine. To do this, place a pillow lengthwise under the chest and abdomen on the side to which the patient normally turns towards. This elevates the upper thoracic spine on the ipsilateral side, thereby rotating it in the same direction as the cervical spine. The patient can facilitate this rotation by abducting the ipsilateral shoulder and hip. Rotational stress diminishes with this method, as does stress due to excessive extension. Another technique is to place a pillow lengthwise under the torso and another cross-ways underneath the chest. This will form a "T".[140] Again, the end result is less extension and rotation.

Sidelying

Sleeping in sidelying can be harmful to the body as well, depending on the patient's positioning. First of all, it is important that the cervical and lumbar spines do not fall into misalignment in the coronal plane. If inadequate support is given to either the cervical or lumbar spine to prevent "sagging" towards the mattress, strain will result. This strain may involve contractile or non-contractile tissues. Contractile tissues are overworked while trying to keep the vertebrae in neutral alignment. Non-contractile tissues may be compressed or stretched, depending on their side of the spinal curvature. On the convex side, tissues including joint capsules are under constant stretch and may develop laxity. On the concave side, tissues including nerves may become compressed by contracted muscles and narrowed intervertebral foraminae.

For both areas of the spine the solution is to provide outside support. A commercial pillow (or strategically placed towel roll) that gives direct support to the cervical and lumbar spines helps eliminate compensation by contractile tissue and the mechanical deformation of non-contractile tissue. To protect the cervical spine, McKenzie advocates the use of a cervical night roll.[141] This is described as a cylindrical-shaped pad that can fit inside the pillowcase to provide direct support to the cervical spine. Mulligan suggests creating a soft collar by folding a pillowcase lengthwise and then fastening the ends with a safety pin.[142]

To provide support to the lumbar spine, similar methods are used. Place a small pillow directly under the lumbar spine to prevent sidebending towards the bed. McKenzie suggests using a lumbar night roll.[143] Like the cervical night roll, the lumbar night roll is a cylindrical-shaped foam pad that is wrapped around the lumbar spine. To substitute for this commercial product, the patient can make a similar roll with a rolled-up beach towel. He suggests making this approximately 3" in diameter, then fixing the ends with a safety pin.

Another way the lumbar spine is affected is by the position of the lower extremities during sleep. Of special concern is the position of the uppermost hip, which will strain the lumbar spine if it falls into excessive adduction. To prevent this, many people already sleep with a pillow between their knees. This appears to be a good idea, as it helps to prevent lumbar sidebending (convex side towards the ceiling). However, caution must be exercised in the patient with a tight/facilitated iliotibial band, as this only promotes further shortening.[144] Another option is to place a body pillow in front of the patient. The flexed knee and leg can now rest on this pillow, as can the patient's arm. This prevents twisting of the spine as well as excessive adduction of the hip.[140]

Besides the mechanical benefits afforded to the patient by modifying his position in sidelying, there is reason to believe that suggesting the patient lie on his right side instead of his left may extend an even greater therapeutic effect. Research shows that lying in the right lateral decubitus position leads to greater cardiovagal modulation than lying supine or in left lateral decubitus position. This has been confirmed not only in normals, but also in patients with systemic lupus erythematosus and congestive heart failure—both patient populations with a lot to gain by optimizing autonomic nervous system function.[145,146,147]

Supine

Sleeping in the supine position is generally thought of as being relatively benign. This is probably true, but there are ways we can help facilitate relaxation.

As mentioned previously, we want to support the cervical spine. If the lumbar spine does not appear to be supported by the bed, we can support it as well with a small pillow or the lumbar night roll. Next, place the hips in slight flexion by pulling a pillow up the posterior thighs until it approximates the ischial tuberosities. These steps will help relax the entire spine. Now, place a small pillow underneath the scapulae. This allows the pectoralis minor and other scapular muscles to shut-off. Finally, place a pillow under the patient's flexed elbows (hands resting on the abdomen). This prevents the shoulder joint from falling into extension, which is worse if the scapulae are protracted.[140]

Telephone Use

Talking on the telephone can be very stressful for the cervical spine/shoulder complex. This is because using a telephone requires the user to use his/her scapular elevators, deltoid, and rotator cuff to elevate the phone to the ear and hold the position for great periods of time. Added to this, the user often sidebends the cervical spine towards the phone, thus compressing structures on the ipsilateral side and stretching those on the contralateral side. More stressful than this is when the user does not use his/her hands to hold the phone. Instead, he pins the phone between the scapula and skull. This requires a strong, sustained contraction of the scapular elevators and cervical/capital sidebenders. To make matters worse, people often have a habit of using the phone more on one side than the other. If the person tends to write or use a mouse while on the phone, the phone will be pinned to the ear on the non-dominant side on a frequent basis.

There are several simple solutions to this problem. The first is to encourage use of a headset. This immediately takes strain off the neck and shoulder. If this is not an option for someone, he or she should be encouraged to switch ears as often as possible. Pinning the phone should be strongly discouraged.

REPETITIVE MOTION

For the purpose of this text, repetitive motion is defined as any motion repeated over and over. While we typically think of repetitive motion as occurring only at work, repetitive motions actually occur every day at home as well. In the sections Sitting and Standing earlier in this chapter we discussed several examples: shaving, ironing, brushing teeth, and combing hair to name a few. Other activities at home requiring repetitive motion are eating, writing, typing, manipulating a computer mouse, and vacuuming. Again, these are important because everyone does them. This does not even include job-related duties or exercise, which can be major perpetrators of repetitive motion injury. There are several reasons why repetitive motions are so harmful.

The first reason is that specific contractile tissues are used over and over. This is stressful by itself and is significantly worsened when combined with any other stressor (i.e. poor mechanics). The end result is the typical conditions seen with contractile tissues, such as soreness, tendonitis, tendonosis, and muscle/tendon tear. Non-contractile tissues in the area are affected as well. Obviously, the type of problem and the level of involvement are closely related to the specific tissue in question and its role in a particular action. As such, a non-contractile tissue can be subjected to repeated compression, torsion, shearing, or stretching. The various conditions seen in these cases range from inflamed bursae to strained/stretched ligaments to swollen joints to disc problems. Indeed, repetitive motion has the potential to affect almost every tissue in the musculoskeletal system. Besides these results, repetitive motion is famous for causing compression of neurovascular structures. This often results from the combination of swelling, hypertrophy, and adaptive shortening that is the result of repetitive motion. In that sense, the major problem (i.e. median nerve compression) is really just a consequence of the other problems.

Table 8-1 includes activities most people perform on a repetitive basis. This is not a complete list, but it should get the reader thinking about how many repetitive motions we perform each day. Addressing these motions is done in a similar way as the static postural stressors. The first step is identifying them. Obviously, because most of these activities are performed only at home, the clinician must make an effort to seek out any faults in the person's technique.

TABLE 8-1 Common Repetitive Motions. Note that walking is a very important stressor. Please see Chapter 4 for a thorough discussion.

1	Writing.
2	Typing.
3	Eating.
4	Brushing teeth.
5	Shaving.
6	Brushing hair.
7	Ironing.
8	Walking.

This can be done through questioning and having the patient "act" these motions out.

The principles behind treatment are much like those for the static stressors. Namely, any modification that improves biomechanical status will be helpful and should be employed. For the most part, this means the body must be in optimal alignment while performing the activity. Also helpful is educating the patient in general body mechanics and ergonomic principles so that she can make improvements on her own. That way, the patient will be able to handle any new activities and/or make any changes to their current ones.

Not to be ignored in treatment is the most helpful modification of all—rest. Ask the patient to break up any long tasks by taking a break. The same goes for repetitive motion on the job. A short break gives the person time to stretch the muscles and put them through their full range of motion. This helps prevent adaptive shortening and adhesion formation. It also helps improve circulation to the affected limb. Together, little breaks along with changes in ergonomics can help break the cycle of pain. Or, in other words, these alterations bring the person back to the asymptomatic side of the symptomatic threshold.

9 The Common Pattern

THIS CHAPTER IS DEDICATED TO ONE OF THE MOST FASCINATING TOPICS IN THE FIELD OF MANUAL therapy, the common pattern. In Chapter 2 we introduced the common pattern and established the neurological basis for its development. We also discussed its connection to the stress response, thereby tying it in to anything which alters homeostasis. With this foundation already in place, our aim in this chapter is different. It is to describe this pattern down to the smallest detail so that the practitioner can see how many of his patient's problems are related to the pattern. This relationship may be a direct or indirect one. A direct connection between the pattern and the problem means that the common pattern caused the patient's problem. This is very common, as the pattern invokes great mechanical strain upon the system. It causes uneven wearing on the joints and forces added responsibility on the soft tissues for support, mobility, etc. It also causes certain muscles to go weak while facilitating others. This causes problems for both muscles. The weak ones are overloaded by average tasks. The facilitated ones never get to rest, stretch out, or repair themselves. This combination also changes the dynamics of the joints to which the muscles attach, causing subluxations, joint hypermobility and joint hypomobility.

The common pattern may also influence the patient's problem indirectly. This relates to a problem not directly caused by the common pattern but instead is aggravated, irritated, or perpetuated by it. Unfortunately, this influence can be substantial and far-reaching. This is for the same reasons mentioned in the paragraph above: alterations in biomechanics, neurology, and movement patterns create harmful forces throughout the body. This often leads to symptoms in distant joints and soft tissues.

On a broader scale, we must also remember that a dominant common pattern compromises the entire system. For instance, it drains the body of vital recuperative energy, as it must work harder than normal to walk, stand, or perform any other task. Biochemically, there is a greater build up of lactic acid and other metabolic waste products due to constant muscle contraction. Neurologically, the central nervous system is not receiving the proper mechanoreceptor input to perform its functions, including dampening nociceptive afferent input. Pulmonary function is impaired as well (due to mechanical positioning and altered movement patterns), leading to suboptimal oxygen saturation and even a less efficient vascular pump.

These are just a few of the implications of a dominant common pattern. Altogether, they serve as the reason to treat this pattern. Listed below are the components of the common pattern broken up region-by-region. Along with each component is a summary of each profession or approach which recognizes the pattern. Also included are the muscular, articular, and neurological implications for each component of the pattern.

Forward Head Posture

Description:

The head is held anterior to the rest of the body. This fault also includes occipital extension, flattened (or reversed) cervical lordosis, rounded shoulders, and posterior-superior mandibular displacement because of its close connections to these structures.

Recognized By:

This finding is possibly the most well-accepted, widespread finding in all of manual therapy. Mechanically-based approaches, neurologically-based approaches, and movement pattern-based approaches not only recognize its significance, but also attribute its occurrence to a problem involving their respective primary factor.

Implications:

Forward head posture has implications for almost every system in the body. Mechanically, it sets the stage for local strain and for compensatory curves throughout the rest of the spine. Neurologically, it robs the CNS of much-needed afferent mechanoreception coming from the most mechanoreceptor-rich area of the body, the mid-cervical spine.[148] This sets the stage for sympathetic nervous system dominance, as discussed previously. Among other things, it is even believed to cause adverse tension of the spinal cord itself. This affects the entire system for obvious reasons.

Traditional thinking holds the belief that mechanical factors such as poor posture create the forward head posture. This is certainly a feasible theory. After all, we in the Western world spend *way* too much time in a flexed posture. This allows certain soft tissue structures to lengthen and others to shorten resulting in the forward head carriage. It seems to make sense.

On the other hand, there are some who propose that the forward head posture is the result of adverse neural activation, and is not merely the cause of it. Take Hanna and Alexander's work, for instance. Both men describe the contraction of the sternocleidomastoids and upper trapezius as resulting in a habitual forward head posture. As highlighted in Chapter 2 these muscles can elevate the shoulders and thrust the head forward within twenty milliseconds of exposure to a threatening stimulus. Why is this? Why are these muscles so closely tied-into unconscious nervous system activity? Is it because of the fact that they are innervated by a cranial nerve arising from such close proximity to the most important parasympathetic nerve in the body? Some experts including Iams believe this is the case.[149]

Given this research it certainly seems likely that adverse neural activation leads to forward head posture. Add to this one other incidental theory: our postures are more closely dictated by our personalities than they are by the physical constraints of our occupations. After all, when was the last time you saw an unhappy, anxious, or fearful person walking with outstanding posture? Likely never—no matter whether he stood and walked all day or sat behind a desk all day long. The mental status trumps the occupation, doesn't it? Actually, when we think about it, none of us can tell what a person's occupation is based on his posture, can we? On the other hand, we can make hundreds of judgments of the people around us just by observing the way they carry themselves. Most importantly, we are all pretty good at it.

Whatever theory one subscribes to, we can all agree that forward head posture must be treated! Even if the nervous system is responsible for causing the asymmetry we must treat the mechanical findings as well. And vice versa. That is because the nervous system influences the mechanical system and the mechanical system influences the nervous system. The body's movement patterns and energetic status play into this equation as well, which is why they must all be treated.

Extended Occiput

Description:

The occiput is extended on the capital spine, usually as a result of forward head posture or abnormal reflex activation. Its extended position keeps the eyes level in the case of FHP; otherwise, the anterior displacement would result in the head being directed towards the floor. The position of extension is held in place actively by contraction of the suboccipitals (a very common finding) and/or true joint hypomobility not allowing the occipital condyles to glide posteriorly on the atlas.

Recognized By:

1. Janda. His theories hold that the suboccipital muscles are normally facilitated, whereas the cervical flexors are usually inhibited. Practitioners who follow his recommendations stretch the suboccipitals and try to strengthen the short neck flexors.
2. Alexander Technique. Correcting occipital extension is one of the top priorities of this technique. Patients are taught to do this in a special way, by inhibiting the Downward Pull and by activating the Primary Control. One of the best-known ways this principle is applied is when the person is arising from sitting. It is interesting to note that this technique has been proven successful at inhibiting the SCM.
3. Makofsky. Physical therapist Howard Makofsky invented the Occivator, a device promoting active capital flexion and lower trapezius contraction (actually based on Alexander's teachings). This device is proven to reduce FHP and occipital extension.[150]
4. Somatics. Great emphasis is placed on reducing the effects of the startle reflex for this fault and for ones that follow. In this case, the suboccipitals and sternocleidomastoids are known to contract vigorously, thereby pulling the occiput into extension.
5. McKenzie. This approach places great emphasis on improving posture, especially that of the cervical spine. Chin retractions are taught to patients to help correct FHP.
6. Numerous approaches in chiropractic. In Gonstead technique, this is known as an AS occiput.
7. Hruska. Habitual FHP results in posterior cranial rotation (thus, an extended occiput). Hruska notes that many factors create this, one of them being overuse of the SCM as an accessory respiratory muscle.[59]

Implications:

Muscular: The suboccipital muscles, SCM, and trapezii are under constant tension. This creates myofascial trigger points and tendonitis for these muscles. Opposing muscles become inhibited.

Articular: The extended position of the occiput on the atlas can create local irritation of this joint. It can also easily cause or perpetuate an upper cervical joint dysfunction.

Neural: Some believe that nerves exiting the suboccipital region can be impinged upon by the excessive muscle tightness, particularly the greater occipital nerve which runs to the front of the skull. They believe this is responsible for retro-orbital pain experienced by many headache sufferers. Others believe this is a referred pain mechanism, generated by nociception coming from the upper cervical spine and converging on the trigeminocervical nucleus.[54] Because the trigeminal nerve innervates the face and dura this information is processed as coming from parts of the head instead of from the upper cervical spine. In any event, treating the upper cervical spine and suboccipitals is beneficial.

Posterior Mandibular Displacement

Description:

The mandible is displaced posteriorly, compressing the temporomandibular joint. It is also usually pulled superiorly, thereby compressing the teeth and the temporomandibular joint further.

Recognized By:

1. Physical therapists. Physical therapists and others treat TMD by correcting forward head posture, thereby attempting to improve the position of the mandible.
2. Makofsky. Makofsky reports posterior-superior mandibular displacement is correlated with forward head posture; this makes correction of forward head posture integral in TMJ treatment.
3. Hruska notes superior-posterior mandibular displacement as a consequence of FHP and posterior cranial rotation.
4. The startle response contracts the mandibular elevators and inhibits the suprahyoids.

Implications:

Muscular: While muscle hyperactivity is largely responsible for this abnormal positioning, one must keep in mind that any structural or functional abnormality can have a great impact on the numerous muscles surrounding the joint. Important muscles such as the medial pterygoid are infamous for going into a facilitated state. Not only do they generate pain, but because they attach to the sphenoid, it is thought that they can create disorder throughout the entire body.

Articular: Abnormal mechanics at the TMJ wreak havoc on the integrity of the joint. This results in capsular laxity, capsulitis, synovitis, articular cartilage damage, and even joint degeneration. Keep in mind this only takes minute changes in joint mechanics given the incredible number of times we open and close our mouths each day.

Neural: There is no known nerve impingement resulting from a posteriorly-displaced mandible. However, keep in mind that the stomatognathic system has a tremendous amount of input into the CNS. Joint disorders and/or malocclusion can have detrimental effects on the entire system.

Rounded Shoulders

Description:

The scapulae are displaced anteriorly upon the rib cage. This includes its related positions such as anterior tilting, winging, and protraction. In all cases, the scapula is pulled forward and abducted instead of being pulled backward. This has implications for both the shoulder and the cervical spine.

Recognized By:

1. Orthopedic medicine and traditional physical therapy recognize this faulty position due to the faulty mechanics it creates. It affects the rotator cuff because it brings the head of the humerus and the undersurface of the acromion closer together. This is especially harmful when the arm is elevated above shoulder height. For the cervical spine, the rounded shoulder position is stressful because the scapula is no longer supported by the rib cage. Instead, the scapular elevators must work hard to support it. This strains them and pulls downwards on the skull and cervical spine.
2. Somatics. The rounded shoulder position is attributed to the startle reflex.

3. Janda. His upper crossed pattern involves hypertonicity of the anterior structures (scapular protractors) and inhibition of the posterior structures (scapular retractors), leading to forward movement. Many physical therapists follow his lead and train patients to activate the rhomboids and the lower/middle trapezius to bring the scapula medially and out of an anteriorly-tilted position.
4. Partridge. Physical therapists including Partridge teach that the scapula's position is important to the function of the rotator cuff complex. She and others encourage taping the scapula with several different methods. In common with each one is that the scapula is pulled medially and/or more vertically.
5. Alexander Technique. One of the benefits of lengthening the spine with the Alexander Technique is that it helps the client to bring the scapulae down so they can rest atop the ribcage.
6. Yoga. Yoga practitioners teach their clients to drop the shoulders back and down during many different poses.
7. Pilates. The Pilates method recognizes the frequency of the rounded shoulder posture and teaches its clients exercises to recruit the middle and lower traps, thereby correcting this malposition.[151]
8. Rolf. Ida Rolf spoke about the problems with scapular stability, particularly "winging" as a result of weak rhomboids.

Implications:

Muscular: The pectoralis minor and upper trapezius are facilitated in these cases. The lower and inferior trapezius and serratus anterior are usually inhibited and cannot keep the scapula in a biomechanically-advantageous position. This problem results in rotator cuff dysfunction due to the lack of proper biomechanical advantage needed by these muscles. Additionally, this positioning allows the head of the humerus to slide out of the glenoid fossa and go anteriorly and/or inferiorly. This forces the surrounding musculature to contract constantly in order to stabilize it. Note that the upper trapezius and levator scapula are forced to work extra hard in these cases to support the scapula. This is because the scapula is not well-supported by the rib cage when it has gone too far anterior.

Articular: Poor positioning of the scapulae often creates irritation of the rib angles and alters the biomechanics of the glenohumeral joint.

Neural: Excessive winging or abduction of the scapula has been blamed for traction injury to the supraspinous nerve. It is also plausible that this position places extra strain on all nerves running to the upper extremity, particularly those traveling posterior to the humerus.

Anteriorly Displaced Humeral Head

Description:

The head of the humerus is displaced anteriorly in the glenoid fossa. This often follows the anterior scapular deviations; the head of the humerus "falls off" the shelf normally provided by the glenoid.

Recognized By:

1. Orthopedists. They recognize this condition and attribute it to several factors, including laxity of the anterior capsule. This is combined with the tightening of the posterior capsule, particularly in throwing athletes. According to these practitioners, this positioning is at least partially responsible for the lack of dominant shoulder internal rotation in this patient population.
2. Mulligan. His mobilization with movement and taping technique for the shoulder each involve a posteriorly-glided pressure upon the head of the humerus.
3. Partridge. Partridge notes that the scapula's anterior tilting causes the head of the humerus to rest on the anterior capsule, thereby causing chronic irritation. She speculates that this is one factor which can eventually lead to adhesive capsulitis.[152]
4. Chiropractic Medicine. The most popular adjustment for the glenohumeral joint is the posterior thrust to correct for an anterior humeral head. Several approaches use this technique as the primary adjustment for shoulder problems.

Implications:

Muscular: Altered biomechanical advantage for the rotator cuff muscles. These muscles are forced into prolonged contraction to provide stability.

Articular: Altered positioning of the humeral head sets the stage for irritation of the supraspinatus tendon and osteophyte development. Additionally, the continuous anterior glide irritates the glenoid labrum and further stretches out important stabilizing tissues of the anterior shoulder.

Neural: Same as for rounded shoulders.

Cubital Valgus

Description:

This is excessive abduction of the ulna and radius upon the humerus. The normal angulation, or carrying angle, is approximately 11–14 degrees in males and 13–16 degrees in females.[153]

Recognized By:

1. Orthopedists. Orthopedists find that a carrying angle over 14 degrees for males and 16 degrees for females is associated with a higher incidence of elbow problems.
2. Osteopathy. This profession recognizes the abduction ulnohumeral lesion, wherein the ulna is forced into a position of increased valgus. The radius then migrates distally, creating altered mechanics at the wrist joint as well.
3. Chiropractic. Hearon's adjusting protocol calls for adjusting the proximal ulna laterally because it typically subluxates medially. If this does not normalize the post-adjustment examination (strength testing the brachioradialis) it is then adjusted medially.
4. Mulligan. His MWM entails gliding the proximal ulna laterally. This technique is used to treat cases of elbow pain including lateral epicondylitis.

Implications:

Muscular: Altered elbow biomechanics cause poor biomechanical advantage for the surrounding muscles. In addition to this, the wrist extensors are notorious for being facilitated in cases of pain. This sets the stage for overuse syndromes including lateral epicondylitis.

Articular: Stretching of ulno-humeral ligaments and compression of the radio-humeral joint.

Neural: The ulnar nerve is excessively stretched in this position. Excessive muscle contraction about the elbow also has the potential to impinge the radial (via the supinator) and median nerves (via the pronator teres), especially if predisposed by the patient's anatomy.

Kyphotic Thoracic Spine

Description:

This refers to the excessive kyphosis of the thoracic spine. It is often associated with forward head posture.

Recognized By:

As with forward head posture, most approaches recognize this fault. They also believe their particular philosophy best explains the occurrence of this fault. The mechanically-based practitioners believe excessive thoracic kyphosis is due to purely mechanical factors, whereas the neurologically-based practitioners blame the nervous system. The movement therapists believe faulty movement patterns are to blame. Please note that some approaches, especially in chiropractic, find many people have excessive kyphosis in the superior portion of the thorax while demonstrating diminished kyphosis in the middle thorax.[154] Be sure to thoroughly examine the patient to determine which pattern he/she displays.

Implications:

Muscular: The thoracic muscles are often stretched and over-worked in these cases. This involves the medial muscles of the thoracic spine and can go as far lateral as the iliocostalis. Anteriorly, the approximation of the sternum and pubic symphysis secondary to this postural disorder results in diminished function of the diaphragm, thereby reducing respiratory capacity.

Articular: Excessive stress and strain on the thoracic vertebrae and ribcage. This stress often peaks at the apex of the patient's curve. As mentioned above, other vertebrae may become extended in order to compensate. This creates extension lesions in the mid-thoracic region. In both cases the excessive muscular contraction helps maintain dysfunction.

Neural: No known implication.

Anteriorly Tilted Pelvis

Description:

This refers to the anterior tilting of the innominate bones, usually present in the standing position. This fault is viewed as a result of several factors including boney structure, muscle weakness, and muscle hyperactivity.

Recognized By:

1. DonTigny. His central theory on low back pain centers on his perception that the pelvis' boney structure leads to anterior tilting over time. In fact, he attributes the majority of insidious-onset low back pain to an anterior pelvic tilt.[155]
2. Pilates. Joseph Pilates stressed the importance of a placing the pelvis in a neutral position. This normally requires correcting an anterior pelvic tilt; thus, he stressed a program to strengthen the abdominal muscles and gluteus maximus while stretching the low back muscles.[156]
3. Traditional physical therapy. Anterior pelvic tilting and the swayback posture are considered irritating factors. The popular posterior pelvic tilt exercise addresses this positional fault while helping to strengthen the core muscles (when the proper muscles are recruited).
4. Somatics. Hanna recognized the anterior pelvic tilt and excessive lumbar lordotic posture as a result of two different reflexes: the startle response and the Landau reflex.
5. The Alexander Technique. This method looks for and corrects excessive lumbar paravertebral muscle contraction, excessive lumbar lordosis, and anterior pelvic tilting when arising from sitting. When present, these findings are attributed to creating low back pain.
6. Janda's lower crossed syndrome involves an anterior pelvic tilt and lordotic lumbar spine. This is due to weakness of the abdominals and gluteus maximus and facilitation of the iliopsoas and lumbar erector spinae.
7. Rolfers place great importance on correcting the anterior pelvic tilt. Cottingham et al. have published several studies demonstrating the efficacy of Rolfing in correcting this postural fault.[157] Along with this structural improvement, the researchers also noted that vagal tone was improved. It is unknown whether this improvement was due to the soft-tissue work itself or the structural correction. In either case, the capacity for soft-tissue work

and pelvic mobilization to increase parasympathetic nervous system activity must be appreciated.

Implications:

Muscular: Constant contraction of the lumbar paravertebral muscles, piriformis and iliopsoas creates local pain and trigger point development. It also forces the hamstring muscles to work constantly in opposition. For this reason, anterior pelvic rotation is implicated as a cause of repeated hamstring strains.

Articular: This position creates sacroiliac instability, alters the weight-bearing surface of the hip joint, places great strain on the lumbosacral junction, and forces the lumbar vertebrae into excessive extension. This causes and/or perpetuates dysfunction at these joints due to physical forces. Surrounding muscle tension helps maintain joint dysfunction already present. This tilt also pushes the center of gravity anteriorly, thereby exacerbating most of the postural faults mentioned in this pattern.

Neural: Decreased diameter of the intervertebral foraminae can impinge upon lumbar nerve roots. Femoral internal rotation and piriformis contraction also compress/stretch the sciatic nerve.

Lordotic Lumbar Spine

This fault is typically associated with an anteriorly titled pelvis. This combination is normally found/noticed in standing or when the patient is arising from sitting. Please see Anteriorly Tilted Pelvis above for a full description.

Implications:

Similar to those for Anteriorly Tilted Pelvis.

Kyphotic Lumbar Spine

Description:

This fault refers to the reversal of the normal lordotic curve of the lumbar spine. This position is typically found/recognized in the sitting posture instead of the standing position. It is believed to cause problems for the low back as well as the upper body.

Recognized By:

This fault is recognized by almost all practitioners utilizing a mechanical approach. This is due to its effect on the disc as well as the slouched position it creates for the rest of the body. Included in this group are chiropractors, orthopedists, physical therapists, occupational therapists, and ergonomists. It is probably safe to say that McKenzie has brought the most attention to this topic, as his theories on disc derangement center around restoring the lumbar lordosis in order to reduce the posterior HNP.

Hip Internal Rotation and Adduction

Description:

The hips are often observed to be adducted and internally rotated, especially in individuals with ligamentous laxity. This position has been implicated in causing hip conditions including bursitis and joint degeneration. Because its position also changes the position of the knee joint, it is also blamed for creating certain knee-related problems.

Recognized By:

1. Orthopedists, physical therapists, and podiatrists. They recognize this fault as a mechanical issue, often stemming from faulty foot mechanics or weak hip abductors. They also consider skeletal abnormalities including femoral anteversion as possible causative factors. In comparison to males, females are believed to demonstrate greater hip adduction because they have a wider pelvis.
2. Physical Therapists. Strength testing in patients with patellofemoral syndrome reveals weakness consistent with the pattern described; the hip abductors and external rotators are often weak and inhibited.[158] Strengthening these muscles results in improved biomechanics and reduction in symptoms.[159]
3. Somatics. The startle reflex contracts the hip internal rotators and adductors.
4. Janda. As part of Janda's lower crossed syndrome, the hip adductors and tensor fascia lata are facilitated and the abductors are inhibited.
5. Hruska. His product, the Protonics brace, works to correct hip internal rotation by posteriorly rotating the pelvis. This brace is most commonly used to treat patello-femoral syndrome.

Implications:

Muscular: Contraction of the piriformis and iliopsoas occurs as part of the lower crossed syndrome, helping to counter hip internal rotation. The hip abductors are also overworked in an attempt to stabilize the joint. Each of these muscles is prone to developing myofascial trigger points and tendonitis. The iliotibial band is tractioned over the greater trochanter, leading to irritation of the band and the underlying trochanteric bursa.

Articular: Altered joint mechanics, especially coxa vara, result in weight-bearing on the superior-lateral acetabulum. This surface is smaller than it is medially (where weight bearing normally occurs), thereby leading to degeneration over time. Also note that constant contraction of the piriformis alters the biomechanics of the sacroiliac joint. At the knee, altered structure and muscle strength may produce PFS.

Neural: Femoral internal rotation and piriformis contraction can impinge the sciatic nerve.

Genu Valgus

Description:

Genu valgus refers to the excessive outward angulation of the tibia upon the femur. As with cubital valgus, a certain amount of this angulation is considered normal. This angle, called the Q (quadriceps) angle, is normally 13-18 degrees with males closer to 13 degrees and females closer to 18 degrees.[160] When this angle is too great it creates problems. This is because it alters the weight-bearing relationship between the femur and tibia. It also changes the mechanics of the patello-femoral joint, in turn drawing much blame for creating patello-femoral dysfunction and patellar tendonitis.

Recognized By:

1. Orthopedists, physical therapists, and podiatrists. As with the hip pattern, these professions often attribute genu valgus to mechanical factors or skeletal abnormality. Included as mechanical reasons for this pattern are hip abductor weakness, ligamentous laxity, and excessive pronation. These professions also recognize the mechanically-mediated effects of this pattern on the tibio-femoral and patello-femoral joints.

2. Somatics. During the startle reflex there is contraction of the hip adductors, thereby pulling the femur medially.
3. Janda. Janda's lower crossed syndrome recognizes an excessive genu valgus.

Implications:

Muscular: Look for stabilizing muscles to be problematic in cases of genu valgus. Also look for patellar tendonitis to result from the constant medial tractioning during tibial internal rotation. Adding to this disadvantage is inhibition of the quadriceps and facilitation of the hamstrings.

Articular: Excessive coronal plane deviation compresses the lateral meniscus and osseous components. Excessive tibial internal rotation (as well as greater velocity into internal rotation) shears the medial meniscus. Patello-femoral dysfunction is also a common result of this fault. This can be due to several factors, including lateral patellar translation and recurrent tractioning upon the patellar ligament during tibial internal rotation.

Neural: No known implication.

Posterior Fibular Head

Description:

Just as it sounds. The fibular head tends to migrate posteriorly more than any other direction.

Recognized By:

1. Mulligan: His taping technique for patellofemoral syndrome involves wrapping around the posterior fibular head and pulling anteriorly before going across to the anterior-medial femur.
2. Chiropractic. Chiropractors frequently find the fibular head is subluxated posteriorly and perform an adjustment to bring it anteriorly.

Implications:

Muscular: This dysfunction changes the length-tension relationships of virtually all muscles of the leg. It also affects the biceps femoris, which attaches directly to the fibular head. This is important because the fascia of the biceps femoris is continuous with that of the sacrotuberous ligament, which can also blend into the deep laminae of the multifidus.[161]

Articular: This subluxation may cause pain at the proximal tib-fib joint.

Neural: No known neural impingement results from this dysfunction, although one could assume that abnormal fibular position places increased stress upon the peroneal nerve.

Pronated Feet

Description:

This portion of the common pattern does not fit the neurological patterning described in Chapter 2 at first glance. But in actuality it does. That is because the common pattern for the foot is forefoot or rearfoot varus, both of which are evident in the pronated foot when it is examined in non-weight bearing. As a result of this posturing upon heel strike, the subtalar joint goes through

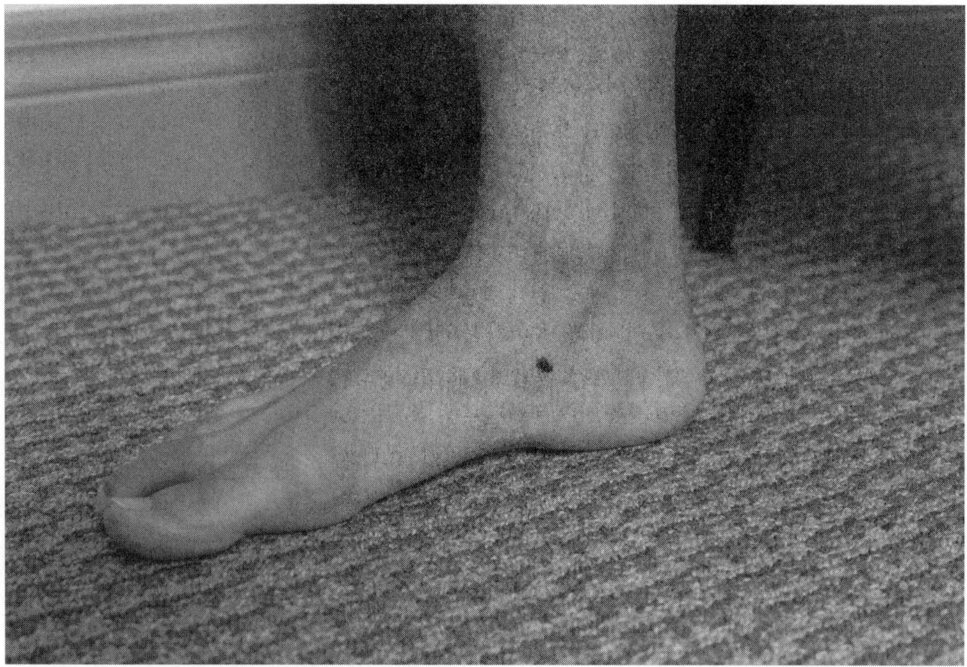

Fig. 9-1 The foot in non-weight bearing.

excessive pronation in order to sustain a normal gait pattern. The rest of the foot follows suit. Over the course of time the ligaments may creep or fail altogether. This gives the foot the characteristic flat foot or pes planus appearance. Despite this etiology, most professions only consider the end result of the compensation—which is the excessive pronation.

Recognized By:

1. Orthopedists and Podiatrists. Both professions recognize the strain excessive pronation causes the foot and knee. However, podiatrists are probably more liberal in their view of this fault's effects in that they would treat pronation in an attempt to reduce hip and/or low back symptoms.
2. Physical Therapists and Chiropractors. As with orthopedists and podiatrists, these professionals consider excessive pronation to be partially due to mechanical insufficiency. However, in addition to this, they also recognize the connection running in the opposite direction: from the top to the bottom. Therefore, treating pronation can be approached by treating the pelvis and hip (usually correcting anterior pelvic tilt and hip internal rotation/adduction) so

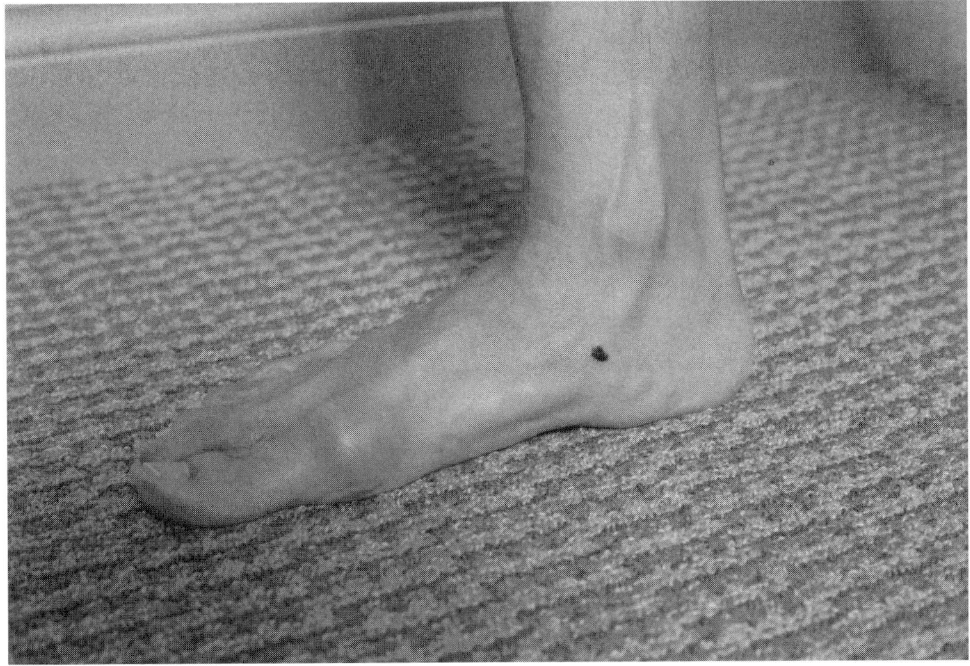

Fig. 9-2 The same foot in weight-bearing. Note the significant drop of the navicular bone.

that weight is brought laterally and the tibia is rotated externally. This brings the subtalar joint closer to supination which provides greater support.

3. Myers. Myers links excessive pronation to looseness of the Spiral Band. He believes this slack is produced by anterior pelvic rotation and reduced with neutral pelvic rotation.[162]
4. Rothbart. His view is different from these others in that he considers the neurological effects from faulty foot mechanics. According to his model, a foot type termed the Rothbart foot (similar to a Morton's foot) is capable of creating a neurological chain reaction which fails to activate vital postural muscles. Treatment differs from traditional methods in that he does not attempt to support the entire foot. Instead, his goal is to partially support the first ray. He believes that this support activates the proper postural musculature throughout the body, thereby optimizing structure. Without this stimulation the body sustains a "bio-implosion," creating FHP, rounded shoulders genu recurvatum, and excessive pronation.[48]
5. Startle Reflex. The startle reflex causes a varus positioning of the foot, which is consistent with the most common foot posture involved with excessive pronation during gait. Only in the presence of severe neurological damage (i.e. TBI, CVA) is this pattern strong enough to resist pronation during gait.

Implications:

Muscular: Excessive tractioning on the plantar fascia occurs with excessive pronation. This creates plantar fasciitis and potentially osteophyte formation at the medial calcaneal tubercle. In addition to this, the excessive calcaneal eversion and inefficient Windlass mechanism resulting from excessive pronation overworks the plantarflexors and may result in Achilles tendonitis.

Articular: Hallux valgus with bunion formation as well as osteophytic formation on the 1st MTP joint are common sequelae of excessive pronation.

Neural: Morton's neuroma can result from excessive shearing between the medial and lateral columns (between the 3rd and 4th metatarsals) of the foot, thereby irritating the interdigital nerve. The medial and lateral plantar nerves can become impinged during excessive pronation as well, leading to sensory changes and pain in the medial and lateral foot, respectively.

Please note: There are many more implications of excessive pronation than those listed. These implications are found throughout the entire body, as the progression of pronation along the kinetic chain can result in all of the lower extremity, scapular, and spinal column distortions listed previously. In addition to this, an excessively pronated foot does not afford the shock-absorptive function it was designed for. One can imagine how the repetitive microtraumas resulting from this will affect the entire body.

THEORETICAL IMPLICATIONS

The common pattern is very important to the manual therapist. First and foremost, knowing about this pattern helps him or her recognize which bodyparts are naturally more prone to breakdown and dysfunction. This helps the clinician narrow things down when looking at the entire body. This does not mean he should use a cookbook approach to evaluation, but it definitely makes the process easier. It also helps remind us to not limit our treatment to a single bodypart when more than one region is affected. Consider the case of 'miserable malalignment.' This structural fault involves excessive pronation, genu valgus, and hip internal rotation. What would happen if just one of these areas was addressed? Or if just the site of symptoms was treated? Most likely, the patient would not receive long-term benefit from such limited care.

Assessing the common pattern also helps the clinician gauge the level of involvement of the stress response. Much of this can be achieved by observing the patient's posture. As Hanna points out, one's emotions can cause long-term postural changes. For instance, he even goes so far as to say that the normal pattern of aging isn't really the aging process itself. Instead, the hunched-over pattern we see in the elderly is the long-term result of the startle and Landau reflexes (these are largely driven by emotions).

Philosophically, we can also learn a lot from these patterns. It is interesting to note the amount of similarity between many of these seemingly different approaches. This should be surprising to the reader, given that these findings not only arise from different professions but are also explained using separate theoretical concepts. For these particular patterns, it seems that every conceivable theory has been proposed to explain their existence. Likewise, countless methods have been devised to try to "correct" them.

As alluded to, the common patterns experience a cross-over into several different theoretical backgrounds. This includes the explanation and treatment rationale for each pattern by neurological, mechanical, and movement pattern theories. Frequently, proponents of each field believe there is enough evidence to explain a specific pattern without the inclusion of these other factors. For instance, some practitioners explain the prevalence of the forward-head posture solely by mechanical theory. Others might point to neurological factors as the cause of this pattern, while some may claim faulty movement patterns are responsible. In any event, this cross-over into multiple professions again demonstrates the frequency of each pattern. Not only is each pattern identifiable within the context of each field, but logical theories are available to explain their existence and potential treatment. This strengthens the argument that therapy should follow a holistic approach.

IMPLICATIONS FOR TREATMENT

Treatment of the common pattern can start at the site of the patient's symptoms, though it must expand beyond that. That is because many of the patterns involving each joint are related to the adjacent joints. These joints are then related to the joints near them, and so on. Besides this, we need to keep in mind that something created the common pattern in the first place. In other words, the common pattern itself is an effect with a knowable cause. It is our job to find and address the cause(s).

Treating the common pattern *and* its cause is absolutely necessary if we want to change it. For instance, if postural stress is causing the common pattern, then the pattern will continuously be reinstated no matter what we do (manually) to the person. By the same token, if we just remove the pattern's causative factor(s), there is little chance the body will spontaneously revert back to normal. This is especially true if adaptive shortening and muscle atrophy have taken place, both of which act as mechanical obstacles to normal posture. Indeed, this is one case where therapy implemented on the right side of the continuum is absolutely necessary to affect long-term change.

Treatment also must be thorough in the *way* it treats, not just in *what* it treats. This means we must involve the neurological, mechanical, and movement pattern systems in order to be successful. Please note that this does not mean we should exclude the energetic system. It is just that at this time diagnostic technology has not caught up with energy medicine. We will find many more reasons why these patterns occur once we have a better understanding of the body's energy system.

THE RIGHT-LEFT PATTERNS

In addition to the common pattern, there are several documented patterns which involve laterality as an important variable. These patterns wreak havoc on the musculoskeletal system just as the common pattern does. Additionally, many of these patterns add a rotational (transverse plane) stress upon the body, thereby placing extra strain on the system.

While a definitive cause for these patterns is lacking at this time, we must consider the strong possibility that something is driving the asymmetries we see on a daily basis. For instance, why do 98-99% of cases of idiopathic scoliosis present with a right thoracic curvature? Is the nervous system responsible for this? Possibly. Or, is the asymmetry of the internal organs the cause? Possibly. In any event, it is valuable for the clinician to be aware of these patterns. In some cases it may be necessary to try to intervene and lessen their effects. In other cases it may be more valuable to do nothing, understanding that this pattern is present in many individuals and is not always responsible for their symptoms. These decisions then are dependent on the pattern involved, the severity of the pattern, the clinician's personal experience and other factors. The reader is urged to consult the works of Greenman, Schamberger, Hruska, and Kippenbrock for more information on these patterns.

10 Treatment

THE FOLLOWING CHAPTERS ARE SET-UP AS TECHNIQUE ATLASES SPECIFIC TO THE DIFFERENT REGIONS of the body. Please note that these chapters do not include details on general anatomy and pathology. It is assumed that the reader already has a general knowledge of these topics. It should also be noted that this list of techniques is not comprehensive—there are literally thousands of manual therapy techniques in existence. Instead, these chapters are streamlined to address the most frequently encountered disorders found at each region. This follows the common pattern in the majority of cases. Other techniques added to this list are ones the author has found especially beneficial, although their relationship to the common pattern is not specific.

Keep in mind that no technique is intended as a stand-alone therapy, and they are not meant to be chosen in an a-la-carte fashion. Instead, these techniques are meant to be used under the theoretical framework outlined throughout this text. Now, within this framework, there is certainly value in using local techniques to treat a given condition. Likewise, there are also regional and global treatments which will benefit the patient. Altogether, treating the entire body with methods involving all 4 primary factors and addressing the secondary factors is the basis of the Complete Manual Therapy approach. It is this approach which addresses all causes of dysfunction and facilitates the body's natural healing processes.

11 The Cervical Spine

THE MANUAL THERAPIST MUST BE ADEPT AT TREATING BOTH MAJOR REGIONS OF THE CERVICAL spine: the upper cervical spine and the middle/lower cervical spine. Remember from Chapter 3 that both regions are considered high-yield components of the global scan. Therefore, they are very important to the health of the individual and must be addressed on *every* patient.

UPPER CERVICAL SPINE

Successful management of the upper cervical spine begins with a thorough, accurate assessment. Presented below are multiple ways to accomplish this. The practitioner is urged to utilize several examination methods to ensure a clear diagnosis before rendering treatment.

Suboccipitals. Palpate these muscles for hypertonicity, fascial adhesions, tenderness, and trigger points. Utilize soft tissue techniques including myofascial release, sustained pressure and ischemic compression to address the findings. Post-isometric relaxation stretching is also useful in reducing tone (Fig. 11-1 to 11-3).

> *Suboccipital facilitation and shortening is prevalent in almost all patients. This worsens and perpetuates FHP and the common pattern while also creating localized joint dysfunction. Upledger writes that these muscles also have a strong influence over the craniosacral system, thus making their influence even more widespread. Manual therapists have recognized the importance of treating these muscles for a*

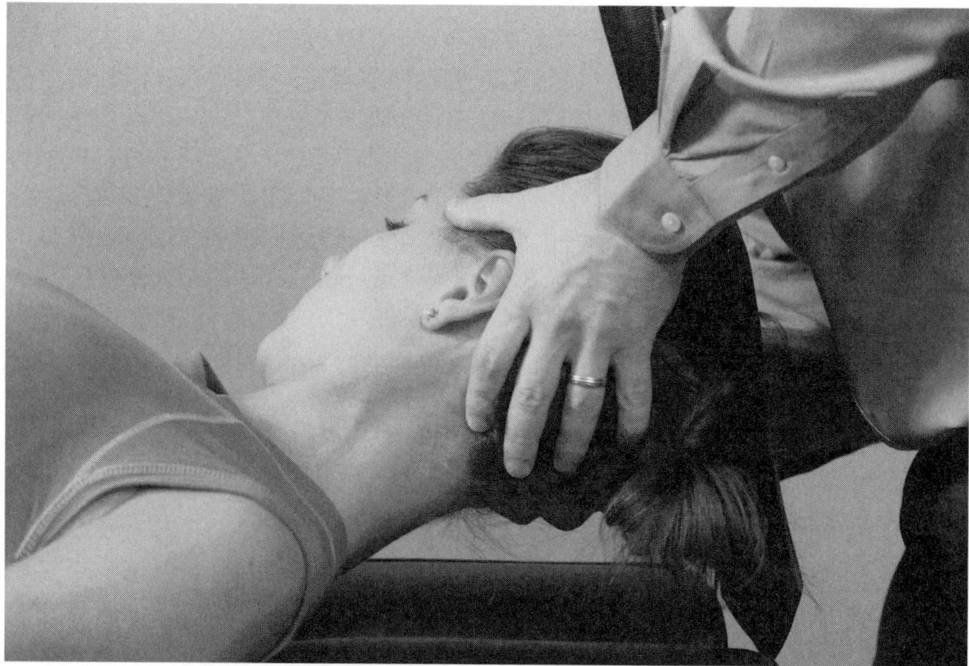

Fig. 11-1 PIR stretching of the rectus capitus posterior. Have the patient gently extend, rotate and sidebend the head ipsilaterally. Upon relaxation, stretch the occiput into flexion, left rotation and lateral flexion.

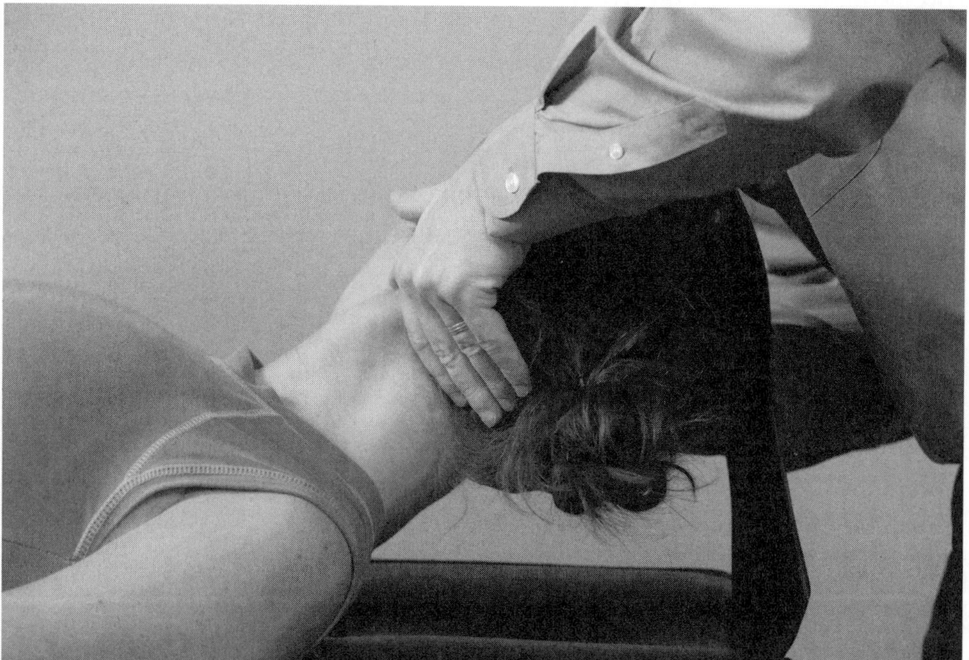

Fig. 11-2 PIR stretching of the inferior oblique. Have the patient gently extend and rotate the head ipsilaterally. Upon relaxation, stretch the atlas into flexion and contralateral rotation.

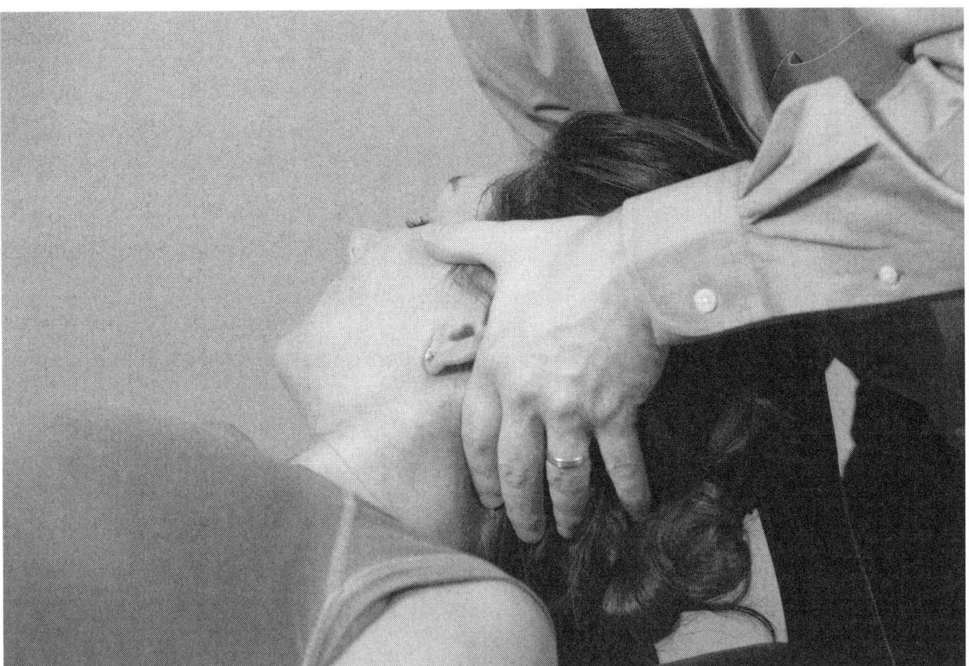

Fig. 11-3 PIR stretching of the superior oblique. Have the patient extend, rotate ipsilaterally and sidebend contralaterally. Upon relaxation, stretch the occiput into flexion, contralateral rotation and ipsilateral sidebending.[163]

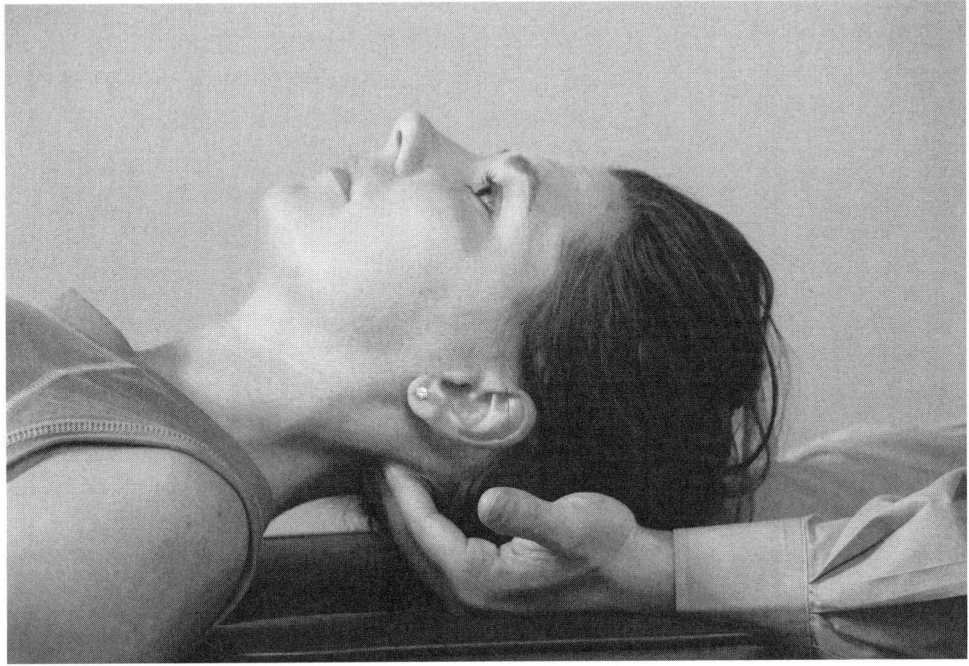

Fig. 11-4 Suboccipital release. The clinician's fingertips support the patient's head and neck just below the occiput. Allow the tissues to relax for 1–2 minutes and then gently traction superiorly. This induces slight flexion of the occiput on the atlas. Continue this maneuver until no further releases occur.

long time, as there are multiple techniques in use to address this dysfunction. The reader is urged to learn as many of these techniques as he/she can, as altering this pattern is of the utmost importance.

Sternocleidomastoid. Palpate the muscle for hypertonicity, fascial adhesions, tenderness, and trigger points. Utilize soft tissue techniques including myofascial release, sustained pressure, strumming and ischemic compression to address the findings. Post-isometric relaxation stretching is also useful in reducing tone and improving flexibility (Fig. 11-5).

The sternocleidomastoid is facilitated as part of the common pattern. By its attachment to the mastoid process, this causes compression of the occipitoatlantal joint. This can be bilateral or unilateral. Working bilaterally, this causes an extended occiput. Unilaterally, this causes ipsilateral sidebending and contralateral rotation of the skull. According to Upledger, hypertonus also causes posterior rotation of the temporal bone.

The sternocleidomastoid is also overworked in cases of dysfunctional breathing. In this pattern, it is repetitively contracted to help raise the ribcage. This causes strain of the muscle itself and negatively impacts the cervical spine. Look for this breathing

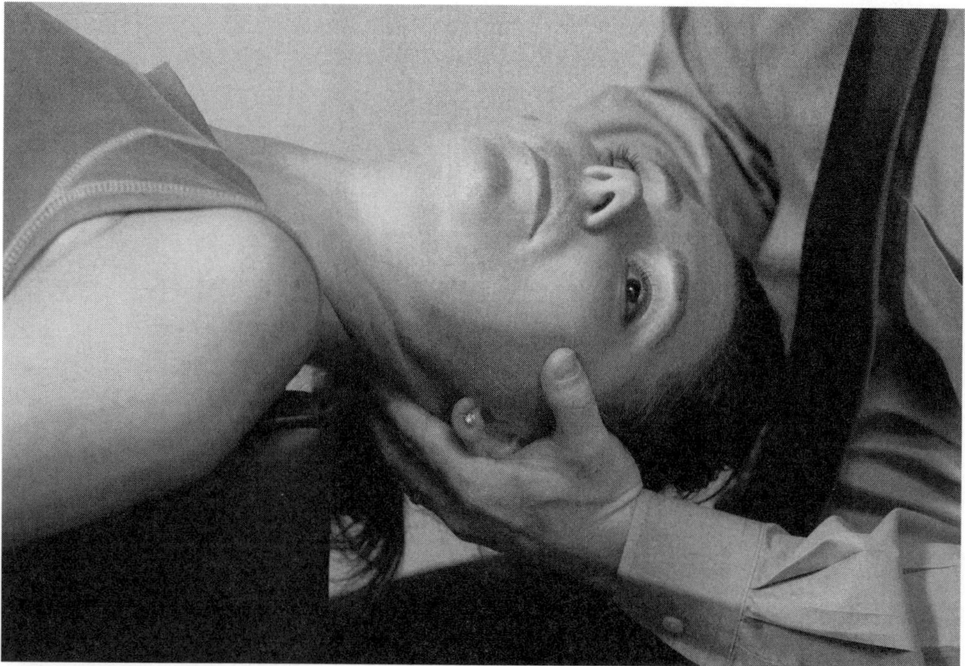

Fig. 11-5 PIR stretching of the sternocleidomastoid. Have the patient gently flex, sidebend ipsilaterally, and rotate contralaterally against the therapist's resistance. Upon relaxation, stretch the patient further into extension, contralateral sidebending, and ipsilateral rotation.

pattern and address if present. Expect trigger points in this muscle to refer pain to the ipsilateral head, forehead, and face.

Upper Trapezius. Palpate the muscle for hypertonicity, fascial adhesions, tenderness, and trigger points. Utilize soft tissue techniques including myofascial release, sustained pressure, strumming and ischemic compression to address the findings. Post-isometric relaxation stretching is also useful in reducing tone and improving flexibility (Fig. 11-6).

The upper trapezius and sternocleidomastoid are closely related. They have the same innervation and are both involved in the startle response. They are also active in most people. Be sure to search both muscles thoroughly for trigger points. Trigger points in the upper trap will refer pain to side of the head and neck, while trigger points in the SCM refer pain to the lateral head, forehead, and face.

Semispinalis Capitis, Splenius Capitis, Longissimus Capitis. Palpate these muscles for hypertonicity, fascial adhesions, tenderness, and trigger points. Utilize soft tissue techniques including myofascial release, sustained pressure, strumming and ischemic compression to address the findings.

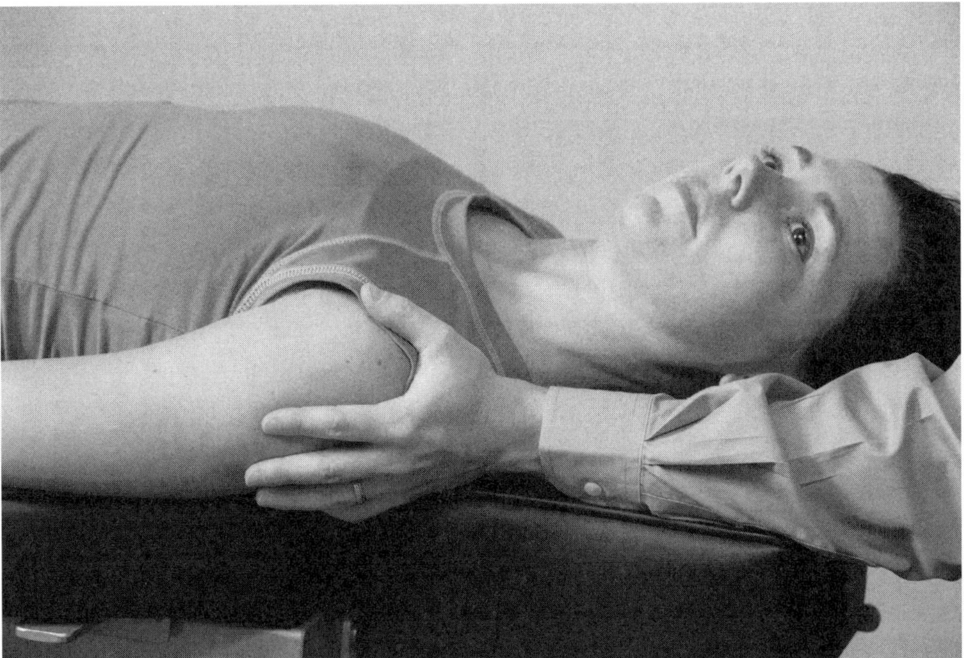

Fig. 11-6 PIR stretching of the upper trapezius. Have the patient shrug the shoulder, ipsilaterally sidebend, and contralaterally rotate the head against resistance. Upon relaxation stretch the patient into shoulder depression, contralateral sidebending and ipsilateral rotation.

MUSCLE STRENGTH

Muscle strength assessment and treatment techniques are presented in the Mid- and Lower Cervical Spine sections.

SEGMENTAL MOBILITY

The assessment and treatment of segmental mobility plays an important role in the management of cervical spine syndromes. This should be obvious to the reader, given the fact that professions including chiropractic are practically based on correcting segmental dysfunction. With this in mind, it should also be obvious to the reader that he/she must be skilled in one of the many segmental assessment and treatment approaches in order to effectively serve his or her patients. It is out of the scope of this text to provide the reader with the necessary details and hands-on instruction necessary to master any of these techniques, so no attempt will be made to do so. This especially applies to those techniques requiring high levels of skill and practice, such as upper cervical technique, Gonstead technique, or the motion palpation approach. Instead, the instruction provided in this section is focused on more simple techniques virtually any manual therapist can perform. For this specific region of the body, strain/counterstrain has been added to aid the clinician in diagnosis. This is because the upper cervical spine is not only very complicated and difficult to assess, but also because it is arguably the most important region of the body and deserves a precise examination.

STRAIN/COUNTERSTRAIN IN DIAGNOSIS

Strain/counterstrain is helpful in the upper cervical spine not only as a treatment technique, but also as diagnostic tool. This is because Jones' points diminish in tenderness as the subluxation is *exaggerated*. Thus, these points help us determine what position a vertebra is "stuck" in. This knowledge can then be used to treat the segment directly or indirectly.

Treating a segment indirectly is especially helpful when a condition is acute and the clinician does not want to exacerbate the patient's problem. It is also useful when the practitioner is not experienced in mobilization or manipulation. The common strain/counterstrain points are presented in the figures below.[164] Remember to use these findings as an adjunctive diagnostic tool to blend with other examination methods, especially those presented in the following sections.

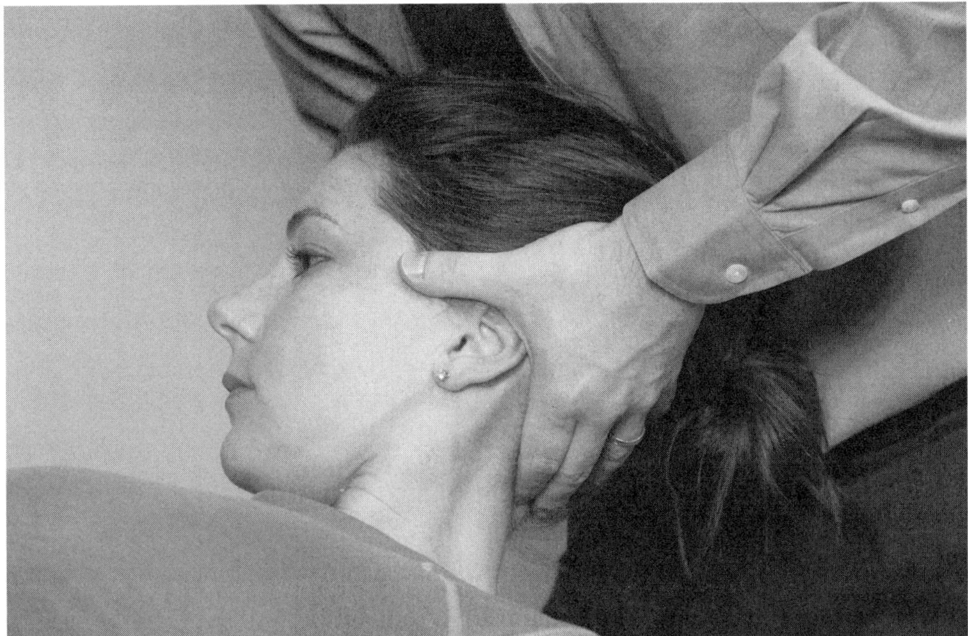

Fig. 11-7 Posterior First Cervical-Flexion. Involvement of the rectus capitis anterior. The tender point is located 3 cm inferior to the EOP just lateral to midline. Treat the tender point by markedly flexing the occiput, slightly sidebending towards and rotating away from the point.

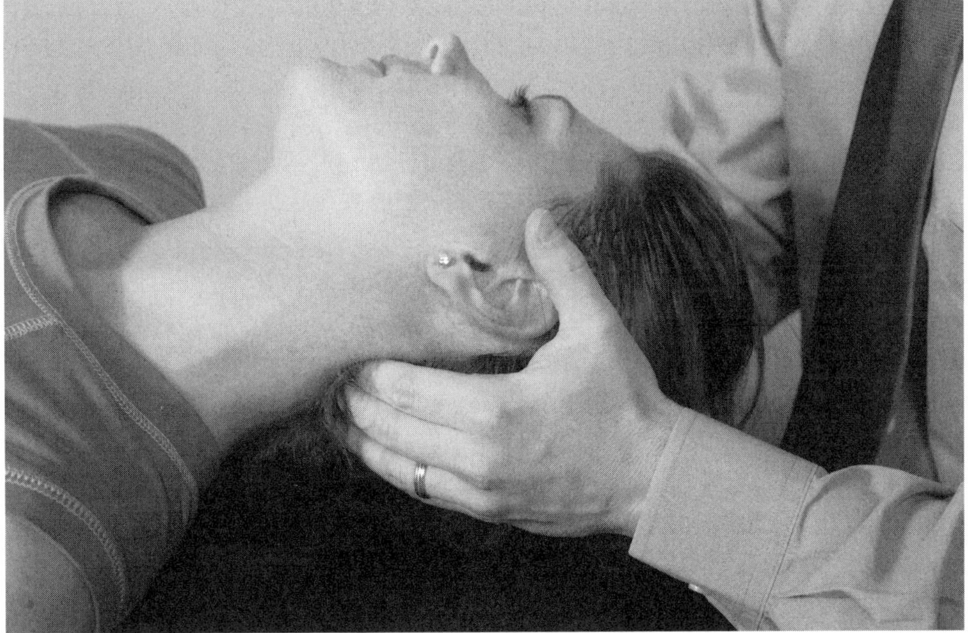

Fig. 11-8 Posterior First Cervical-Extension. The tender point is found 1 to 1.5 cm medial to the mastoid process. To treat this point, extend the occiput and add moderate contralateral rotation and sidebending.

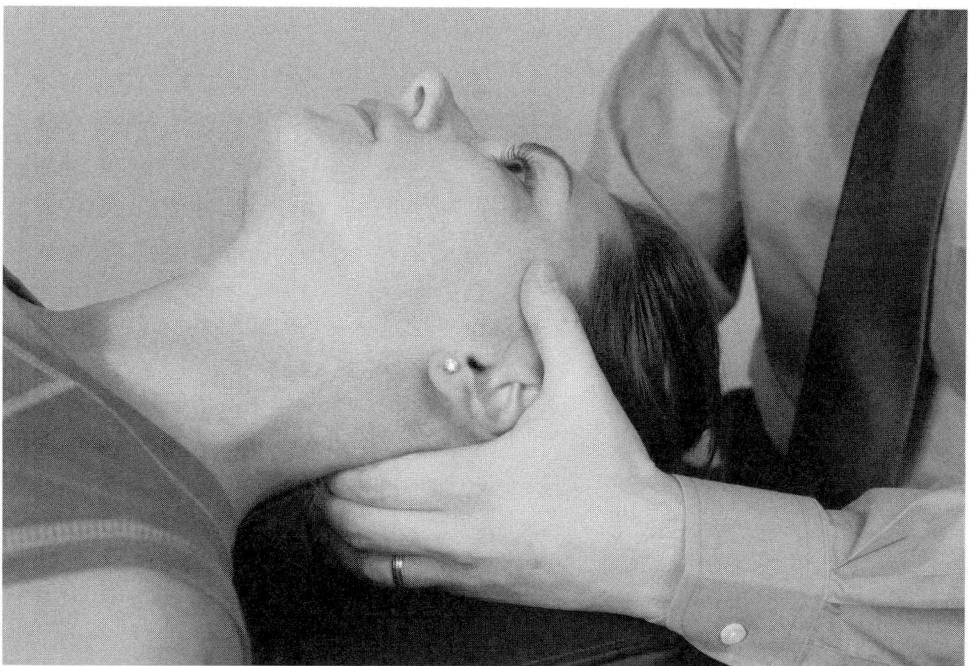

Fig. 11-9 Posterior Second Cervical. Involvement of the rectus capitis posterior major/minor. The tender point is found lateral to the insertion of the semispinalis capitis. Treat this point by extending the occiput and adding slight contralateral sidebending and rotation.

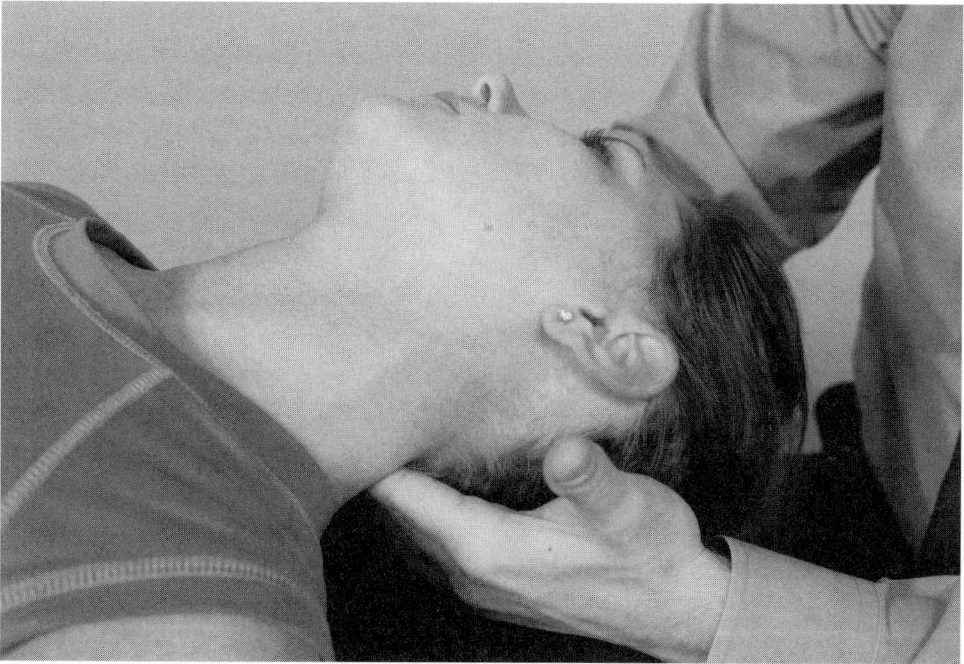

Fig. 11-10 Posterior Third Cervical. Involvement of the rotators, multifidus, interspinalis. The tender point is found on the inferior surface of the C2 spinous process or on the articular process of C3. To treat these points, extend the neck and then laterally flex and rotate to the opposite side.

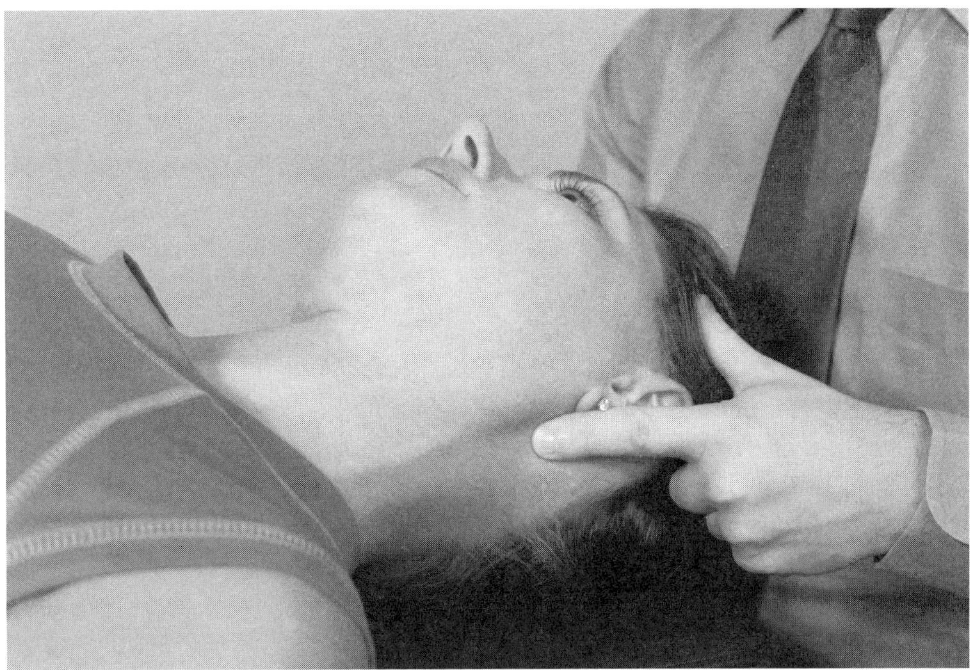

Fig. 11-11 Lateral First Cervical. Involvement of the rectus capitis lateralis. The tender point is found on the lateral aspect of the C1 TVP. To treat this point, laterally flex the head toward or away from the tender point side.

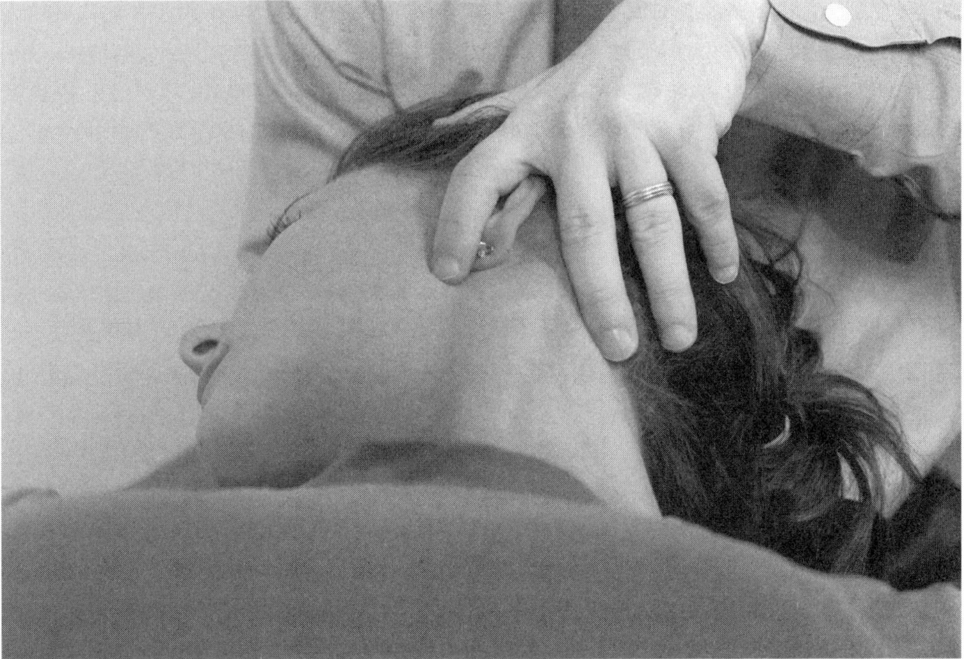

Fig. 11-12 Anterior First Cervical. Involvement of the rectus capitis anterior. The tender point is found on the posterior aspect of the ramus of the mandible. Treatment involves marked contralateral rotation of the neck.

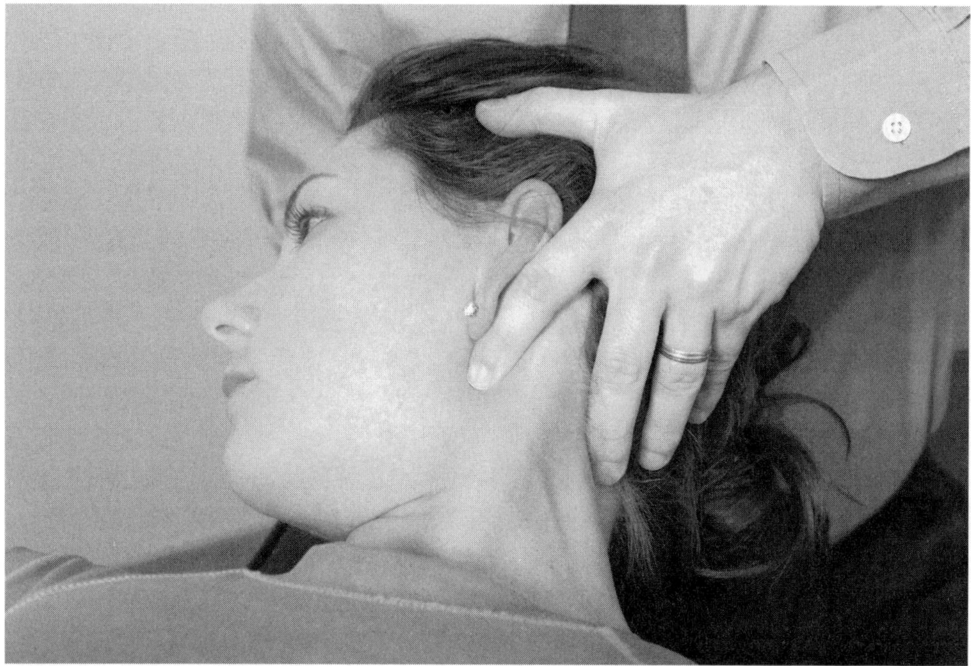

Fig. 11-13 Anterior Second Cervical. Involvement of the longus colli. The tender point is found anterior to the C2 TVP. To treat this point markedly rotate the head to the opposite side and add slight flexion.

THE OCCIPUT

There are many methods available to test the occipitoatlantal joint. A simple one from the Thompson technique is presented below. It is based on neurology and leg length testing. Although it is a scan for a specific occipital subluxation, clinically it is very helpful.

Thompson's Bilateral Cervical Syndrome (Extended Occiput). Begin by checking the prone patient's leg lengths. Then, have him rotate his head to one side. The leg on the side he turned to will shorten. Now, have him turn to the opposite side. The other leg will now shorten.

Treatment via the Thompson technique is a superiorly-directed thrust to the base of the occiput. This is done on a drop table. If the clinician does not have a drop table he can use a prolonged stretch or just mobilize in this position (Fig. 11-14).

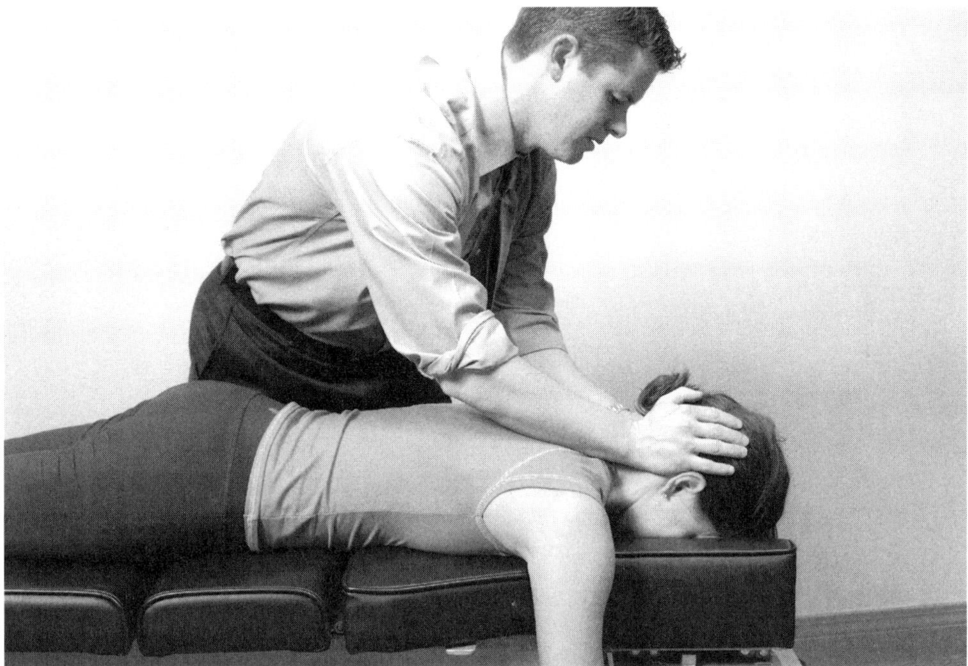

Fig. 11-14 Apply a prolonged stretch to decompress the posteriorly-displaced occiput.

THE ATLAS

There are a myriad of ways to assess the atlas. Upper cervical practitioners take specific x-rays to determine its exact position. (This is the most accurate method, although it takes specialized training and equipment to practice this approach.) Other doctors challenge the atlas, looking for changes in leg length or weakening of a strong indicator muscle. Both methods are valuable tools and are worth learning, but each is out of the scope of this text. Instead, atlantoaxial evaluation is presented from the physical therapy perspective.

Physical Therapy Approach. There are two simple physical therapy techniques to assess and treat the atlantoaxial articulation. The first method begins by assessing the patient's cervical rotation. In general, this indicates the functional mobility of the C1-2 articulation. If motion is restricted in one direction, the clinician palpates for tenderness/tautness at the C1-2 junction on the side of restriction. If a problem is present at C1-2, this tenderness will worsen when the patient rotates the head ipsilaterally. Treatment for this finding is simple. Mobilize the C1-2 joint in a posterior-anterior direction with the head rotated 30 degrees ipsilaterally (Fig. 11-15). The reader is urged to treat gently and evaluate the effects of mobilization to ensure he/she has chosen the proper technique.

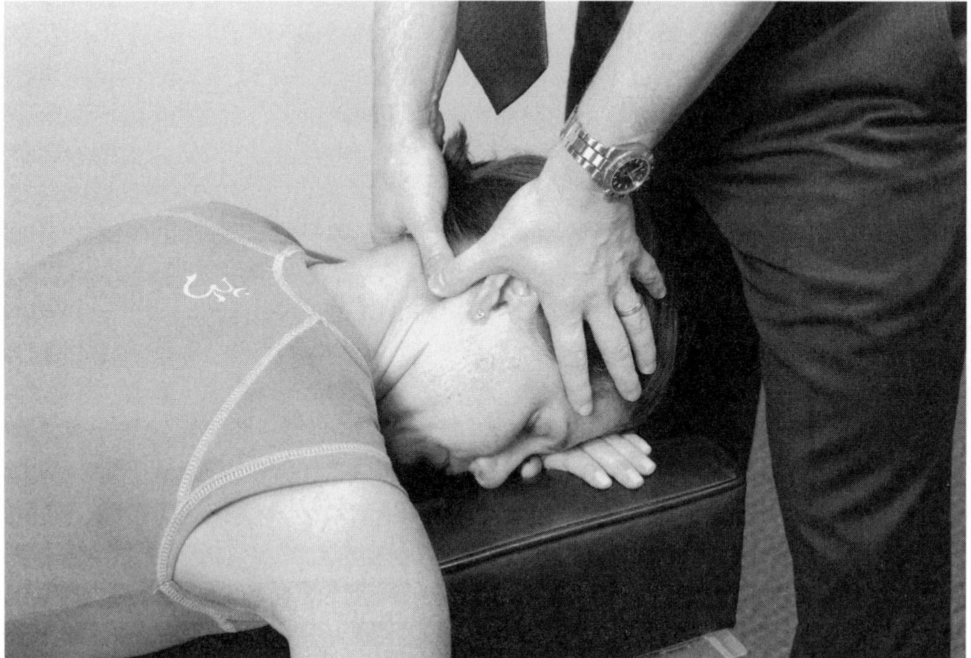

Fig. 11-15 C1-2 rotation restriction. Mobilize the lateral junction of C1-2 with the head rotated 30 degrees ipsilaterally. The glide should be directly P-A.

A second effective technique for the atlas is presented by Mulligan. He starts with assessing the atlas' rotation with conventional methods. If motion is limited, have the patient use a thin band (or the edge of a towel) to help push the transverse process forward during the motion.[165] For instance, if the patient has limited rotation to the left, have him contact the posterior aspect of the right transverse process. Holding this pressure from the start to the end of the range of motion will help increase range of motion if the technique is indicated. Repeat ten times as a treatment modality.

THE AXIS

As with the atlas, there are many ways to assess the axis. A simple approach from physical therapy is presented below.

Physical Therapy Approach. We can use the same assessment technique as was described above for the atlas. In this instance, however, the axis is incriminated when the patient's tenderness at C1-2 is not worsened with ipsilateral head rotation. Treatment is a posterior-anterior mobilization of C2 with the head in neutral (Fig. 11-16). Post-mobilization assessment will demonstrate increased ipsilateral neck rotation.

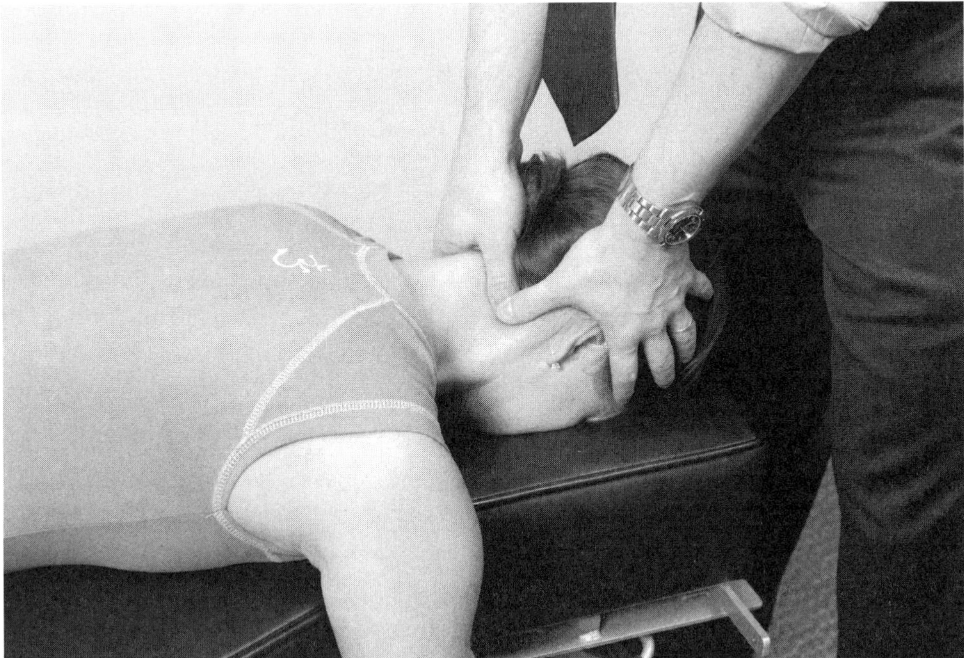

Fig. 11-16 C2 rotation restriction. Mobilize the junction of C1-2 posterior-anterior with the head in the neutral position.

MOVEMENT PATTERNS

The predominant movement pattern disorder here is excessive suboccipital muscle contraction. This causes problems locally. It also sends the spine into a massive compensatory pattern.

Alexander referred to the suboccipital contraction as the downward pull. He understood how harmful this was to the body and how important it was to break-up this pattern. Employing what he called the Primary Control helps do this. Please review Chapter 6 for details on this technique. Remind the patient to use it whenever he/she performs any action that causes contraction of these muscles.

ENERGY-BASED APPROACHES

Auricular Acupressure. Gently squeeze the point corresponding to the neck with two fingers. Hold for 5 seconds, then relax 5 seconds. Increase the amount of pressure with each cycle for a total time of one minute (6 cycles). Do this initially on the ear on the involved side only; treat the opposite ear as well if the patient does not improve.

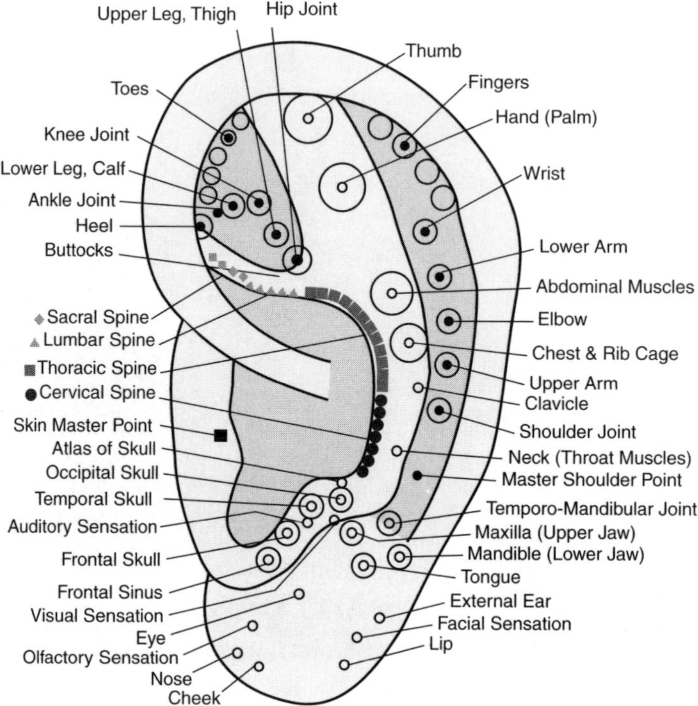

Fig. 11-17

Foot Reflexology. Begin by massaging the entire foot. Walk up the foot with the thumbs along the five zones. Treat both the plantar and dorsal surfaces. Work the toes as well. Spend extra time on the medial border of the foot corresponding with the spine. Also, work on areas associated with different organs needing an extra "boost." Following this long warm-up, massage the area on the foot corresponding with the cervical spine.

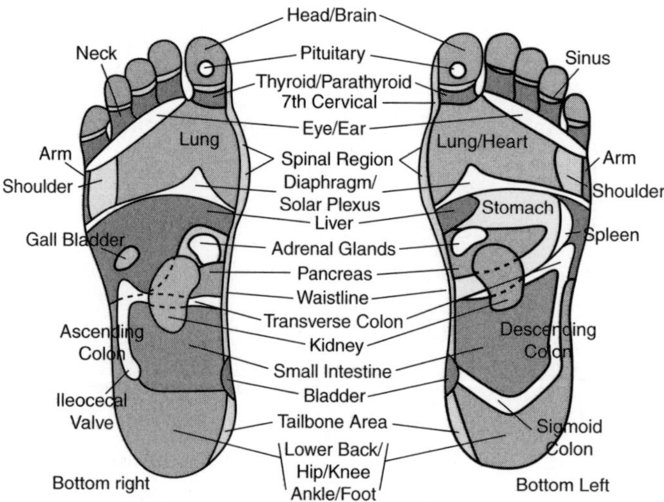

Fig. 11-18

HIGH-YIELD SCAN

Perform a scan of the high-yield elements of the body including:

- Gait
- Posture
- Sit-to-Stand
- Miniature Squat
- Respiration
- Romberg Test
- Fukuda's Test
- Lower Cervical Spine
- TMJ
- Pelvis
- Feet
- Stress Screen

EVALUATION AND TREATMENT OF THE SECONDARY FACTORS

Sleeping. Remember from Chapter 8 that improper sleeping posture is stressful on the cervical spine. Most harmful is prone sleeping with full rotation. If the patient sleeps in this position he must be strongly urged to change.

Posture. Assess the patient's posture in sitting and standing. Also, inquire about his posture at work and home. Specifically, ask him to emulate his typical posture when he is on the job or relaxing at home. Ascertain his exact position while on the phone, the computer, and on the sofa. Screen for habits or environmental factors which reinforce a negative postural pattern, such as a poorly placed computer screen or a deep sofa. Help the person modify these environmental factors to reduce cervical strain.

MIDDLE AND LOWER CERVICAL SPINE

Scalenes. Palpate these muscles for hypertonicity, fascial adhesions, tenderness, and trigger points. Utilize soft tissue techniques including myofascial release, sustained pressure, strumming and ischemic compression to address the findings. Post-isometric relaxation is also useful in reducing tone and improving flexibility.

The scalenes are facilitated as part of the common pattern. Compounded with this, they are used to elevate the ribcage in cases of dysfunctional breathing. Together, this means the scalenes are contracted in most individuals. Contracted, dysfunctional scalenes will cause a variety of symptoms. Trigger points in these muscles refer pain down the radial aspect of the forearm into digits one and two, mimicking cervical radiculopathy. These muscles may even cause thoracic outlet syndrome by compressing the brachial plexus and subclavian artery. Lastly, they may lead to chronic 1st rib subluxations due to constant pulling. Screen for all of these problems.

Levator Scapula. Palpate the muscle for hypertonicity, fascial adhesions, tenderness, and trigger points. Utilize soft tissue techniques including myofascial release, sustained pressure, strumming and ischemic compression to address the findings.

The levator scapula is inhibited as part of the common pattern. However, it is frequently a pain generator, as it is stretched and overworked in cases of poor posture. Manual techniques are typically helpful in the short-term; long-term improvement requires changing the patient's posture and movement patterns.

Longus Capitis and Longus Colli. Palpate these muscles for hypertonicity, fascial adhesions, tenderness, and trigger points. Utilize gentle soft tissue techniques including myofascial release, sustained pressure, and strumming to address the findings (Fig. 11-19).

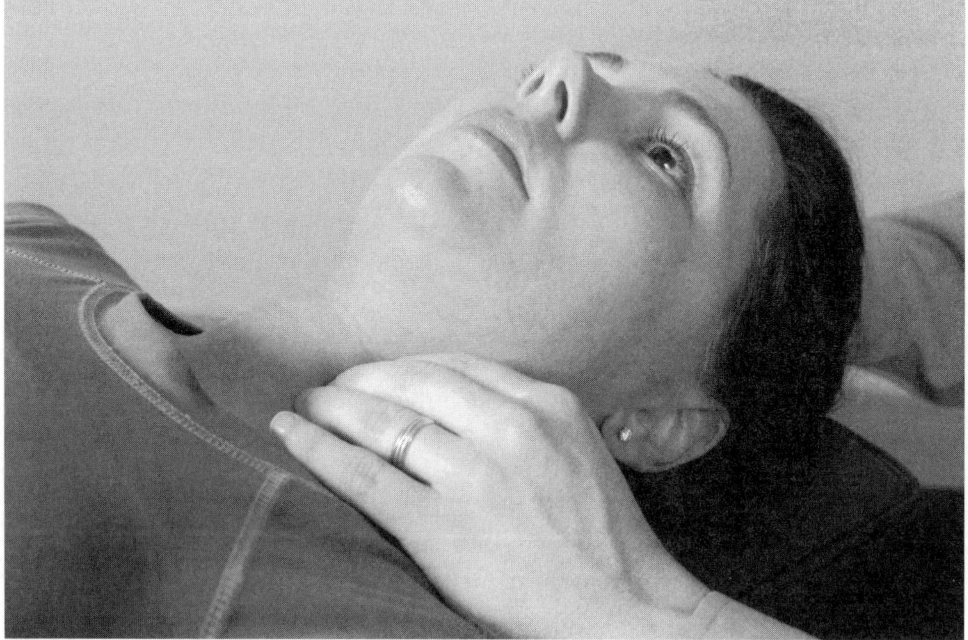

Fig. 11-19 The clinician can apply MFR or sustained pressure in this position.

The longus capitis and colli are inhibited as part of the common pattern, so the typical focus is on their recruitment and strengthening. The longus colli frequently acts as a pain generator, as it is strained in whiplash injuries. Keep in mind that these muscles rarely produce pain in the front of the neck; it will surprise the patient when palpation proves them to be tender to the touch. This tenderness is a sure sign that they are involved to some extent and should be treated with manual methods.

STRENGTH TESTING

Evaluate the strength of the neck muscles with traditional methods. Make sure to assess both their ability to initiate a contraction as well as their sheer strength. Most often, what we perceive as weakness is more a matter of inhibition. This will follow the common pattern and/or be due to local or segmental dysfunction. Treating the causative factor restores normal strength in these cases. In cases of true muscle weakness, such as those involving muscle atrophy, remedial strengthening is indicated.

The most common finding in cases of cervical dysfunction is short neck flexor weakness. One can screen for it by having the supine patient first tuck the chin. Then have him slightly lift the head off the table. He should be able to do this in a slow, controlled manner without losing the chin tuck position. Ideally, one should not see marked recruitment of the sternocleidomastoids or platysma either.

Remedial strengthening for short neck flexor weakness is through repetition. The patient can begin this exercise in the sitting position, which is easiest. He can then progress to prone or quadruped and then to supine as strength improves. From here, have him increase the number of repetitions and holding time until he can hold it for at least 30 seconds without difficulty. For more advanced methods of neck flexor strength assessment and therapy, the reader is urged to consult the work of Gwendolyn Jull. She promotes the use of a pressure biofeedback unit to objectively define the patient's current level of strength and to gradually progress him in a controlled exercise regimen.

One can expect weakness of the spinal intrinsics in addition to the short neck flexors. These muscles are vital for stability and intricate movement of the spinal vertebrae. Strengthening these muscles is best accomplished with activities which stress the patient's balance. Specialized exercises to activate these muscles are presented in Chapter 6, Movement Pattern Considerations.

STRAIN/COUNTERSTRAIN

As in the upper cervical spine, we can use strain/counterstrain as a stand-alone treatment or in an effort to aid segmental diagnosis. D'Ambrogio[164] and Jones[178] describe these individual points and give the name for each point. In general, diagnosing the positional fault and/or applying treatment revolves around a few simple rules:

1. Rotate the spine to the side opposite the tender point.
2. If the tender point is anterior, add a degree of flexion.
3. If the tender point is posterior, add a degree of extension.
4. The more lateral the tender point, the more rotation is added.
5. The closer the tender point is to midline, the more flexion or extension necessary.

SEGMENTAL MOBILITY

As noted above, the assessment and treatment of segmental mobility is beyond the scope of this text. In its place are several very simple techniques virtually any manual therapist can perform. These techniques are presented below.

Thompson Technique

The Thompson protocol provides a quick, easy way of finding localized segmental dysfunction. Begin by assessing the patient's leg lengths in the prone position. Next, have him turn his head to one side. Re-check the leg lengths. Then, have him turn to the opposite side. Re-check the leg lengths. A positive finding is when head rotation to one side causes a short leg to lengthen. This happens when the patient turns away from the dysfunctional side. In essence, this is because the involved facet is unweighted and irritation to the system is removed. Thompson calls a positive finding with the knees extended a Unilateral Cervical Syndrome.

This assessment is repeated with the knees flexed 90 degrees. A positive finding in this position is called an X-Derifield Cervical Syndrome. In both cases, the practitioner palpates the side opposite to the head rotation which caused the short leg to even. He will find a tender nodule at the level of involvement.

Treatment is simple. Under the Thompson protocol, the practitioner uses a drop table. He contacts the tender nodule with the patient's head rotated away from the tender side. He thrusts anteriorly and superiorly in the upper cervical spine, straight anteriorly in the middle cervical spine, and anterior and inferior in the lower cervical spine. This causes the legs to go even and the nodule to disappear.

Without a drop table the clinician can use these same principles to apply a manipulation or mobilization. Strain-counterstrain may also be applied.

Australian Approach

This approach is a simple, effective way of vertebral examination and treatment. In a nutshell, examination begins by finding the direction wherein cervical motion is painful and limited. Treatment is even more simple: mobilize or manipulate the spine in the opposite direction. Rotation or lateral flexion is usually used with this technique. Another excellent technique is the cervical lateral glide, which basically involves imparting a lateral glide towards the pain-free side. Although these techniques sound too simple to be effective, they really work. Both of them usually cause an immediate reduction in pain and an increase in range of motion.

In addition to these methods, the facets are palpated for tenderness. Typically, one finds tenderness on the same side as the motion restriction. Once again, treatment is simple. Use the thumbs to mobilize the tender facets anteriorly. Re-examination shows increased pain-free motion.

Clinical reasoning plays a big role in this approach. Mobilizing or manipulating in the direction opposite the limitation (an indirect approach) is most effective when the patient is in the acute and subacute stage. It is actually just like a strain-counterstrain technique in that it places hypertonic muscles on a slack. This indirect approach is less effective when the patient's motion limitation is due to true adaptive shortening, capsular tightness, or adhesion formation. In these cases, a direct approach is utilized. This can be with mobilization or manipulation as with the indirect approach. It can also include prolonged stretching into the limitation or repetitive patient-induced movements into the restriction. Keep in mind that the direct approach is prone to causing pain. Normally, this is localized and resolves when the stretching ceases. Other times the pain may linger for a little while after therapy has stopped. At no time should the technique cause referred or radiating pain or any other neurological symptoms.

(Author's note: This approach is presented in several manual therapy textbooks, including those by Maitland,[166] Murtagh and Kenna,[167] and Maigne.[67] The author is not sure it is called the "Australian Approach," though for the purpose of this text that is how it is named).

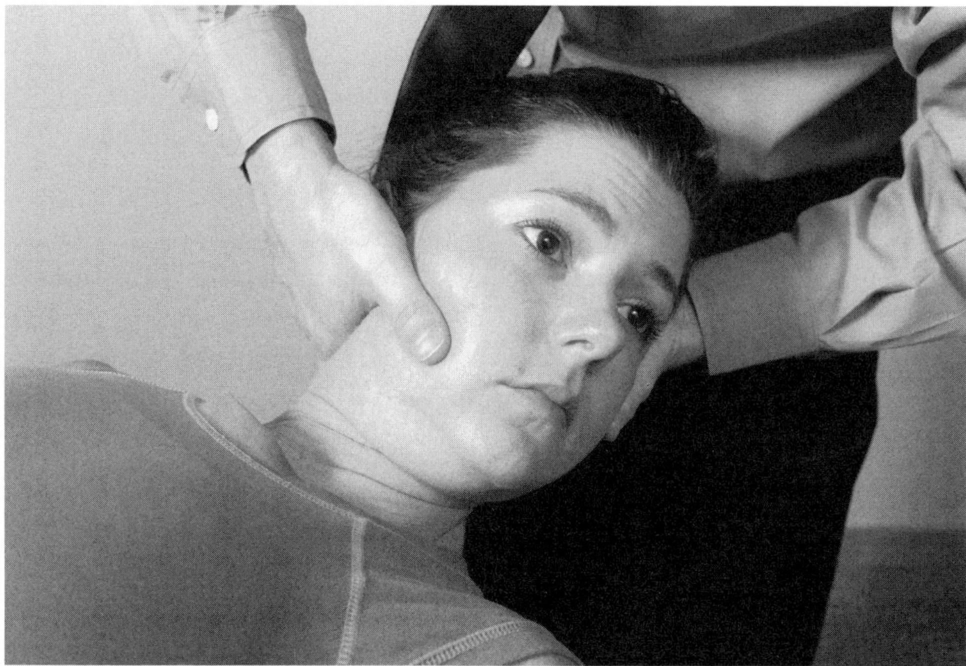

Fig. 11-20 Treatment for right rotation restriction. Rotate the patient into left rotation, taking care to first localize the affected segments with flexion and ipsi- or contralateral sidebending. Apply overpressure with the radial aspect of the 2nd metacarpalphalangeal joint to the posterolateral aspect of the articular pillar.

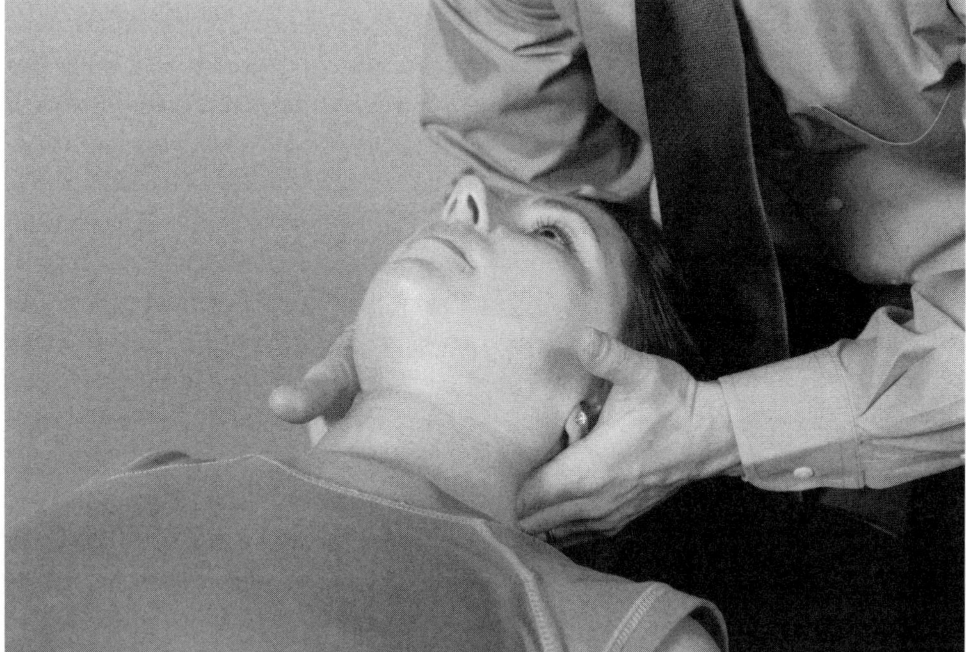

Fig. 11-21 Cervical lateral glide. Contact the C5/6 region and glide the vertebrae in the direction opposite the side of symptoms. This technique has been proven to effectively treat neurogenic cervicobrachial pain[168] and lateral epicondylalgia,[169] among other conditions.

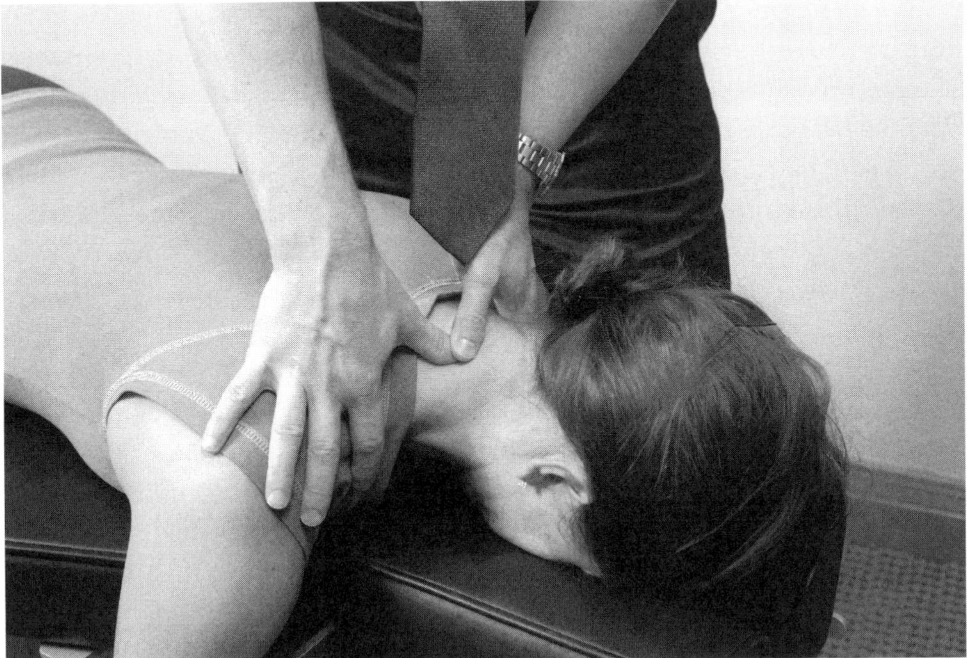

Fig. 11-22 Treatment for right facet dysfunction. Place the thumbs close together and contact the affected facet joint. Mobilize P-A for 30 seconds.

Mulligan Technique

Physical therapist Brian Mulligan's techniques for the cervical spine are both easy to implement and quite effective when they are indicated.[142] To perform his SNAG technique, begin by finding the direction of limited motion (restricted rotation responds especially well to this technique). Then, apply a superior and anterior directed pressure upon a facet where the patient complains of pain. This is usually also on the side to which motion is limited. Re-test rotation to that side. If the technique is indicated and the therapist is on the right level, the patient will demonstrate increased pain-free rotation while the pressure is held.[170] If the range of motion does not change or changes very little, the therapist is to move up or down a level and try again. Treatment consists of repetitive movement into the restricted direction while pressure is applied. As with other Mulligan techniques, remind the patient to only move as far as possible without causing pain. Repeat this ten times.

CERVICAL SPINE POSTURE

Examine the general contour and shape of the cervical spine to determine its curvature (or lack thereof) in the sagittal plane. Typically, one finds a diminished cervical lordosis in the lower and middle cervical spine before it is forced to compensate by extending in the upper cervical spine. As mentioned previously, a great deal of importance is placed on this hypolordosis. A substantial amount of research has been performed to study its neurophysiological and mechanical implications—and they are very negative. A strong case has been made that this deformity places excessive tensile force on the spinal cord itself. Equally strong research proves that the abnormal curvature robs the central nervous system of valuable mechanoreception. Together, these two consequences spell trouble for the patient's body in many different ways.

Restoring the normal cervical lordosis is the primary goal for practitioners of several chiropractic techniques, including Chiropractic Biophysics. These chiropractors perform adjustments with the intent being to normalize the structure of the spine, and add specialized traction with extension and compression to help support the process. Overall, their main treatment approach is to mechanically treat the spine in order to benefit the nervous system.

Given the amount of research and science behind the importance of improving/restoring the cervical lordosis, the reader is urged to address this finding in his/her patients. The Chiropractic Biophysics approach and the Pettibon approach have excellent tools for doing so. At the same time, the reader is also urged to not limit his treatment to the mechanical system. Certainly, it is involved in most cases of forward head posture and cervical hypolordosis. Adaptive shortening has surely occurred to some extent. But what about the nervous system's influence including the startle response and upper crossed syndrome? We have seen how stress activates the sternocleidomastoid and upper trapezius, thereby pulling the head down and forward. One just has to look at an anxious person to see a textbook example of poor posture including FHP and cervical hypolordosis. So, given this, we must also do what we can to affect the person's emotions, movement patterns, occupational habits, and any other aspect driving the forward head posture in the first place.

With all of the attention paid to sagittal plane posture, clinicians often forget to look at transverse and coronal plane alignment. Deviations due to vertebral malalignment or scoliosis will create cervical spine asymmetry and add a great deal of stress to this region. Look for the cause of any asymmetry all the way down to the feet, as compensations from leg length deformity may be seen up at the occiput.

MOVEMENT PATTERNS

Assessment of movement pattern disorders in the middle and lower cervical spine begins as it did in the upper cervical spine—looking for excessive suboccipital contraction. Following this, the clinician should observe the way the patient's neck moves. Does it move smoothly, with isolated, segmental motion? Or, does it move in an en-bloc fashion, with multiple segments moving all at once?

Moving outside the neck, observe the influence of the upper crossed syndrome on the individual. As discussed previously, this pattern alters the posture, structure, and biomechanics of the middle and lower cervical spine and must be addressed in treatment. Next, assess the movement capacity of the rest of the spine. If the thoracic and lumbar spines are hypomobile, the cervical spine will be forced to compensate. Consequently, treatment should involve therapies to improve thoracic and lumbar motion. Additionally, the patient should be instructed to emphasize thoracic and lumbar motion as much as possible in order to reduce cervical strain.

ENERGY-BASED TECHNIQUES

Auricular Acupressure. Perform as described in Upper Cervical section.

Reflexology. Perform as described in Upper Cervical section.

HIGH-YIELD SCAN

Perform a scan of the other high-yield elements of the body including:

- Gait
- Posture
- Sit-to-Stand
- Miniature Squat
- Respiration
- Romberg Test
- Fukuda's Test
- Upper Cervical Spine
- TMJ

- Pelvis
- Feet
- Stress Screen

EVALUATION AND TREATMENT OF THE SECONDARY FACTORS

Look into all secondary factors with a focus on sleeping and postural habits (Same as for upper cervical spine).

12 The Temporomandibular Joint

ANYONE WONDERING WHETHER OR NOT THE TEMPOROMANDIBULAR JOINT PLAYS AN IMPORTANT role in the body's overall functioning needs only read Dr. A.C. Fonder's writings on the Dental Distress Disorder. In this dissertation, Dr. Fonder outlines copious amounts of research linking dental malocclusion with systemic problems. He also outlines the neurological connections explaining why malocclusion is so harmful to the CNS. Briefly stated, this is because the TMJ is rich in joint receptors, and the numerous muscles attaching to it are equally rich in muscle spindle cells. Therefore, with any disruption, a huge nociceptive barrage is inflicted on the CNS. This activates Selye's General Adaptation Syndrome, as Fonder points out. Thus, by activating the stress response, one can clearly see how malocclusion and TMJ malalignment lead to countless acute and chronic conditions.

Research on the musculoskeletal effects of malocclusion substantiates Fonder's proposal that malalignment in this area has an effect on the entire body. Two studies demonstrating this connection are as follows:

1. Bergamini et al. found that correcting malocclusion reduced mean voltage in the sternocleidomastoid, soleus, and lumbar erector spinae.[171]
2. Sforza et al. found that using occlusal plates not only normalized SCM activity but also reduced body sway with the eyes open and the eyes closed.[172]

Not only do these studies prove there is a strong link between dental alignment and the rest of the body, but they also show how optimizing alignment within this complex can benefit the musculoskeletal system as a whole. Namely, reducing tone in postural muscles such as the SCM, lumbar erector spinae, and the soleus is often of clinical value. So is improving our patients' balance and motor control. For these reasons, the reader is urged to assess the TMJ in all patients, even if there is not a clear connection between the person's presenting complaint and this joint. Author's Note: Assessing occlusion is a job for the dentist. However, misalignment or dysfunction of the TMJ directly affects occlusion and *can* be assessed by the manual therapist.

Several basic examination and treatment techniques are presented in this chapter, but note that these are merely an introduction to TMJ care. Specialists in temporomandibular dysfunction look at many more factors influencing this region and are therefore qualified to implement more intensive treatment than what is presented. With this being said, the goals of this chapter are to give the reader several tools so that he/she can help optimize TMJ function—without harming the patient whatsoever. Therefore, the main crux of assessment/treatment here is on soft tissue work, gentle mobilization, and postural correction to help normalize TMJ mechanics. Again, the emphasis here is on simplicity. The reader is encouraged to follow-up with other resources for information on pathology and advanced examination and treatment techniques.

EXAMINATION AND TREATMENT OF THE PRIMARY FACTORS

Lateral Pterygoid. Palpate the muscle for hypertonicity, fascial adhesions, tenderness, and trigger points. Utilize soft tissue techniques including myofascial release, sustained pressure, strumming and ischemic compression to address the findings (Fig. 12-1). Strain/counterstrain is useful in reducing tone (Fig. 12-2).

The lateral pterygoid plays a very important role in the creation and/or perpetuation of temporomandibular dysfunction. Facilitation of this muscle not only alters joint mechanics but it also leads to trigger point formation. Trigger points within this muscle refer pain to the temporomandibular joint and maxilla. Upledger stresses the influence of the lateral pterygoid on the craniosacral system. He points out that this is due to its broad attachment to the sphenoid.

Medial Pterygoid. Palpate the muscle for hypertonicity, fascial adhesions, tenderness, and trigger points. Utilize soft tissue techniques including myofascial release, sustained pressure, strumming and ischemic compression to address the findings (Fig. 12-3).

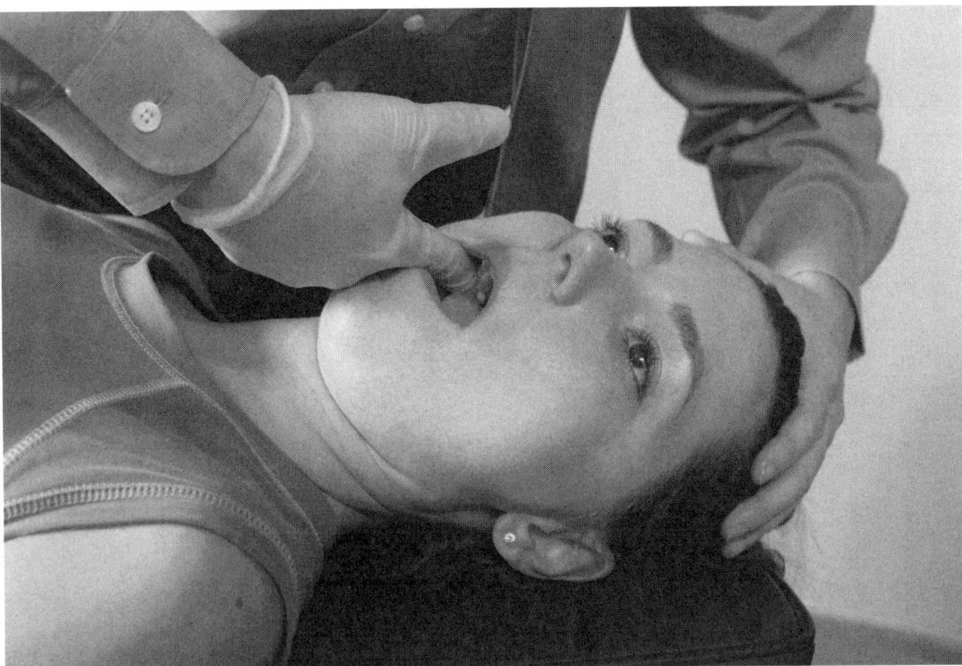

Fig. 12-1 The clinician can apply MFR, sustained pressure, strumming and ischemic compression in this position.

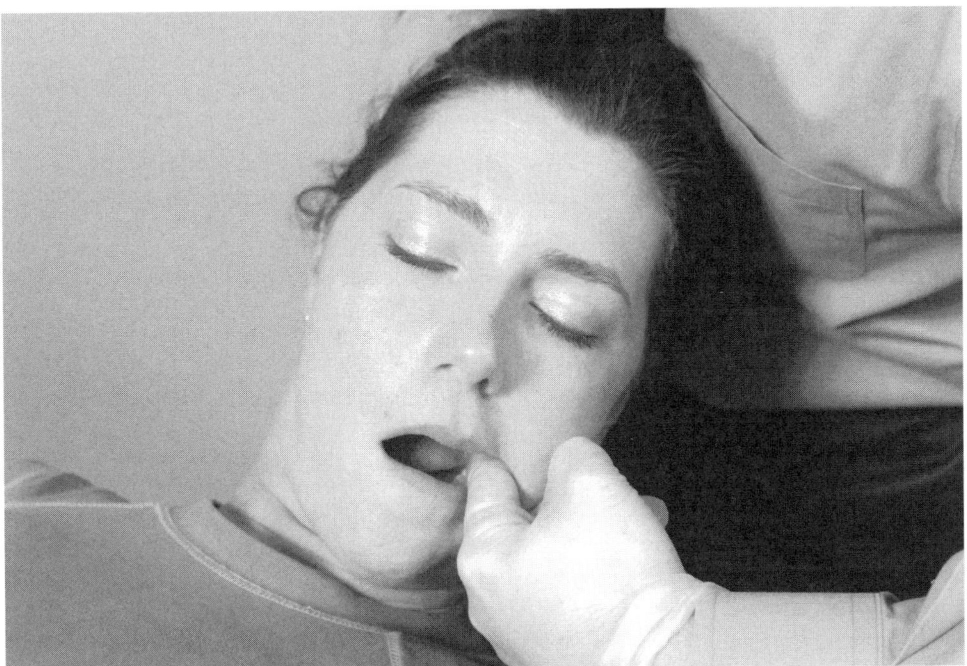

Fig. 12-2 Strain-counterstrain of the pterygoids. Walther suggests cervical flexion, ipsilateral side bending and rotation while monitoring the pterygoid pocket for changes in tone. This method is useful for both the lateral and medial pterygoids.[14]

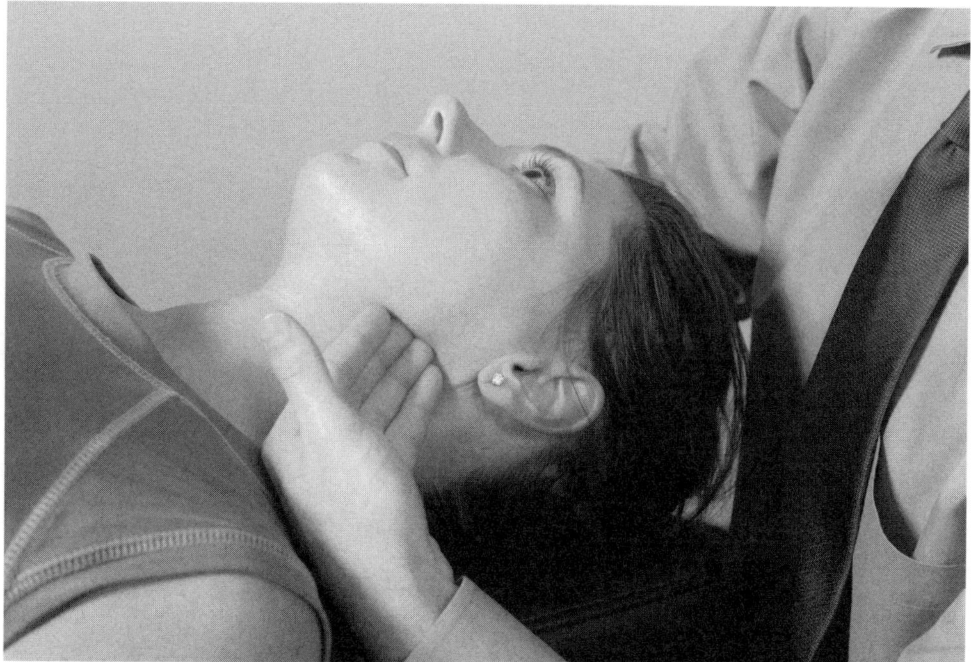

Fig. 12-3 The clinician can apply MFR, sustained pressure, strumming and ischemic compression in this position.

The medial pterygoid is facilitated as part of the common pattern. This alters joint mechanics and leads to trigger point formation. Trigger points within this muscle refer pain to the TMJ itself, the ear, and towards the back of the mouth. Travell and Simons note that trigger points in this muscle may also cause the symptom of stuffiness in the ear.[31]

Upledger stresses the importance of the medial pterygoid's insertion onto the sphenoid, the palatine bone and the tuberosity of the maxilla. This means its influence can be difficult to predict, given that it has the potential to affect the "keystone" of the craniosacral system.[70]

Masseter. Palpate the muscle for hypertonicity, fascial adhesions, tenderness, and trigger points. Utilize soft tissue techniques including myofascial release, sustained pressure, strumming and ischemic compression to address the findings (Fig. 12-4).

The masseter is facilitated as part of the common pattern. This lends itself to trigger point formation. Look for trigger points in this muscle to refer pain to the maxilla, eyebrow, ear, molars, and the TMJ.[31]

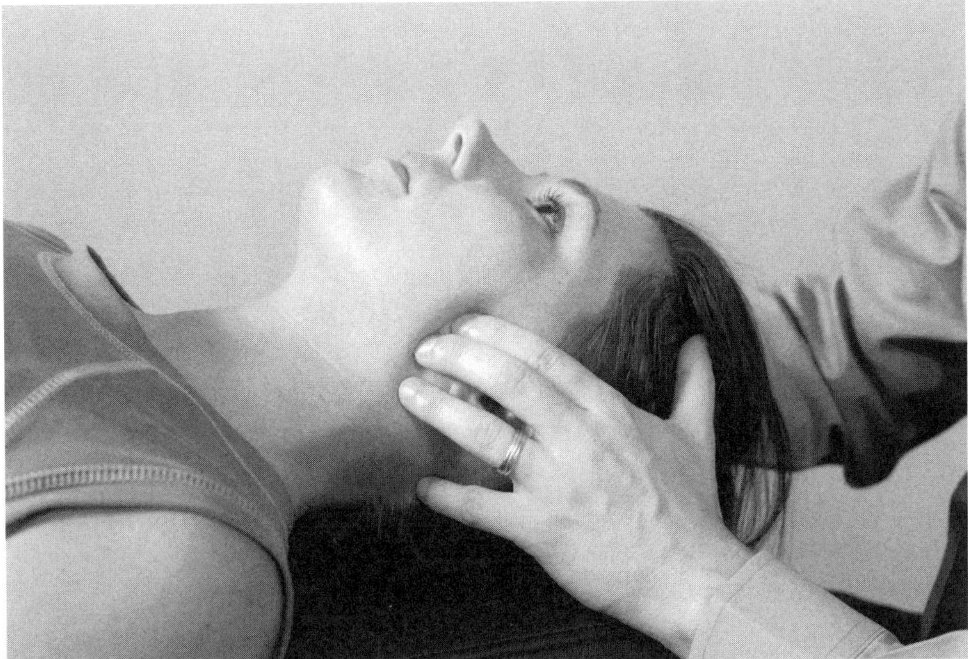

Fig. 12-4 The clinician can apply MFR, sustained pressure, strumming and ischemic compression in this position.

Temporalis. Palpate the muscle for hypertonicity, fascial adhesions, tenderness, and trigger points. Utilize soft tissue techniques including myofascial release, sustained pressure, strumming and ischemic compression to address the findings (Fig. 12-5).

The temporalis is facilitated as part of the common pattern. This added tension pulls the mandible superiorly and posteriorly, thereby changing mechanics at the TMJ. It is also prone to trigger point formation, which will refer pain to the TMJ as well as the maxillary teeth and even above the eyebrow.[31]

Upledger stresses the importance of this muscle due to its attachments on the sphenoid, parietal, and frontal bones in addition to the insertion on the mandible. These multiple attachment points give the temporalis the potential to influence a great part of the craniosacral system.

Additional Muscles. There are many other muscles in the head and neck region, including the digastrics, the suprahyoids, the infrahyoids, the platysma,

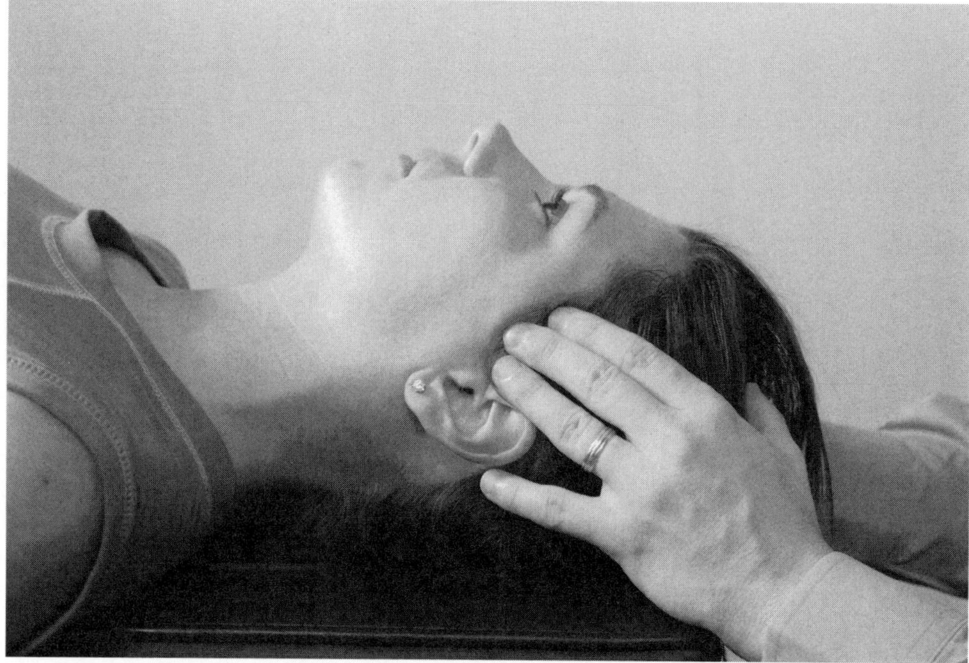

Fig. 12-5 The clinician can apply MFR, sustained pressure, strumming and ischemic compression in this position.

and the omohyoid. Many of these muscles are important given their influence on the stomatognathic and craniosacral systems. See Walther[173] and Upledger for further details.

MUSCLE STRENGTH

Begin by testing jaw strength in all planes. Be sure to assess both the ability to initiate a contraction as well as sheer strength. Most often, what we perceive as weakness is more a matter of inhibition. This will follow the common pattern and/or be due to local dysfunction. Treating the causative factor restores normal strength in these cases. In cases of true muscle weakness, remedial strengthening is indicated. This can be accomplished by giving light resistance to motion in the affected plane. Another option is to incorporate rhythmic stabilization exercises. Not only do these exercises promote muscle strengthening, but they also enhance coordination and the patient's ability to recruit muscles in isolation. Please see Figure 12-6 for further details.

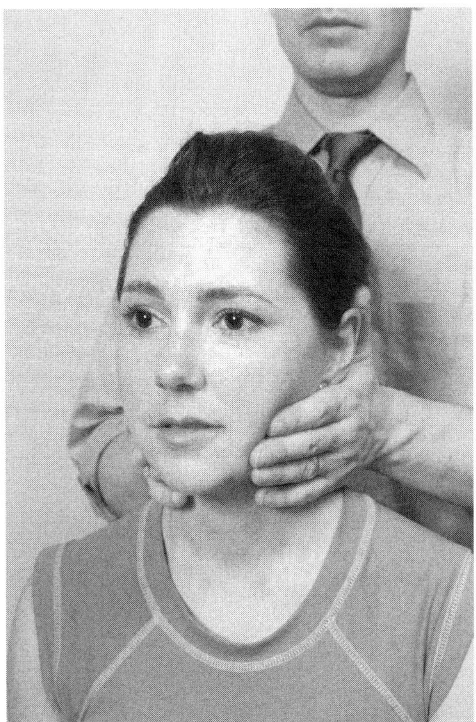

Fig. 12-6 Rhythmic stabilization exercises. Have the patient hold the jaw in neutral while pressure is applied to the mandible from all directions. It is helpful to have the patient look in the mirror to assure proper alignment is maintained throughout this exercise.

JOINT MOBILITY

Mobility testing of the temporomandibular joint begins by examining the gross movements of the jaw. To do this, have the patient depress, laterally deviate, and protrude the mandible. Ideally, there should be approximately 40–50 mm of depression, 8 mm of lateral deviation, and 8 mm of protrusion—each performed with symmetry, smoothness of movement, and without crepitus, clicking, or popping in the joint. Restricted motion in any of these planes suggests hypomobility. The cause for this may be muscular shortening/facilitation, capsular thickening, or joint derangement. Muscular shortening or hypertonicity should be treated with the techniques described in the previous section. This will improve jaw motion, optimize biomechanics, and lead to a reduction in symptomatology.

Capsular thickening, when present, will display a very distinctive pattern. With unilateral involvement expect to see decreased jaw depression with ipsilateral deviation, decreased lateral excursion to the opposite side, and decreased protrusion along with ipsilateral deviation. With bilateral involvement expect to see limited motion in all planes, but without any deflection or deviation. Confirm these restrictions by testing joint play. Perform long-axis distraction, lateral glide, and anterior glide techniques (Fig. 12-7 to 12-9). Expect capsular shortening to create limited joint play motion, and for there to be a firm end-feel associated with these limitations.

Makofsky states that a non-reducing disc derangement must be differentiated from capsular shortening as a cause of hypomobility.[174] This is because this form of joint derangement prevents normal jaw motion—causing pain and muscle splinting. The manual therapist will find that the non-reducing disc displacement creates a more firm end-feel than capsular shortening. With capsular shortening there is an appreciable creep to the tissues, whereas disc derangement is less yielding to pressure. In addition to this, Makofsky remarks that assessing the joint's response to distraction manipulation is especially helpful. For the deranged joint there will be a substantial increase in range of motion after

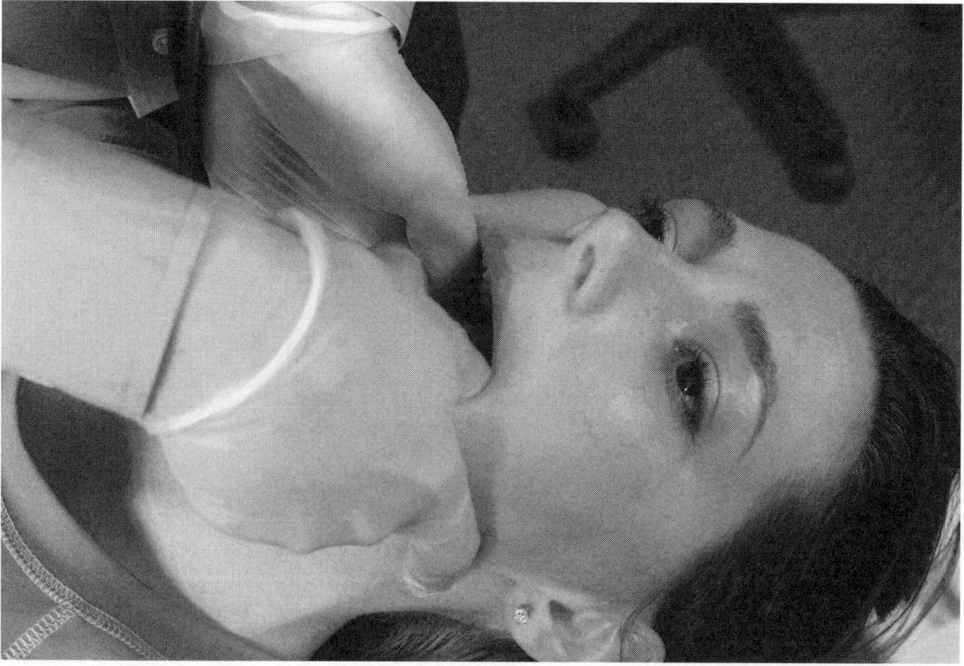

Fig. 12-7 Long-axis distraction of the temporomandibular joint.

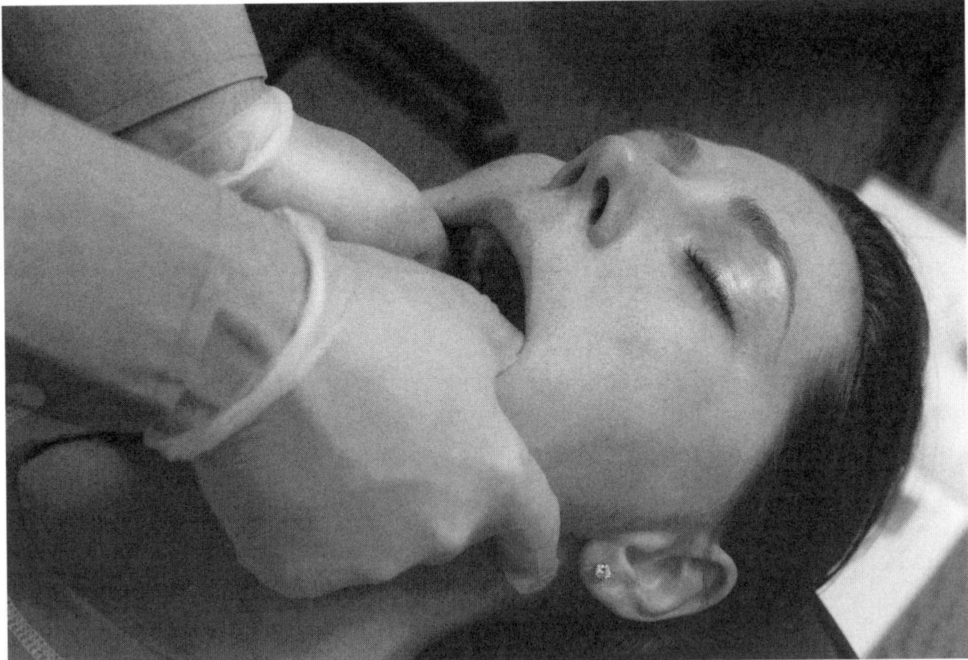

Fig. 12-8 Lateral glide of the temporomandibular joint.

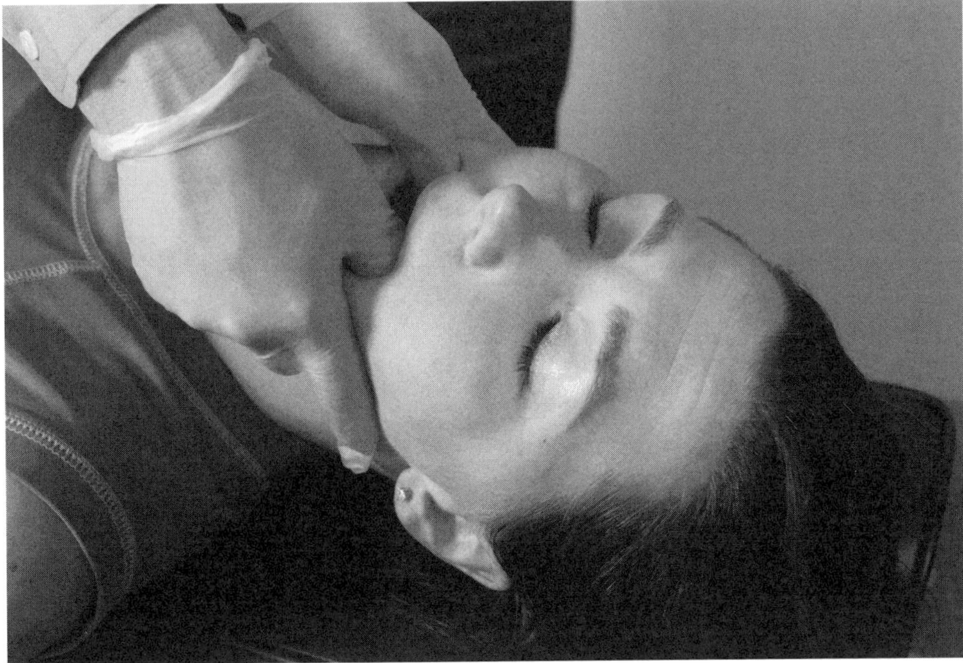

Fig. 12-9 Anterior glide of the temporomandibular joint.

manipulation. Conversely, there will only be minor improvement with manipulation in a patient with capsular shortening.

With this being said, it is advised that only clinicians with advanced training attempt any manipulative technique on this joint. This is for two reasons. First, the TMJ is a relatively delicate joint. Any aggressive technique improperly performed may cause irreparable damage. Second, the TMJ is most often found to be hypermobile—not hypomobile. Thrusting the joint just to reduce muscle spasm will make it even more hypermobile. For these reasons, the clinician is urged to treat true hypomobility with joint mobilization techniques. To do this, simply apply the joint play assessment techniques in a repetitive fashion. The intensity and duration of these mobilizations should be altered as per the patient's condition and their response to care.

POSTURE

Begin by closely examining the position of the jaw relative to the maxilla. Look for lateral deviation, tilting, protrusion, and retrusion of the mandible. Also look at the distance between the top and bottom incisors. Oftentimes, muscle imbalance and joint hypomobility create an improper resting position of the mandible. Therefore, attempt to correlate any observable malalignment with the patient's other findings (i.e. muscular hypertonicity, capsular shortening). A relationship between the two indicates the need for corrective treatment.

Following this local examination, assess the patient's posture as a whole. Deviation from neutral *will* affect the TMJ. Most notable of these is the harmful effects of forward head posture. Among other things, the forward head, extended occiput malposition creates posterior-superior displacement of the mandible, an altered length-tension ratio in the masticatory muscles, and an improper resting position of the tongue. Together, these sequelae stress the temporomandibular joint surfaces, promote muscle imbalance and trigger point formation, and lead to malocclusion.

Given these relationships it is no surprise that therapy to correct forward head posture is beneficial for all types of temporomandibular dysfunction. Again, it is just one more instance where the common pattern creates localized dysfunction, and treating the pattern leads to resolution of the local problem. In fact, many of the exercises TMJ specialists prescribe—whether they are to address local *or* global dysfunction—overlap with the principles already presented in this text. With this in mind, the reader is reminded to incorporate the global concepts of common pattern correction even when treating a seemingly localized problem like temporomandibular dysfunction.

MOVEMENT PATTERNS

The *way* the person moves his jaw often contributes to temporomandibular dysfunction and should be assessed thoroughly. To do this, closely inspect the tracking of the mandible during elevation and depression. Does it move to one side or the other, or go too far forward or backward? Deviation in any plane is important and should be corrected. This begins with addressing mechanical causes of asymmetrical movement as discussed in the previous sections—muscle imbalance and joint hypomobility. After these things are addressed (if present), the work of re-programming motor patterns begins. Start by informing the patient of their asymmetry. She simply may not realize the jaw deviates more to one side or the other when she opens and closes it. She may not even realize she tends to chew on one side more than the other. Teach her to be cognizant of such asymmetries and to practice opening and closing the jaw in the mirror while keeping the top and bottom incisors lined up. This helps retrain motor patterns and ensures joint receptors and spindle cells on each side are given the same amount of stimulation. In patients with hypermobility and/or disc dislocation it may be helpful to have the person practice this exercise with the tongue touching the roof of the mouth. This helps ensure proper joint mechanics and does not allow excessive movement (translation) which may cause disc subluxation.

On a larger scale look for aberrant movement of the body occurring with mandibular motion. Most commonly, one will see patients extend the head to open the mouth instead of simply dropping the jaw. This leads to neck problems in addition to altering TMJ mechanics. This pattern is consistent with what is expected with the common pattern: the body leads a motion by extending the head. Teach the patient to override this pattern and isolate motion to the TMJ only.

Globally we can expect common movement pattern dysfunction to affect the TMJ as well. Therefore, look for things associated with the common pattern/upper crossed syndrome and correct them with methods already discussed. Optimizing control of weak, inhibited phasic muscles will surely benefit the jaw. After all, the jaw elevators are facilitated as part of the common pattern. By reducing input that perpetuates this, one can expect improved joint mechanics and diminished myofascial pain.

Author's note: Temporomandibular specialists utilize many, many more techniques than those presented here. They analyze and treat virtually every muscle of the face and stomatognathic system while also addressing almost every conceivable activity involving the jaw. The reader is encouraged to look into the works of Walther, Makofsky, and Rocabodo for more information on temporomandibular care.

ENERGY-BASED TECHNIQUES

Auricular Acupressure. Gently squeeze the point corresponding to the TMJ with two fingers. Hold for 5 seconds, then relax 5 seconds. Increase the amount of pressure with each cycle for a total time of one minute (6 cycles). Do this initially on the ear on the involved side only; treat the opposite ear as well if the patient does not improve.

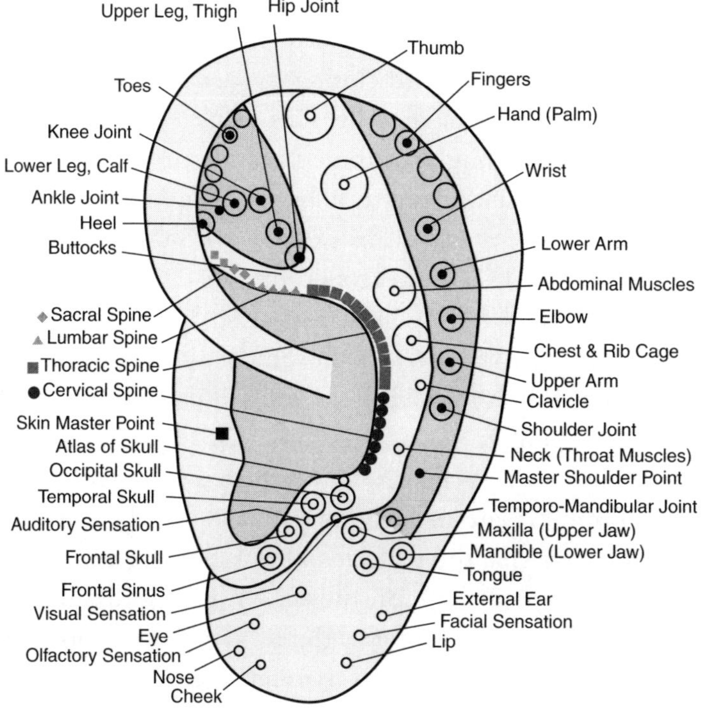

Fig. 12-10

Reflexology. Begin by massaging the entire foot. Walk up the foot with the thumbs along the five zones. Treat both the plantar and dorsal surfaces. Work the toes as well. Spend extra time on the medial border of the foot corresponding

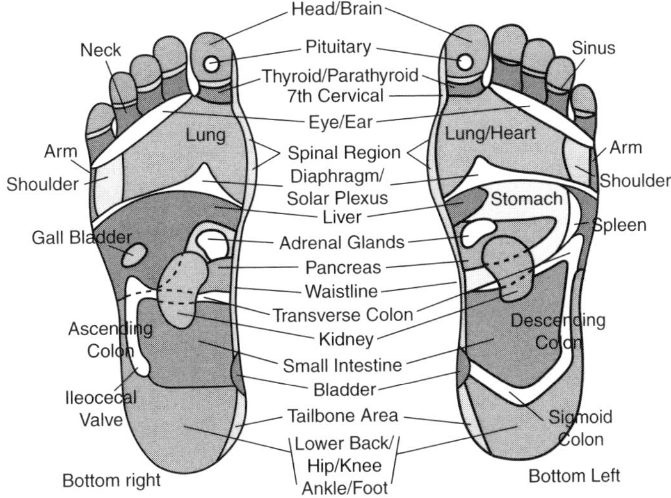

Fig. 12-11

with the spine. Also, work on areas associated with different organs needing an extra "boost." Following this long warm-up, massage the area on the foot corresponding to the temporomandibular joint.

HIGH-YIELD SCAN

Perform a scan of the other high-yield elements of the body including:

- Gait
- Posture
- Sit-to-Stand
- Miniature Squat
- Respiration
- Fukuda's Test
- Turning Test
- Upper Cervical Spine
- Middle and Lower Cervical Spine
- Pelvis
- Feet
- Stress Screen

EXAMINATION AND TREATMENT OF THE SECONDARY FACTORS

Because jaw function is so closely related to cervical spine function, the clinician must address all secondary factors that can influence the TMJ or cervical spine. Listed below are several secondary factors especially detrimental to temporomandibular function. Secondary factors with an impact on the cervical spine were presented in Chapter 11.

Chewing. Many people chew in an asymmetric fashion and do not even realize it. This is potentially very harmful, as it places abnormal stress on the TMJ and surrounding soft tissues while providing the central nervous system with asymmetric afferent input. Take steps to correct this asymmetry with manual methods (if indicated). Perhaps even more important, educate the patient of their asymmetry and teach them to watch themselves chew in the mirror. This habit frequently takes some time to change, so encourage them to be diligent in monitoring their alignment and chewing pattern.

Bruxism. Bruxism is another harmful parafunctional activity. Not only does it stress the TMJ complex immensely, but it is also damaging to the teeth. Ask the patient if he knows whether or not he grinds his teeth. If he does, hopefully he has been given a device to reduce the grinding and protect the teeth at night. The Nociceptive Trigeminal Inhibition (NTI) splint is one such tool. It works on the theory that pressure applied to the lower incisors inhibits jaw elevation. Therefore, this device not only protects the teeth while the patient sleeps, but it also reduces the amount of muscular contraction.

If the patient is unsure whether or not he is a bruxer, be sure to look at his teeth. Flattened, beveled teeth indicate he is most likely a grinder. If this is the case, encourage him to see a dentist to fit him for an NTI splint or another equally effective product. It is readily apparent how grinding one's teeth each night impairs the ability to recover from any form of temporomandibular dysfunction.

Parafunctional Activities. People need to be questioned what type of parafunctional habits they engage in. Do they chew gum? Do they smoke? Do they chew tobacco? Do they bite their fingernails? Each of these activities places added stress on the TMJ complex and is not compatible with optimal TMJ function. Urge the patient to minimize (or eliminate) time spent each day engaging in any of these habits.

Other Activities. Teach the patient to be cognizant of any activity he engages in where he puts added pressure on the jaw. For instance, many people lie prone and prop the jaw up on their hands. Others rest their chin on the forearms while relaxing at an office or school desk. Some people even support their jaw while standing. Each of these activities stresses the joint and should be stopped.

13 The Thoracic Spine

EVALUATION AND TREATMENT OF THE PRIMARY FACTORS

Erector Spinae. Palpate these muscles for hypertonicity, fascial adhesions, tenderness, and trigger points. Utilize soft tissue techniques including myofascial release, sustained pressure, strumming and ischemic compression to address the findings. Post-isometric relaxation is useful in reducing tone and increasing flexibility (Fig. 13-1).

The erector spinae in the thoracic spine are prone to inhibition as part of the common pattern. Consequently, they are frequently strained and cause feelings of discomfort in the midback. Another important thing to remember about this muscle group is that the most lateral portion, the iliocostalis, inserts into the rib angles. This makes it a frequent contributor to the painful symptoms of scapulothoracic syndrome. Be sure to work this muscle throughout its entire course in cases of scapulothoracic dysfunction.

Diaphragm. Palpate the muscle for hypertonicity, fascial adhesions, tenderness, and trigger points. Utilize soft tissue techniques including myofascial release and sustained pressure to address the findings (Fig. 13-2).

The diaphragm is facilitated as part of the common pattern. This goes back to the startle reflex; when a person is scared he breathes in and holds. Over time this mechanism becomes engrained and leads to an obstructive breathing pattern along with overinflated lungs.

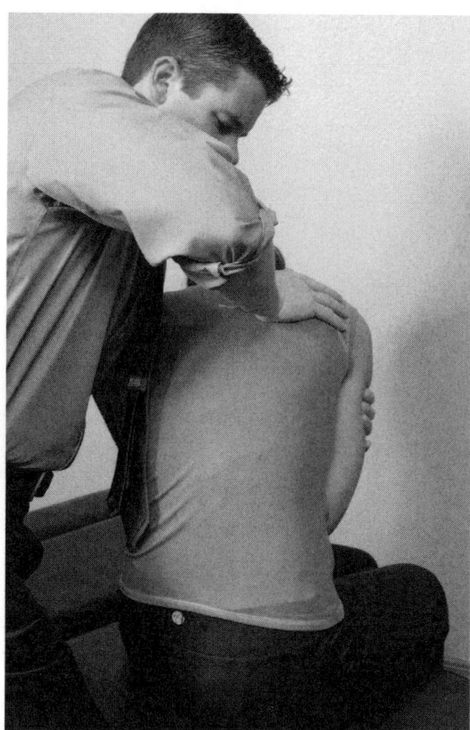

Fig. 13-1 Post-isometric relaxation of the erector spinae. Have the patient gently extend and rotate the spine into resistance. Upon relaxation, stretch her further into flexion and contralateral rotation.

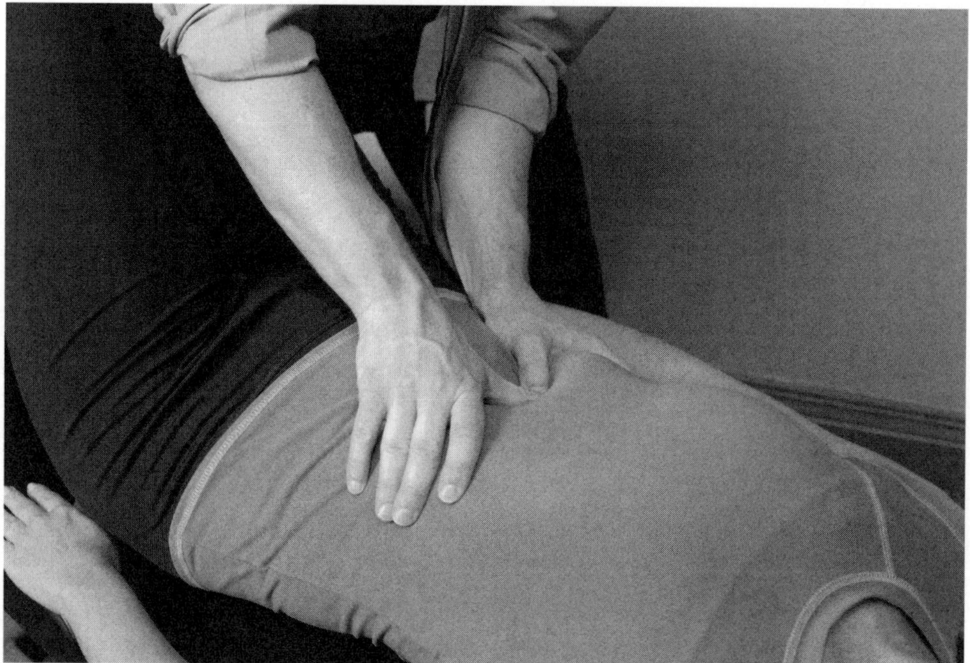

Fig. 13-2 Myofascial release of the diaphragm. The clinician can assess and treat the peripheral aspects of the diaphragm with the thumbs in this position. Treatment is augmented by having the patient take a breath in followed by a deep exhalation, upon which the clinician pulls the diaphragm and ribcage anteriorly. This is repeated for several breathing cycles.

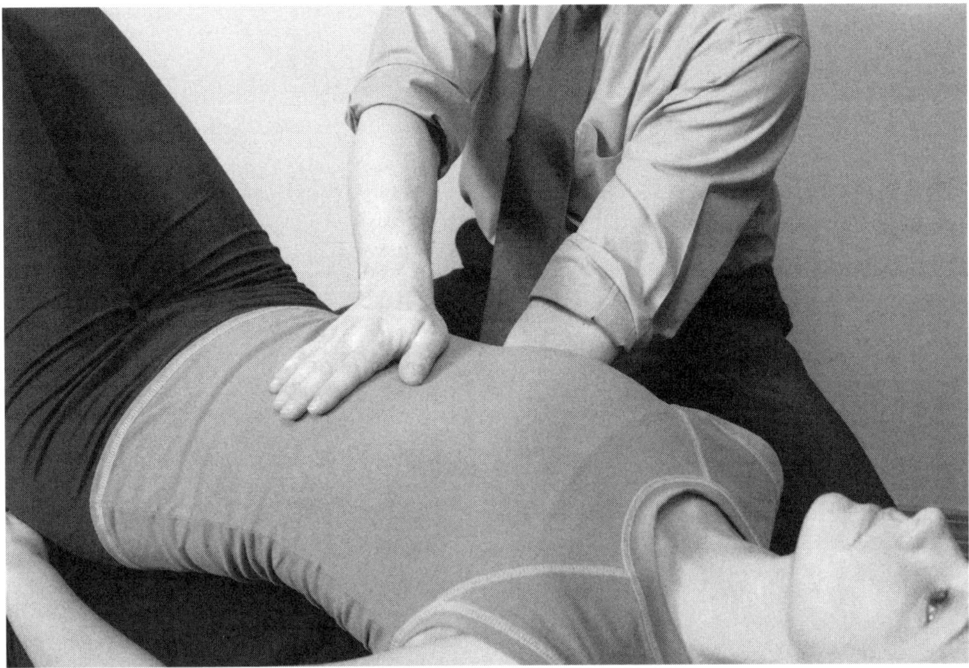

Fig. 13-3 Diaphragmatic release. The clinician contacts the patient's thoracolumbar junction with one hand and the zyphoid region with the other. Next, he *gently* applies a compressive force into the patient's body and waits for a release or subtle unwinding of the tissue. This is followed for several minutes or until motion stops.

This dysfunctional respiratory pattern affects motion of the ribs and thoracic spine, forcing numerous compensatory patterns. This creates gross hypomobility at the levels of the diaphragm's origin. It can also cause trigger point development. If the trigger points are peripherally located, they will refer to the region of the costal margin. If they are centrally located, they will refer to the ipsilateral shoulder near the angle of the neck.[31]

Besides the relationship described above, Hruska points another common problem involving the diaphragm.[59] *He finds that many people utilize their diaphragm as a postural muscle to aid in thoracolumbar stability. This compromises oxygenation, changes posture, and through fascial connections to the psoas and other regions influences will affect the entire body.*

Levator Costarum, Serratus Posterior Superior, Serratus Posterior Inferior. Palpate these muscles for hypertonicity, fascial adhesions, tenderness, and trigger points. Utilize soft tissue techniques including myofascial release, sustained pressure, strumming and ischemic compression to address the findings (Fig. 13-4).

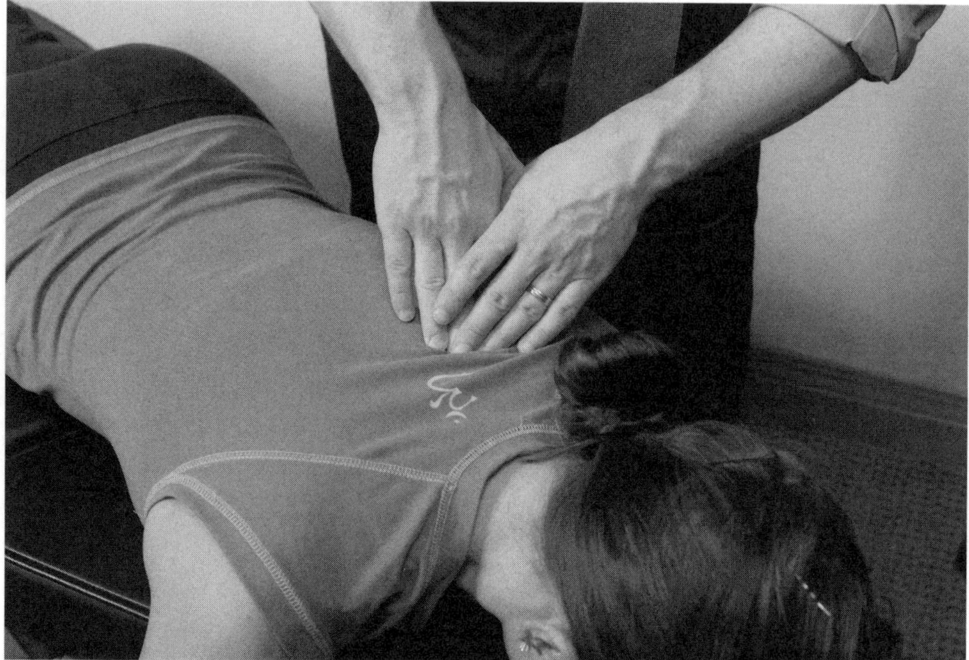

Fig. 13-4 The clinician can apply myofascial release, sustained pressure, strumming and ischemic compression to the levator costarum and serratus posterior superior in this position.

These muscles should be examined in cases of dysfunctional breathing patterns and local pain patterns. The levator costarum, in particular, should also be suspected in cases of chronic thoracic anteriorities.[14] *Trigger points in the serratus posterior superior refer pain to the upper and middle scapula and down the dorsal arm, medial forearm and into the fifth digit. Trigger points in the serratus posterior inferior refer pain locally.*

MUSCLE STRENGTH

Begin by assessing general core strength as described for the lumbar spine. Next, assess the strength of the muscles controlling the thoracic spine with traditional methods. Make sure to assess both the ability to initiate a contraction as well as sheer strength. Most often, what we perceive as weakness is more a matter of inhibition. This will follow the common pattern and/or be due to local or segmental dysfunction. Treating the causative factor restores normal strength in these cases. In cases of true muscle weakness, such as those involving muscle atrophy, remedial strengthening is indicated. This is done with traditional strengthening techniques.

Of the many strengthening exercises to choose from, it is suggested the reader implement the Brügger Relief Position.[75] Not only does this exercise

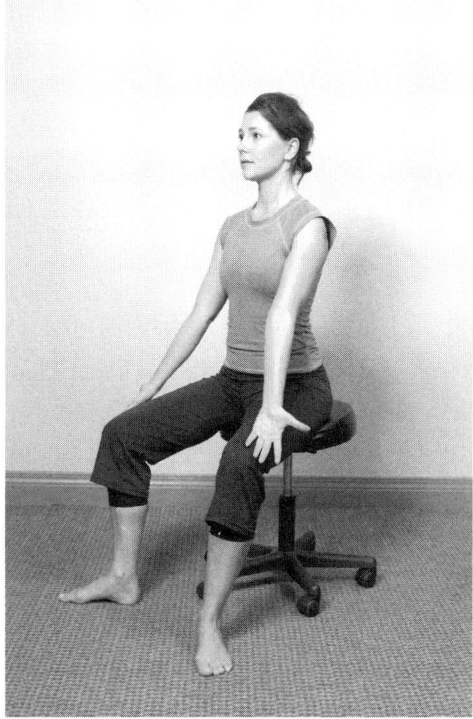

Fig. 13-5 The Brügger Relief Position. The patient sits on the edge of a stool or chair, keeping the hips abducted, feet externally rotated, the shoulders back, the head up, the forearms supinated, and the wrists and fingers extended. Have her perform a sternal lift while actively exhaling. Repeat two to three times and do this several times per day.

strengthen important postural muscles, but it helps inhibit painful, facilitated muscles as well. This makes it valuable in treating almost every area of the body—*not just the thoracic spine.* See Figure 13-5 for details.

SEGMENTAL MOBILITY

Assessment and treatment of segmental mobility plays an important role in the management of thoracic spine syndromes. This should be obvious to the reader, given the fact that professions including chiropractic are practically based on correcting segmental dysfunction. With this in mind, it should also be obvious to the reader that he/she must be skilled in one of the many segmental assessment and treatment approaches in order to effectively serve his or her patients.

It is out of the scope of this text to provide the reader with the necessary details and hands-on instruction necessary to master any of these techniques, so no attempt will be made to do so. This especially applies to those techniques requiring high levels of skill and practice, such as Gonstead technique or the motion palpation approach. Instead, the instruction provided in this section is focused on more simple techniques virtually any manual therapist can perform. These techniques are presented below.

Australian Approach. This approach is a simple, effective way of vertebral examination and treatment. In a nutshell, examination begins by finding the direction in which thoracic motion is painful and limited. Treatment is even more simple: mobilize or manipulate the spine into the opposite direction. This sounds too good to be true, but it works. It usually causes an immediate reduction in pain and an increase in range of motion (See Fig. 13-6).

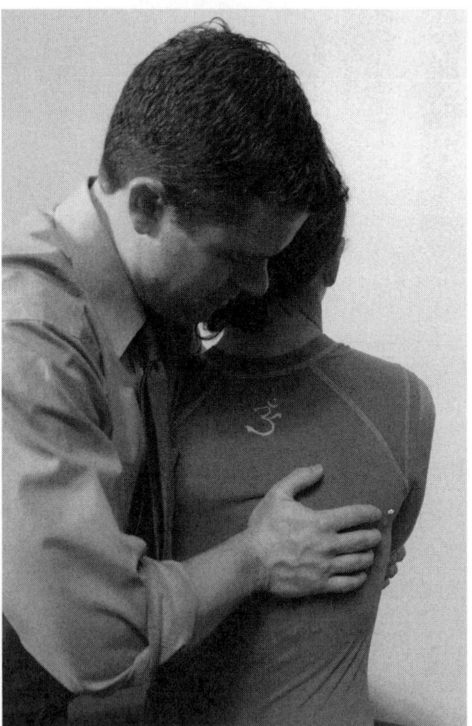

Fig. 13-6 Treatment for right rotation restriction. Rotate the patient into left rotation, taking care to first localize the affected segments with lateral flexion. Apply overpressure with the thenar to the transverse process of the dysfunctional segments.

In addition to this method, the facets are palpated for tenderness. Typically, one finds tenderness on the same side as the motion restriction. Once again, treatment is simple. Use the thumbs to mobilize the facets anteriorly (See Fig. 13-7). Re-examination shows increased pain-free motion.

Clinical reasoning plays a big role in this approach. Mobilizing or manipulating in the direction opposite the limitation (an indirect approach) is most effective when the patient is in the acute and subacute stage. It is actually just like a strain-counterstrain technique in that it places hypertonic muscles on a slack. This indirect approach is less effective when the patient's motion limitation is caused by true adaptive shortening, capsular tightness, or adhesion formation. In these cases, a direct approach is utilized. This can be with mobilization or manipulation as with the indirect approach. It can also include prolonged stretching into the limitation, or repetitive patient-induced movements into the restriction. Keep in mind that the direct approach is prone to causing pain. Normally, this is localized and resolves when the stretching ceases. Other times the pain may linger for a little while after therapy has stopped. At no time should the technique cause referred or radiating pain or any other neurological symptom.

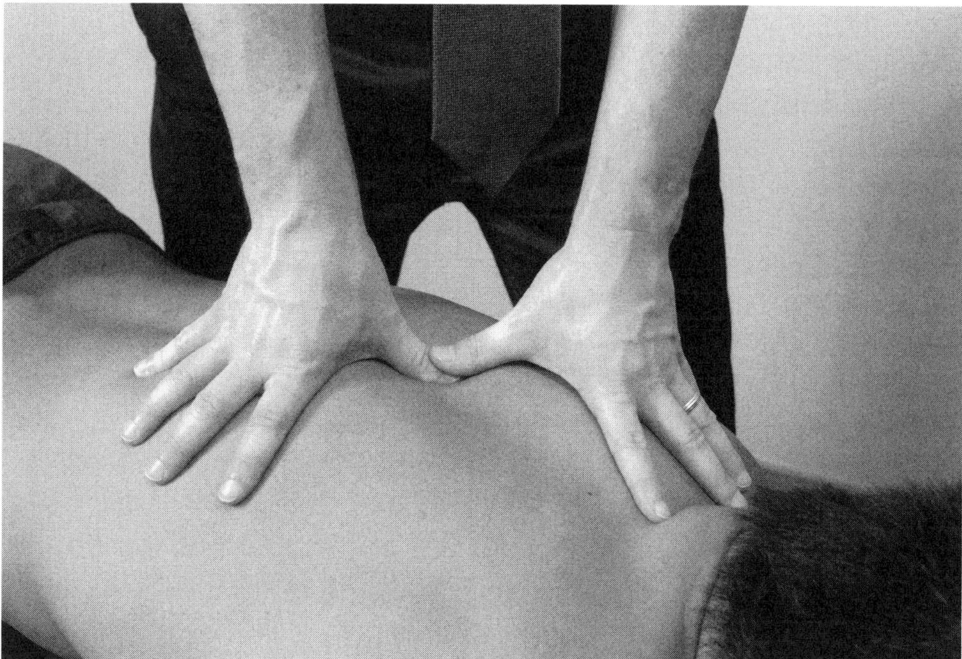

Fig. 13-7 Treatment for left facet dysfunction. Place the thumbs close together and contact the affected facet joint. Mobilize P-A for 30 seconds.

FIRST RIB DYSFUNCTION

First rib dysfunction is exceedingly common. It can be found with two easy methods. The first is to palpate both ribs just anterior to the upper trapezius. Next, have the patient fully inhale and then exhale. Typically what is seen is that one rib is stuck in elevation and does not descend with exhalation. The second examination technique is called the cervical rotation lateral flexion test. For this test, begin by palpating the first rib of the seated patient. Have him then extend his neck, rotate contralaterally, and sidebend to the side in question (in this sequence). Normally, the rib should descend when the patient sidebends the head. If the rib is stuck in elevation, however, the rib will remain elevated and will actually prevent full lateral flexion.

Treatment for an elevated first rib is accomplished with several methods. The most basic is with a general mobilization to drive the rib medially and inferiorly. A manipulative thrust can also be added if the practitioner has experience with this (Fig. 13-8). In addition to this, the clinician must treat the surrounding soft tissues (scalenes) and address the patient's breathing, as each of these factors typically cause the rib subluxation in the first place.

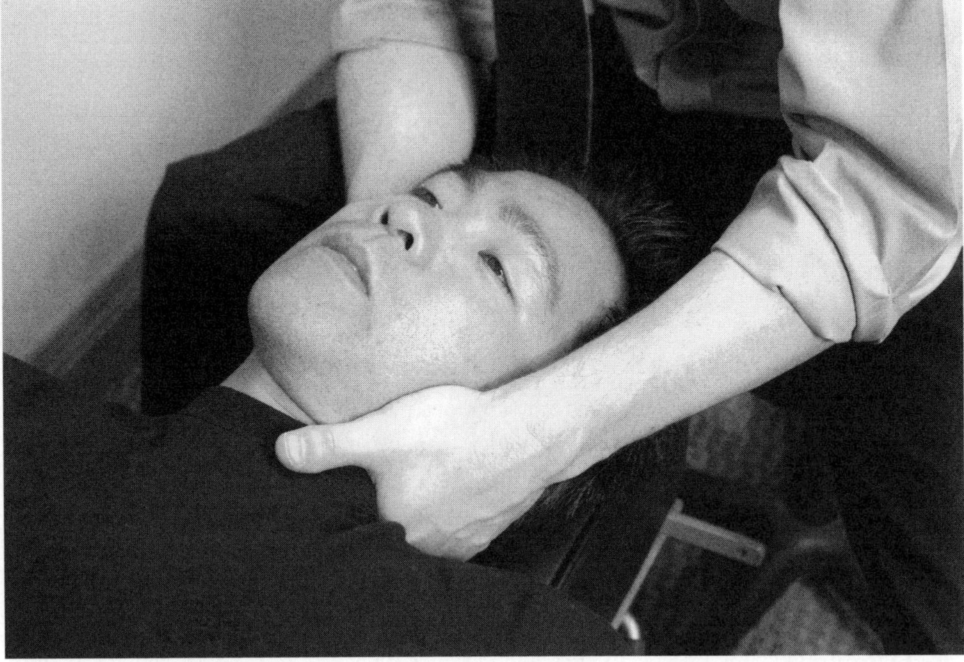

Fig. 13-8 Mobilization/manipulation of an elevated first rib.

RIBCAGE DYSFUNCTION

Subtle ribcage dysfunction is best found with a technique such as the motion palpation or osteopathic approach, as both of these methods are designed to detect small changes in function. Otherwise, when dysfunction here is enough to create symptoms, the practitioner can utilize Mulligan's mobilization with movement technique[142] or general rib mobilization. Simply put, this technique begins by locating the area of pain and the painful, limited plane of motion. Next, gently mobilize the rib in the posterior-to-anterior direction with contact made on the affected rib angle if tenderness is present here. Have the patient repeat the offending movement and re-assess. If pain and motion are not significantly improved, then try the sequence again at a different level. The clinician can even attempt mobilizing the rib from the front, into an anterior-to-posterior direction. Once again, proceed gently and re-assess for changes after each mobilization.

Another technique worth using to treat ribcage dysfunction is strain-counterstrain. Anteriorly, these tender points are found on the superior surface of the ribs just anterior to the midaxillary line. The position of ease for ribs 3-10 is a combination of trunk rotation and sidebending to the ipsilateral side

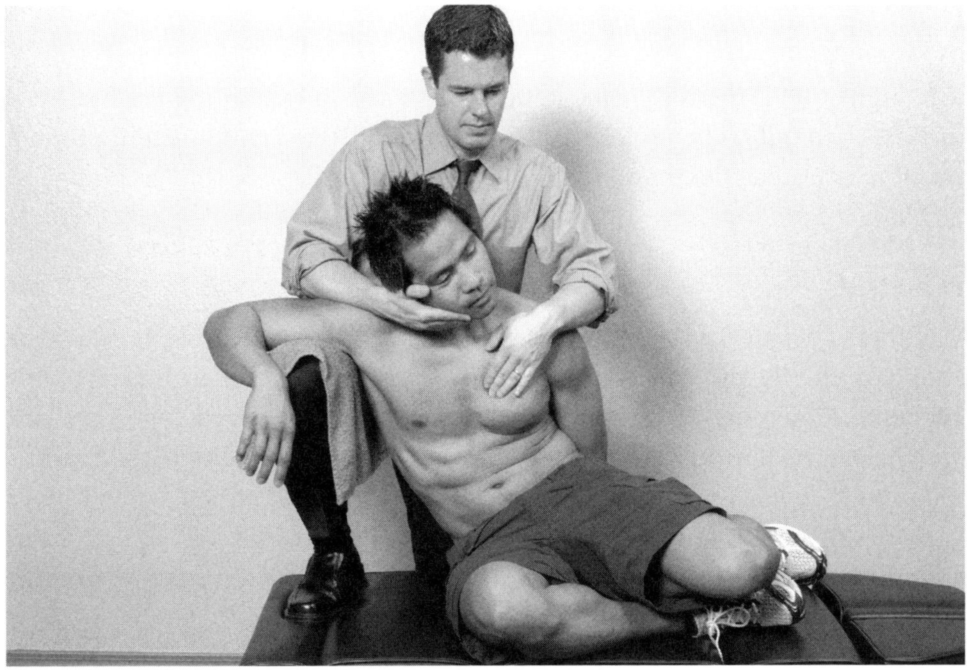

Fig. 13-9 Position of ease for an anterior ribcage tender point.

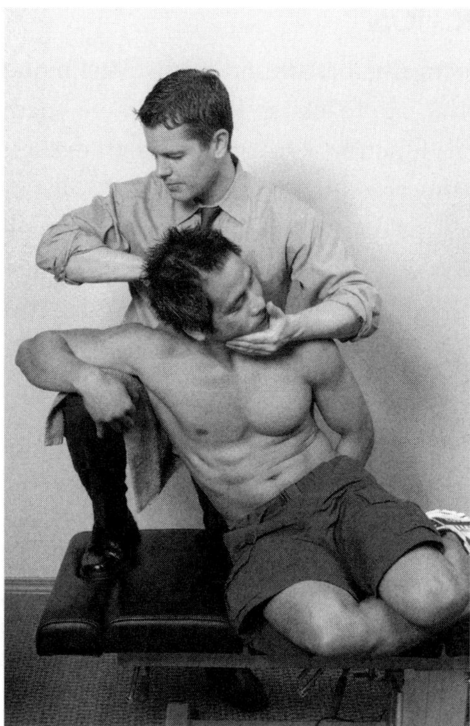

Fig. 13-10 Position of ease for a posterior ribcage tender point.

(See Fig. 13-9). Posteriorly, these tender points are found on the posterolateral surfaces of the ribs. The position of ease for ribs 2-10 is a combination of trunk rotation and lateral flexion to the opposite side (See Fig. 13-10).[164]

POSTURE

The overall posture of the spine will greatly affect the function of its individual segments. Ideally, the patient should demonstrate a smooth, natural kyphotic curvature. Common deviations from this, including excessive kyphosis as seen with Scheuermann's disease or flat-back syndrome due to multiple anteriorities *will* stress individual segments. Select vertebrae are placed at or near end-range in these situations, causing them to be a person's "problem spot." In such cases, lasting correction of segmental dysfunction is dependent on normalizing the curvature of the thoracic spine and ribcage.

In addition to its effects on the vertebrae, an abnormal thoracic curve will also affect the shoulder girdles, the cervical spine, and even the function of the respiratory mechanism (some even say cardiac function is impaired). For each of these reasons it is imperative to optimize the alignment of the thoracic spine.

To accomplish this, begin by restoring normal mobility of the thoracic spine and ribcage. Mobilizing/manipulating specific segments plays a role in this, as do stretching exercises aimed at increasing motion. Two popular stretches are presented in Figures 13-11 and 13-12.

Concurrent with these exercises to improve thoracic mobility, the practitioner must also implement corrective measures for the cervical and lumbar spines. This is important because oftentimes thoracic spine asymmetry is merely a compensation for cervical or lumbar spine dysfunction. For an example of this, just consider what happens to the thoracic spine when a patient has forward head posture, or when he is sitting with his lumbar spine in kyphosis. In these instances the thoracic spine must heavily compensate.

Manual therapy and exercises to help correct cervical and lumbar spine asymmetry are thus helpful to the thoracic spine. So are postural alterations—usually the same ones made for the cervical and lumbar spines. This should include addressing the person's sitting posture first and foremost and ensuring

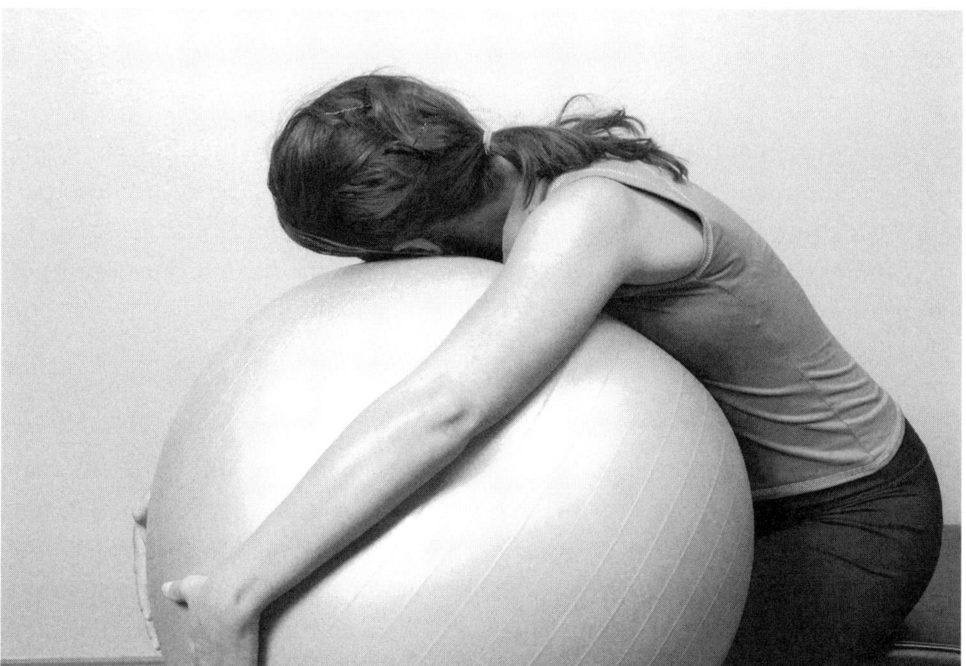

Fig. 13-11 The ball hugging exercise. The patient grabs an exercise ball and flexes forward while then rotating the trunk. This exercise addresses segments stuck in extension.

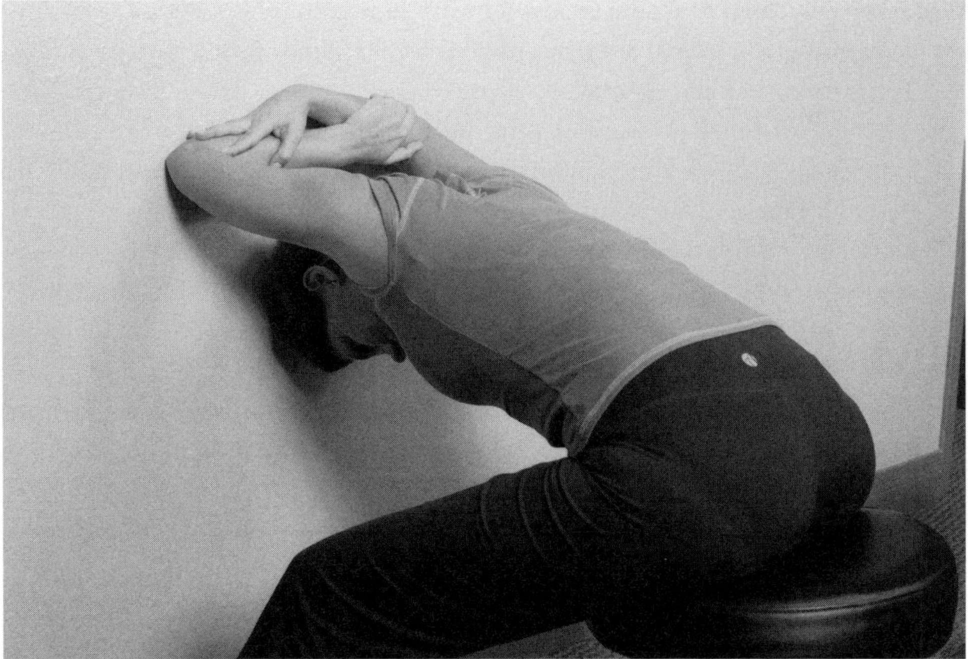

Fig. 13-12 Lewit's wall stretch.[75] Have the patient lean against a wall with their arms folded above the head. As the person breathes out, have them drop the sternum, feeling the extension in the middle and lower thoracic vertebrae. Reinforce the importance of a full exhalation and ask them to cough or forcefully expire if necessary to mobilize these joints.

he has adequate lumbar lordosis at all times. Along with this, the clinician should stress the importance of keeping the head back and avoiding forward head posture. Next, the patient should be urged to keep his shoulders rolled back and his arms and hands near his body when he is working. The further out in front his extremities are, the greater the pull on the thoracic spine.

MOVEMENT PATTERNS

Proper movement patterns are very important to the health of the thoracic spine. Most important of all is the act of breathing—a subject covered extensively in Chapter 6. For the thoracic spine, proper breathing provides constant mobilization as well as reciprocal contraction and relaxation of respiratory muscles. Dysfunctional breathing alters this ebb and flow and disrupts spinal and ribcage motion. It often leads to overuse of accessory muscles such as the sternocleidomastoids and scalenes. Sternocleidomastoid contraction helps pull the head further forward and compromises optimal thoracic alignment. Scalene contraction promotes trigger point formation, localized neck pain, and thoracic outlet syndrome.

On the other hand, relaxed, diaphragmatic breathing helps provide a firm foundation of support for the thoracic spine. It is also associated with decreased stress, which means less of a startle/flexor withdrawal pattern pulling the body forward. All of these things together help pull the head and shoulders back, further lessening stress on the thoracic spine.

In addition to addressing the patient's respiratory pattern, the clinician should also implement the movement pattern principles presented for the low back, neck, and shoulder. Doing this will address common problems such as en-bloc movement and flexor dominance. It will also provide stability for the rest of the spine.

ENERGETIC CONSIDERATIONS

Auricular Acupressure. Gently squeeze the point corresponding to the thoracic spine with two fingers. Hold for 5 seconds, then relax 5 seconds. Increase the amount of pressure with each cycle for a total time of one minute (6 cycles). Do this initially on the ear on the involved side only; treat the opposite ear as well if the patient does not improve.

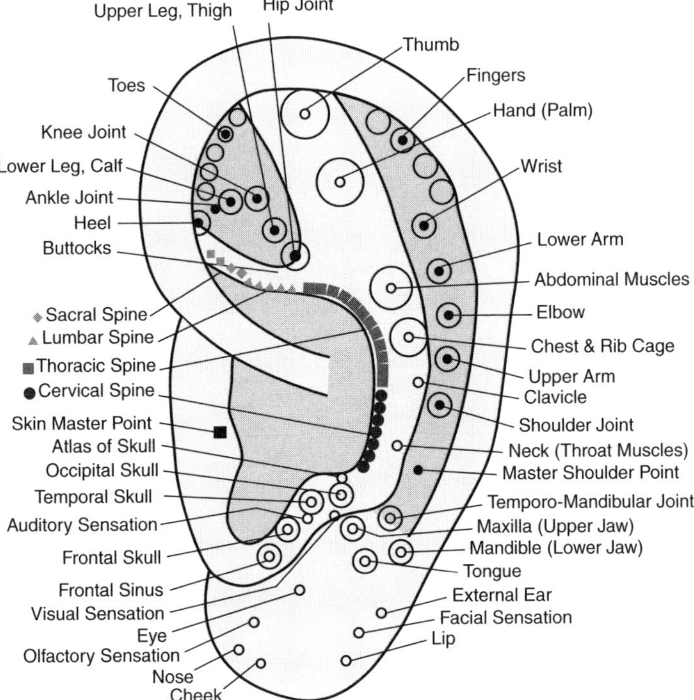

Fig. 13-13

Reflexology. Begin by massaging the entire foot. Walk up the foot with the thumbs along the five zones. Treat both the plantar and dorsal surfaces. Work the toes as well. Spend extra time on the medial border of the foot corresponding with the spine. Also, work on areas associated with different organs needing an extra "boost." Following this long warm-up, massage the area on the foot corresponding to the thoracic spine.

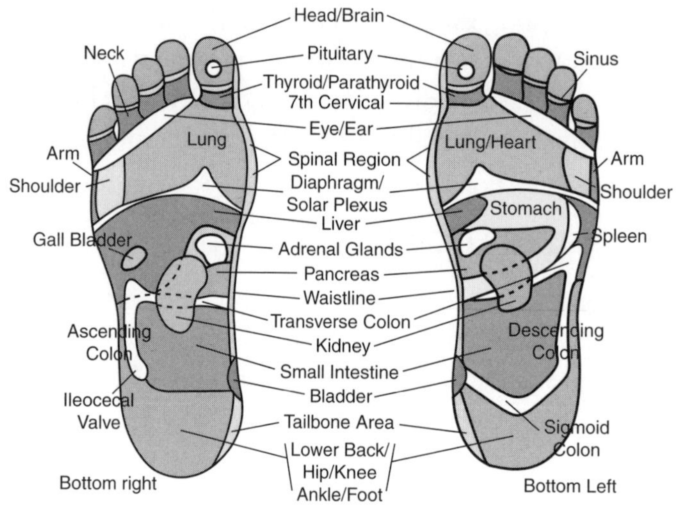

Fig. 13-14

HIGH-YIELD SCAN

Perform a scan of the high-yield elements of the body including:

- Gait
- Posture
- Sit-to-Stand
- Miniature Squat
- Respiration
- Romberg Test
- Fukuda's Test
- Upper Cervical Spine
- Middle and Lower Cervical Spine
- TMJ

- Pelvis
- Feet
- Stress Screen

ASSESSMENT AND TREATMENT OF THE SECONDARY FACTORS

For the most part, postures and activities which place stress on the cervical and lumbar spines will also stress the thoracic spine. Review the corresponding section in Chapters 11 and 14 for detailed information.

14 The Lumbar Spine

EVALUATION AND TREATMENT OF THE PRIMARY FACTORS

Iliopsoas. Palpate the muscle for hypertonicity, fascial adhesions, tenderness, and trigger points. Utilize soft tissue techniques including myofascial release, sustained pressure, strumming and ischemic compression to address the findings. Post-isometric relaxation and strain/counterstrain are also useful in reducing tone (See Fig.'s 16-1 through 16-4).

The iliopsoas has a tremendous influence on the lumbar spine. Due to its attachments it has the capability to alter the overall posture of the lumbar spine. Bilateral contraction causes increased lordosis while unilateral activation causes a lateral curvature. In addition to this mechanical influence, the muscle often refers pain to the low back region due to myofascial problems and/or trigger points.

Besides manual treatment, remember to look for factors which activate the psoas. Prolonged sitting is a frequent cause—it allows the muscle to shorten and lose flexibility. Emotional turmoil—especially fear—is also implicated as a cause of psoas spasm. Koch points out reflex mechanisms behind this relationship.[176] Remember, too, that the psoas is linked to the kidney in Eastern philosophy. Not surprisingly, this meridian is linked to fear.

Quadratus Lumborum. Palpate the muscle for hypertonicity, fascial adhesions, tenderness, and trigger points. Utilize soft tissue techniques including myofascial release, sustained pressure, strumming and ischemic compression to address the findings. Post-isometric relaxation and strain-counterstrain are useful at reducing tone (Fig. 14-1 and 14-2).

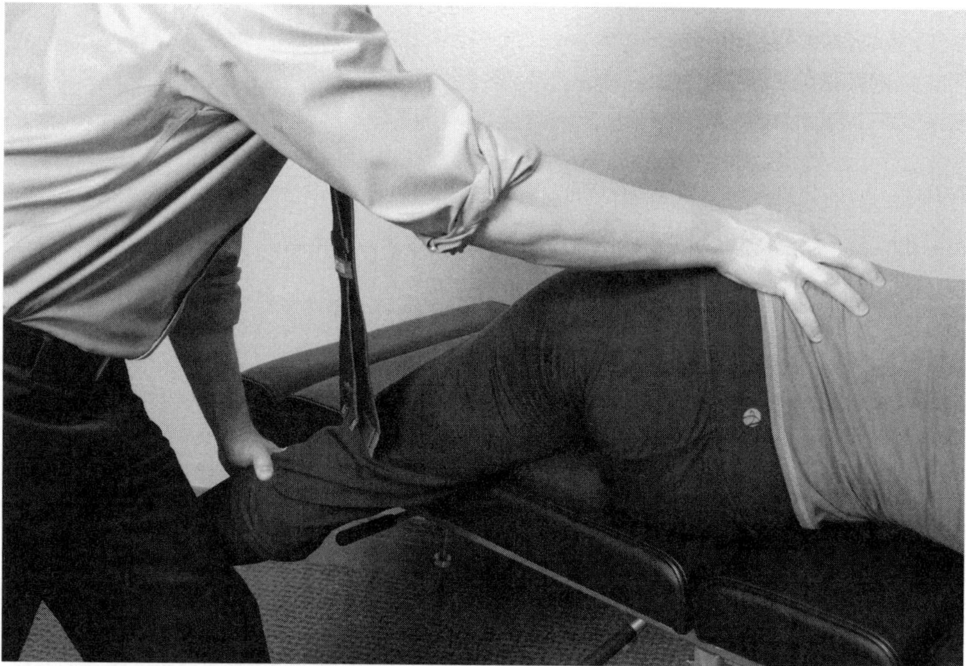

Fig. 14-1 Post-isometric relaxation stretching of the quadratus lumborum. Have the patient in sidelying with the involved side up and the bottom hip slightly flexed. Position the patient toward the back edge of the table so that with slight hip extension the lower extremity will be allowed to fall past the surface of the table. With the clinician's hand on the patient's iliac crest, have her gently contract the QL, pulling the ilium into resistance. Upon relaxation, stretch the ilium inferiorly and encourage the patient to let the entire leg fall towards the floor.

The quadratus lumborum is facilitated as part of the common pattern. This response leads to localized pain and the development of trigger points. Per Travell these may refer pain to the sacroiliac joint, the lower buttock, and sometimes along the crest of the ilium, the greater trochanter, groin, and into the lower quadrant of the abdomen.[68] As is the case with the iliopsoas, the quadratus lumborum is an important player in the development of low back pain and must be examined.

Multifidus (and the spinal intrinsics). Palpate these muscles for hypertonicity, fascial adhesions, tenderness, and trigger points. Utilize soft tissue techniques including myofascial release, sustained pressure, strumming and ischemic compression to address the findings. Strain/counterstrain is also useful in reducing tone (Fig. 14-3).

The most important muscles of the spine from a stabilization and intricate movement perspective are the intrinsics. As part of the common pattern these muscles

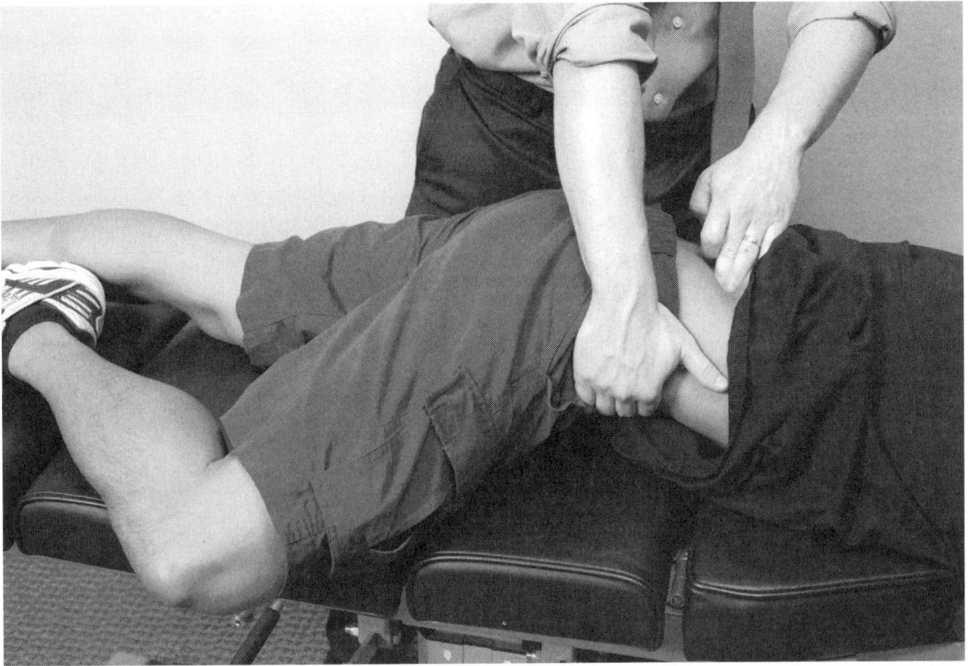

Fig. 14-2 Strain-counterstrain applied to the quadratus lumborum. Find a tender point on the lateral aspect of the transverse processes of L1-5. The position of maximum ease is found by raising the patient's ipsilateral pelvis up and towards the opposite side while the patient's ipsilateral hip is placed in 45 degrees flexion and abduction.

are inhibited, thereby compromising stability of the spine while also resulting in a loss of fine, segmental motion. Research indicates that adequate strength and timely recruitment of these "core muscles," along with the transversus abdominis is vital to successful spinal rehabilitation.

Upledger notes that hypertonus of the multifidi is likely to cause disruption in craniosacral function. Most harmful, he reports, is hypertonus of the bilateral multifidi at the lumbosacral junction. This results in "compression of the atlantooccipital joints and in membranous sphenobasilar joint compression."[70] One of his treatments for this condition is the lumbosacral decompression technique. This maneuver involves the clinician placing her superior hand under the supine patient's lumbar spine while the other hand is underneath the sacrum. Over the course of several minutes, the therapist slowly disengages the sacrum by pulling inferiorly with her inferior hand. Please see texts by Upledger, Manheim, and Barnes for further details on this popular technique.

Erector Spinae. Palpate the muscle for hypertonicity, fascial adhesions, tenderness, and trigger points. Utilize soft tissue techniques including myofascial

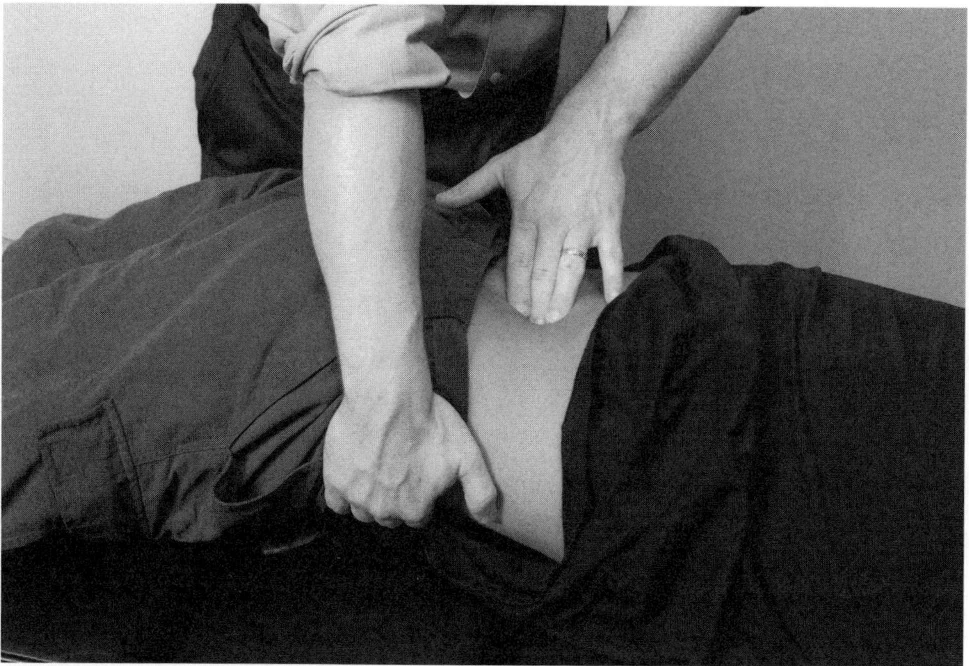

Fig. 14-3 Strain-counterstrain of the multifidus. Find a tender point on the posterior aspect of the L1-5 transverse processes. Raise the ipsilateral pelvis up so that the entire pelvis is rotated approximately 30–45 degrees off the table.

release, sustained pressure, strumming and ischemic compression to address the findings. Post-isometric relaxation is useful in reducing tone and improving flexibility.

The large erector spinae muscle group becomes facilitated as part of the common pattern. This adds to the action of the psoas, resulting in excessive lordosis of the lumbar spine. Deep tissue work affects all muscle layers and is necessary to improve tissue tone and elasticity down to the segmental level. Connections to the sacrum must be evaluated as well, as this is frequently an area full of soft-tissue dysfunction.

MUSCLE STRENGTH

The current trend in rehabilitation is core strengthening. This involves specific exercises to both strengthen and enhance recruitment of the transversus abdominis, the levator ani, and the multifidi/spinal intrinsics. There are several ways to do this. Pulling the navel posteriorly in prone or supine is the easiest way to start this exercise. From here, the patient can practice activating these muscles while sitting, standing, walking, and in quadruped. In fact, he should practice contracting these muscles while performing all movements as a means to protect his spine and also so that the body gets accustomed to activating them. Along with this, any activity which challenges the patient's equilibrium is inherently beneficial. This is because the intrinsic muscles are unconsciously fired by the brain in order to maintain balance. Standing on uneven surfaces, doing exercises on a wobble board, and even sitting on an exercise ball are helpful in this regard.

Overall, strengthening the core helps stabilize the entire body. For the spine, it provides stabilization while also allowing for the fine, intricate movement patterns the vertebrae were designed for. For the extremities, it provides a solid foundation from which to work. This reduces wear and tear on these joints because it provides for optimal leverage. It also helps conserve energy by making appendicular and spinal movement more efficient. Direct strengthening of the multifidus muscles is indicated in all cases of low back pain, as these muscles are proven to quickly atrophy with any low back condition. It has also been shown that even when a patient recovers from a low back condition, without specific strengthening of these muscles, they remain atrophied and leave the person predisposed to another LBP incident. Simple exercises for the multifidus are presented in Fig.'s 14-4, 14-5, and 14-6.[177]

SEGMENTAL MOBILITY

Assessment and treatment of segmental mobility plays an important role in the management of lumbar spine syndromes. This should be obvious to the reader given the fact that professions including chiropractic are practically based on correcting segmental dysfunction. With this in mind, it should also be obvious to the reader that he/she must be skilled in one of the many segmental assessment and treatment approaches in order to effectively serve his or her patients. It is out of the scope of this text to provide the reader with the necessary details and hands-on instruction necessary to master any of these techniques, so no attempt will be made to do so here. This especially applies to those techniques requiring high levels of skill and practice, such as Gonstead or the motion palpation approach. Instead, the instruction provided in this section is focused on more simple techniques virtually any manual therapist can perform. These techniques are presented below.

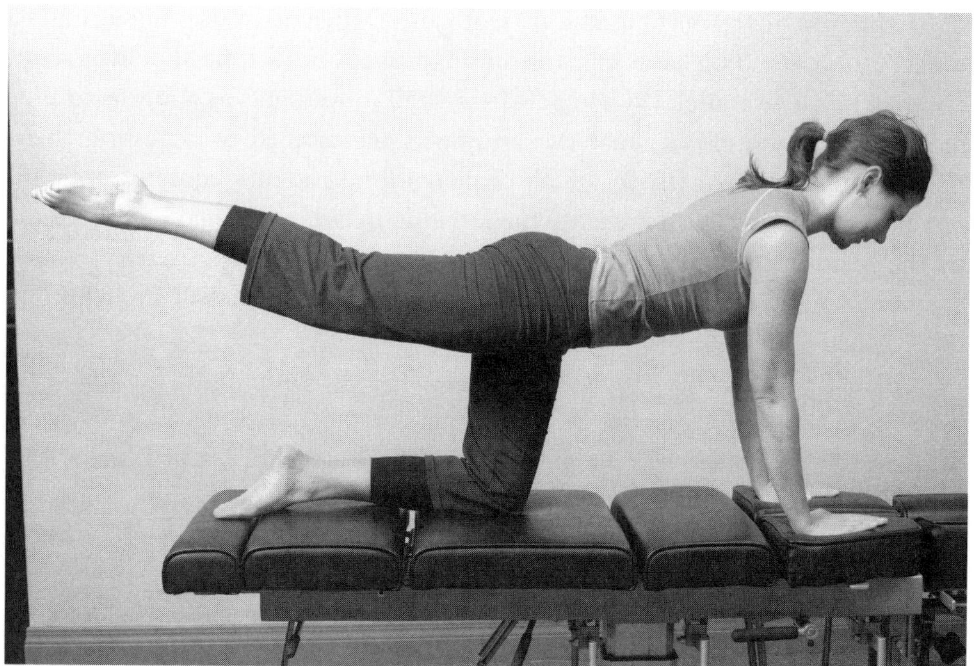

Fig. 14-4 Hip extension in quadruped.

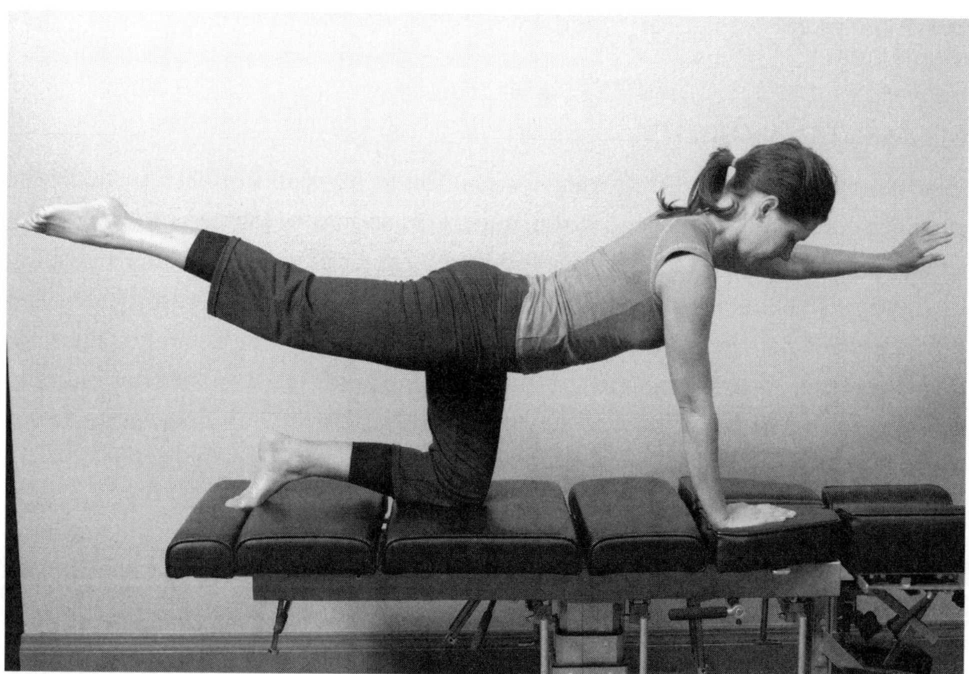

Fig. 14-5 Contralateral hip and shoulder extension in quadruped.

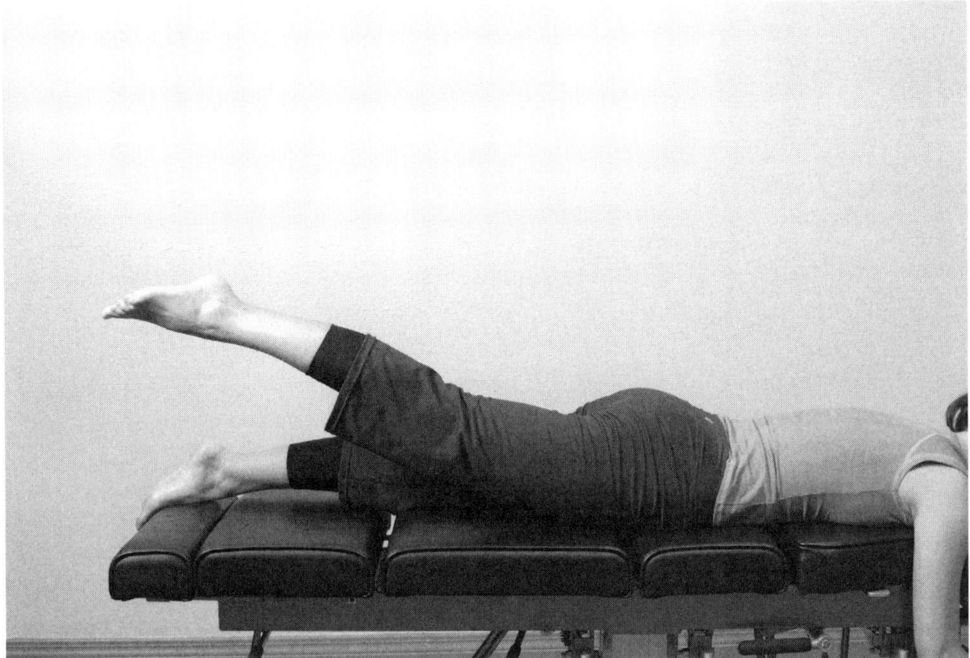

Fig. 14-6 Prone hip extension.

Australian Approach. The basic principles for this approach in the lumbar spine are the same as they were in the cervical spine (see Chapter 11). Side posture mobilization, muscle energy, and manipulation are employed into the direction of least resistance/pain. Segmental mobilization is also applied in this approach as it was in the cervicals. Again, the practitioner places his thumbs on the most tender segment and mobilizes anteriorly (Fig. 14-7).

Mulligan Technique. Mulligan advocates several methods to treat low back dysfunction.[142] One of the most simple yet effective techniques is his "SNAG" technique. This technique begins by testing lumbar range of motion and finding the direction of pain and limitation. Concurrent with this, the patient notes the exact location of pain.

To treat, have the patient seated. Simply place one's hands on the spinous processes at the associated level if the pain is centrally located, or on the corresponding mamillary process if the pain is laterally located. Next, press anteriorly and superiorly to support the segment.[170] Maintain this pressure and have the patient perform the offending movement again. When the technique is indicated this pressure will result in an immediate improvement in pain-free range

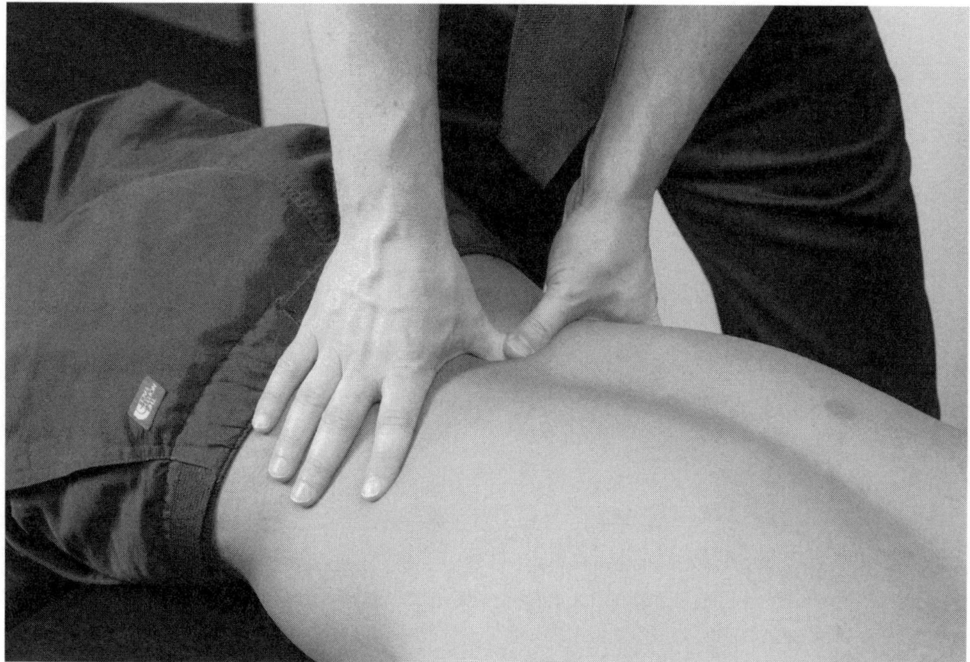

Fig. 14-7 Treatment for left facet dysfunction. Place the thumbs close together and contact the affected facet joint. Mobilize P-A for 30 seconds.

of motion. If the pressure did not create a change, or the improvement is minor, repeat the SNAG at a different level or on the opposite side. Try several levels until one is found which allows greatest pain-free motion. When found, repeat this maneuver at least ten times. Remember, do not have the patient go into pain—it is not a no-pain, no-gain technique. For treatment at home the patient can use his or her thumbs, or the edge of a towel to accomplish a similar effect. Again, stress to him or her the importance of finding the proper vector which gives the greatest relief.

LUMBAR SPINE POSTURE

Most frequently, the lumbar spine falls into a hyperlordotic posture (particularly of the lumbosacral junction). This is especially true in patients who are hypermobile and have an anterior pelvic tilt. This posture is successfully treated by addressing the factors driving the common pattern, releasing hypertonic muscles including the psoas and erector spinae and teaching the patient lumbar stabilization exercises including the posterior pelvic tilt.

In patients who are hypolordotic expect to see a posterior pelvic tilt along with hypomobility. These patients will benefit from therapies to improve mobility and increase lordosis. This helps reduce acute disc protrusions or at the least helps prevent them.

The examiner must also inspect for deviations in the coronal and sagittal planes caused by leg length discrepancy, pelvic asymmetry, and scoliosis. Any asymmetry created by these conditions will place undue stress on pain-generating structures of the lumbar spine. Be sure to address the former conditions as thoroughly as possible with manual therapy and heel lifts. In the case of structural scoliosis the practitioner is encouraged to refer to a clinician specializing in scoliosis treatment.

MOVEMENT PATTERNS

Lumbar spine movement pattern dysfunction can be broken down into two major categories. The first category is the general muscle imbalance and sagittal-plane postural distortion as occurs with the lower crossed syndrome. The second category deals with improper segmental mobility due to dysfunctional recruitment patterns. This results in what is termed "en-bloc" motion. Both categories of movement dysfunction are described below.

Lower Crossed Pattern. The pattern of hypertonic psoas and erector spinae muscles combined with inhibited spinal intrinsics, rectus abdominis, transversus abdominis, and gluteus maximus promote a state of hyperlordosis, chronic muscle contraction and facet compression. This pattern is so evident and pervasive that it seems to serve as the "common ground" for several different techniques—each one identifying the pattern as an important cause of low back pain and aiming to treat it in a similar way.

Among these approaches are Pilates and Alexander Technique. Pilates teaches students to "hollow out" the abdomen. The Alexander Technique teaches its students to lengthen the spine, thereby lessening the lumbar lordosis. Added to this is the fact that physical therapy's most popular lumbar stabilization exercise is the posterior pelvic tilt.

The popularity of this concept is not a surprise; each approach using it works. Not only does it recruit inhibited muscles and inhibit contracted muscles, but it also puts the spine in a more natural lordotic position (relative to a hyperlordotic state). Clinicians should learn these techniques and add instructions to the patient to bring the umbilicus towards the spine. This activates the core musculature as described previously. This combination of altered sagittal plane positioning plus core activation helps guarantee less stress on the lumbar spine.

It is also the clinician's responsibility to teach the patient how to integrate this motor control into his/her daily life. Activities which stress the spine—even ones which appear benign—should be addressed. The Alexander Technique's sit-to-stand drill is a perfect example of this. For instance, most patients with low back pain have increased pain when arising from sitting due to cervical and lumbar hyperextension. However, under guidance the patient can inhibit these muscle groups and effectively "lengthen" the spine. This results in an immediate decrease or elimination of back pain, thereby illustrating how benign daily activities can impact one's condition if left unaddressed. Remember to search for other repetitive, benign activities which can impede the patient's progression through therapy. Then, teach him/her how to stabilize the spine to reduce/eliminate this stress.

En-Bloc Movement. General or localized dysfunction causes en-bloc movement. This refers to the vertebrae moving together as a single unit instead of moving as separate segments. This causes a functional immobility, thereby promoting all of the negative sequelae resulting from lack of motion. Among these are diminished blood flow, decreased imbibition of fluid into the disc, decreased mechanoreception, increased nociception, muscle atrophy, and eventually degenerative changes. In other words, en-bloc movement makes a bad problem worse.

Treatment to restore normal motion is multi-factorial. Any intervention to normalize nervous system function/diminish common pattern dominance is necessary first and foremost. Once the stimulus for this movement pattern dysfunction is eliminated, the practitioner can implement remedial exercises geared at promoting segmental motion. A valuable therapy for these individuals is to introduce them to the concept of awareness. This can be by teaching them to feel the motion in their lumbar spine occurring at each segment instead of as an entire unit. This will take practice at first, as it is not second-nature to most people. Practicing Feldenkrais-type principles to improve awareness may be valuable in many circumstances, as will Hanna's methods to correct what he calls sensory-motor amnesia.

Yet another helpful tip for patients with dysfunctional lumbar movement patterns is to introduce them to the fact that other joints in the area—such as the pelvis and hips—are there to take stress off the low back. Oftentimes, patients are not really aware that their hips can move as they do; some do not even know exactly where these joints are. Training them to utilize their hip joints during rotation and flexion/extension can be invaluable in reducing stress on the low back. This will also help retrain the patient's motor system, helping him realize that he can move a certain way or a certain amount without having the pain associated with it.

TAPING

There are two popular taping techniques available for those with lumbar spine syndromes. Kinesiotaping is one of these. Its primary function is neurological; it reduces abnormal muscle tone and is great for acute lumbar spasm. The other approach to taping is more structural in nature. It is used to help stabilize unstable segments when indicated. Other times, structural taping helps maintain lumbar lordosis. This is helpful in cases of disc herniation, when the patient must maintain a lordotic posture to retain nucleus reduction (Fig. 14-8).

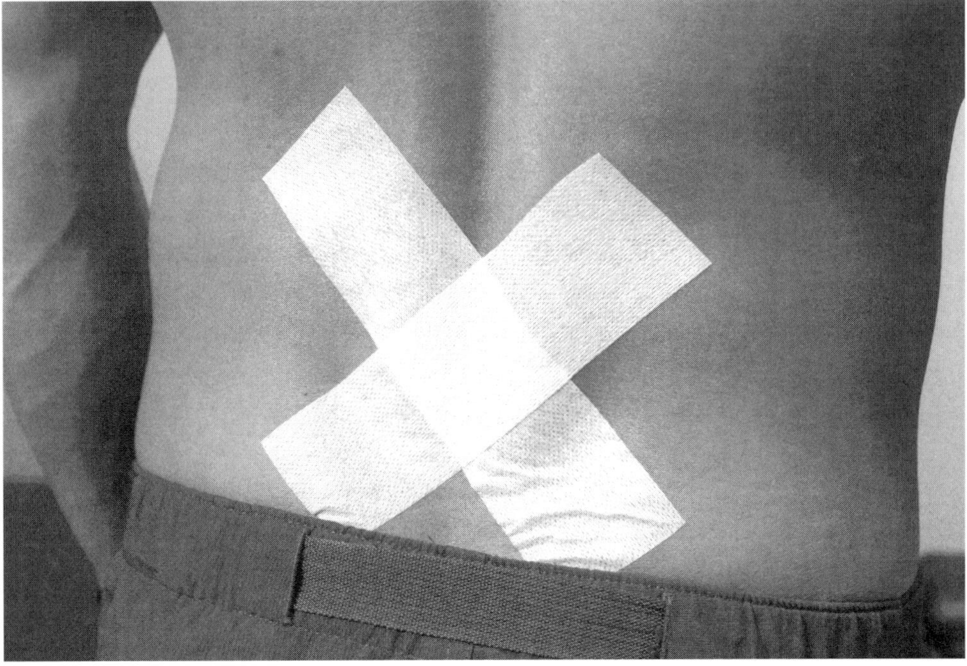

Fig. 14-8 Lumbar taping to stabilize the spine and maintain lordosis.

ENERGY-BASED TECHNIQUES

Auricular Acupressure. Gently squeeze the point corresponding to the lumbar spine with two fingers. Hold for 5 seconds, then relax 5 seconds. Increase the amount of pressure with each cycle for a total time of one minute (6 cycles). Do this initially on the ear on the involved side only; treat the opposite ear as well if the patient does not improve.

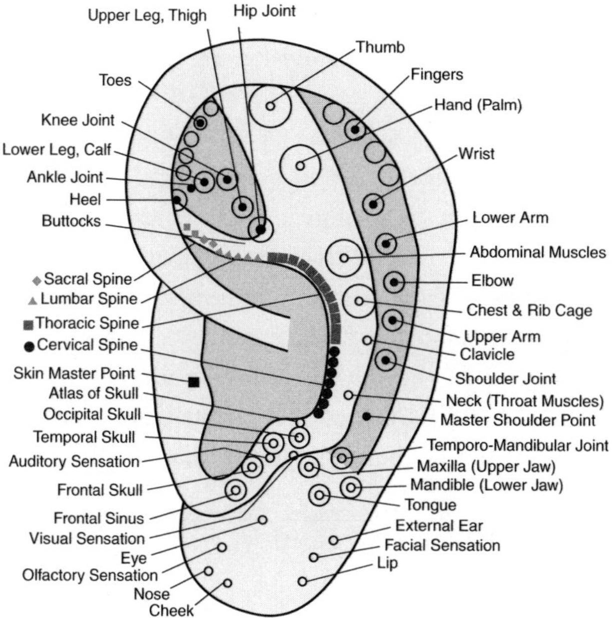

Fig. 14-9

Reflexology. Begin by massaging the entire foot. Walk up the foot with the thumbs along the five zones. Treat both the plantar and dorsal surfaces. Work the toes as well. Spend extra time on the medial border of the foot corresponding with the spine. Also, work on areas associated with different organs needing an extra "boost." Following this long warm-up, massage the area on the foot corresponding with the lumbar spine.

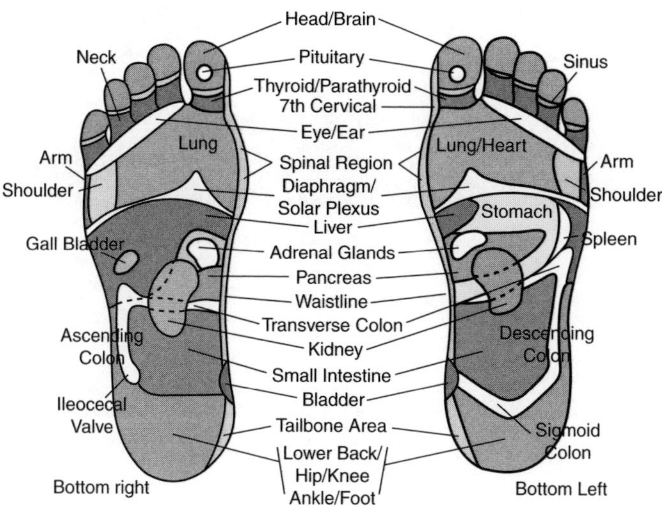

Fig. 14-10

HIGH-YIELD SCAN

Perform a scan of the high-yield elements of the body including:

- Gait
- Posture
- Sit-to-Stand
- Miniature Squat
- Respiration
- Romberg Test
- Fukuda's Test
- Upper Cervical Spine
- Middle and Lower Cervical Spine
- TMJ
- Pelvis
- Feet
- Stress Screen

EVALUATION AND TREATMENT OF THE SECONDARY FACTORS

There are many things which influence the low back. It is the responsibility of the clinician to review each of these with the patient. Of all these causative factors probably the most common mechanical cause of low back problems is prolonged sitting in an improper position. To address this, the patient must first be instructed to reduce his total time sitting, or at least break it up by getting up and walking around. He must also be given advice on proper furniture which promotes a healthy posture while sitting. This is important for all cases of low back pain, and absolutely imperative in cases of disc herniation.

15 The Pelvis

THE PELVIS IS CONSIDERED A HIGH-YIELD REGION OF THE BODY FOR MANY REASONS. MECHANICALLY, its importance is obvious—distortions or deviations from neutral lead to patterns of strain and compensation in the spine and lower extremities. Neurologically its importance is just as great. As a large weight-bearing region, it is responsible for providing the central nervous system with vital afferent information. Thus, deviations from neutral impact the central nervous system on a broad scale.

Besides this mechanical and neurological influence, remember that pelvic dysfunction impacts the myofascial system and the body's movement pattern scheme. Altogether, it is easy to understand why this region should be evaluated on every patient—whether or not a clear cause-and-effect relationship is readily established with the person's presenting complaint.

EVALUATION AND TREATMENT OF THE PRIMARY FACTORS

Piriformis. Palpate the muscle for hypertonicity, fascial adhesions, tenderness, and trigger points. Utilize soft tissue techniques including myofascial release, sustained pressure, strumming and ischemic compression to address the findings. Post-isometric relaxation and strain/counterstrain are also useful in reducing tone (See Fig.'s 16-7 and 16-8).

Levator ani. Palpate this muscle group for hypertonicity, fascial adhesions, tenderness, and trigger points. Utilize soft tissue techniques including myofascial release, sustained pressure, strumming and ischemic compression to address the findings (Fig. 15-1). Strain/counterstrain is useful in reducing tone (Fig. 15-2).

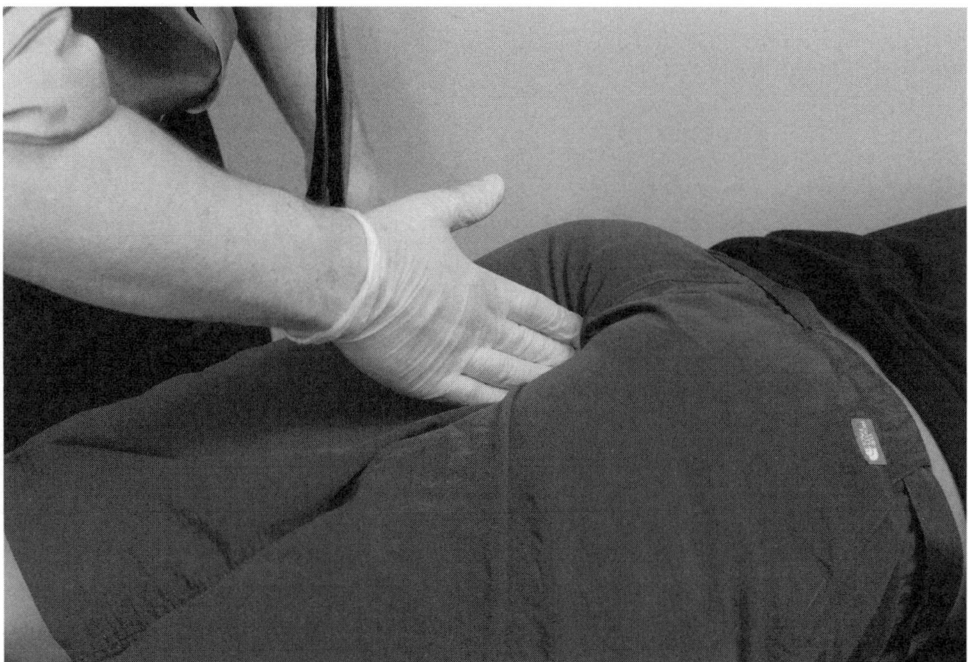

Fig. 15-1 The clinician can apply MFR, sustained pressure, strumming and ischemic compression in this position.

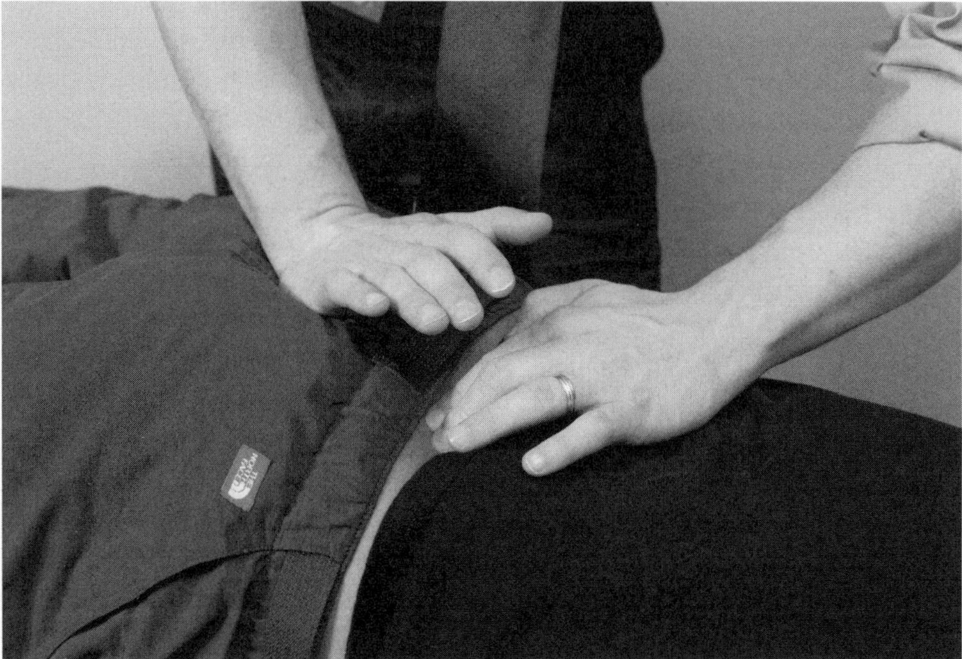

Fig. 15-2 Strain-counterstrain of the levator ani. Tender points are found along the border of the sacrum. The position of ease is found by applying a posterior-to-anterior force on the opposite border of the sacrum in order to pull the affected portion of the sacrum posteriorly.[178]

The levator ani muscle group is inhibited as part of the common pattern. This compromises the stability of the pelvic girdle and lumbar spine. It also compromises the function of the genitourinary systems—particularly in the female. Myofascial trigger points in this muscle will cause pain in the sacrococcygeal region. Expect the presence of soft tissue dysfunction in almost all cases of coccygeal dysfunction or after injury.

Besides the piriformis and levator ani, the clinician should also address any other muscles with an influence on the pelvic girdle. These include, but are not limited to, the hamstrings, iliopsoas, quadratus lumborum, hip adductors, hip abductors, spinal extensors, quadriceps, and abdominals.

MUSCLE STRENGTH

Begin by assessing general core strength as described for the lumbar spine. Next, assess the strength of the muscles controlling the pelvic girdle with traditional methods. Make sure to assess both their ability to initiate a contraction as well as their sheer strength. Most often, what we perceive as weakness is more a matter of inhibition. This will follow the common pattern and/or be due to local or segmental dysfunction. Treating the causative factor restores normal strength in these cases. In cases of true muscle weakness, such as those involving muscle atrophy, remedial strengthening is indicated. This is done with traditional strengthening techniques.

In addition to assessing these muscle groups be sure to assess the levator ani. This group is frequently inhibited and weak and must be strengthened. Traditional exercises for these muscles are called Kegel exercises and are often prescribed to women after childbirth. Several of these exercises are described by Murphy.[54] He suggests having the sidelying patient attempt to pull the pelvic floor towards the head. Once the person is proficient in activating these muscles, he/she can progress to a sitting position. In this position, the patient is taught the "elevator exercise." This involves asking the patient to consider the act of raising the pelvic floor equivalent to raising an elevator. Raising the pelvic floor as much as possible is designated as raising it to the fourth floor. Thus, the distance ranging from the point of relaxation to full contraction can be equally divided into four parts. The patient is instructed to then "raise the elevator" to the first floor, then the second, and so on. She should practice bouncing between different floors to further improve the tone of these muscles.

ARTICULAR MOBILITY

As in the lumbar spine, there are multiple ways to analyze the motion and structure of the pelvic girdle. Presented below are common pelvic misalignments along with methods used in their diagnosis. While there is some overlap between the fields of chiropractic and osteopathy, there are also some differences. The reader is urged to use whatever techniques he/she is most proficient in, and to utilize several examination methods if necessary to confirm a diagnosis.

AS INNOMINATE/ANTERIOR INNOMINATE ROTATION

Diagnosis

Several methods help confirm this diagnosis. In standing, the patient displays an inferior ASIS and superior PSIS on the affected side. The standing forward flexion test is positive on the affected side (Fig. 15-3). The long-sitting test reveals a long lower extremity in supine which shortens when the patient sits up while keeping the knees extended (Fig. 15-4). In prone, the patient displays a long leg on the affected side which shortens when the knees are flexed to 90 degrees (Fig. 15-5). There is often a tender nodule in the gastrocnemius on the affected side. Note: this nodule often disappears immediately following successful treatment.

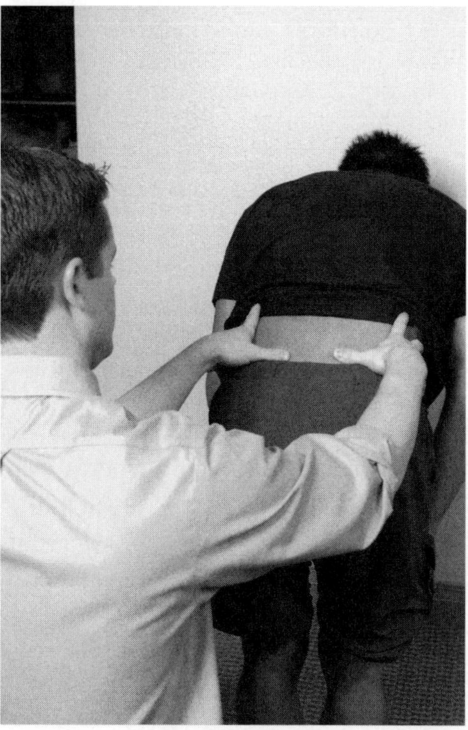

Fig. 15-3 The Standing Forward Flexion test. With the examiner's thumbs on the PSIS's, have the patient bend forward. The PSIS and thumb that move first indicate the side of iliosacral involvement.

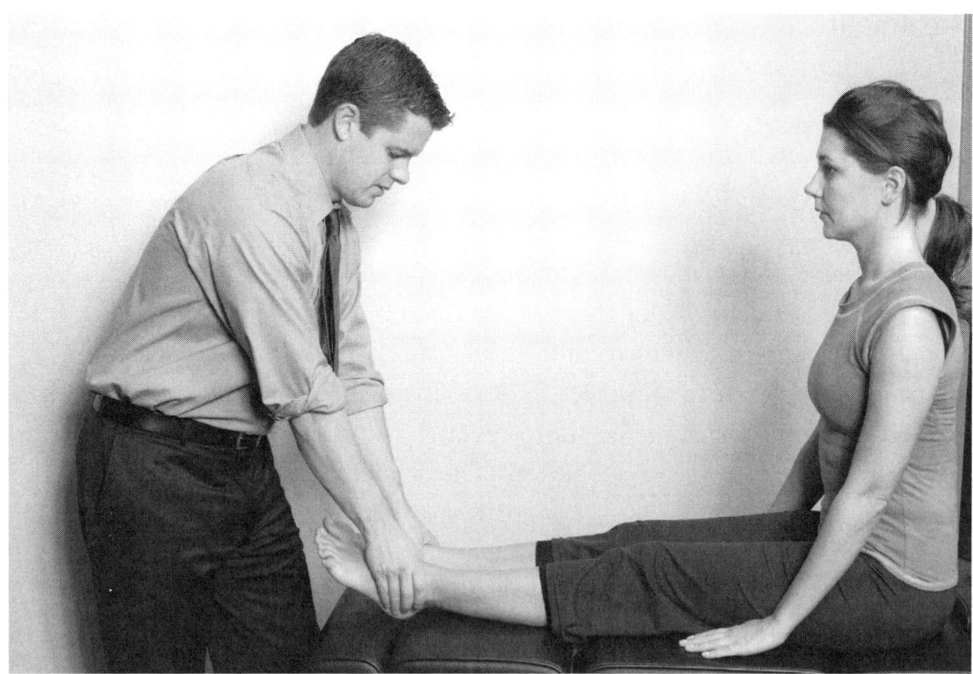

Fig. 15-4 The long sitting test. The long leg will shorten when sitting up from a supine position.

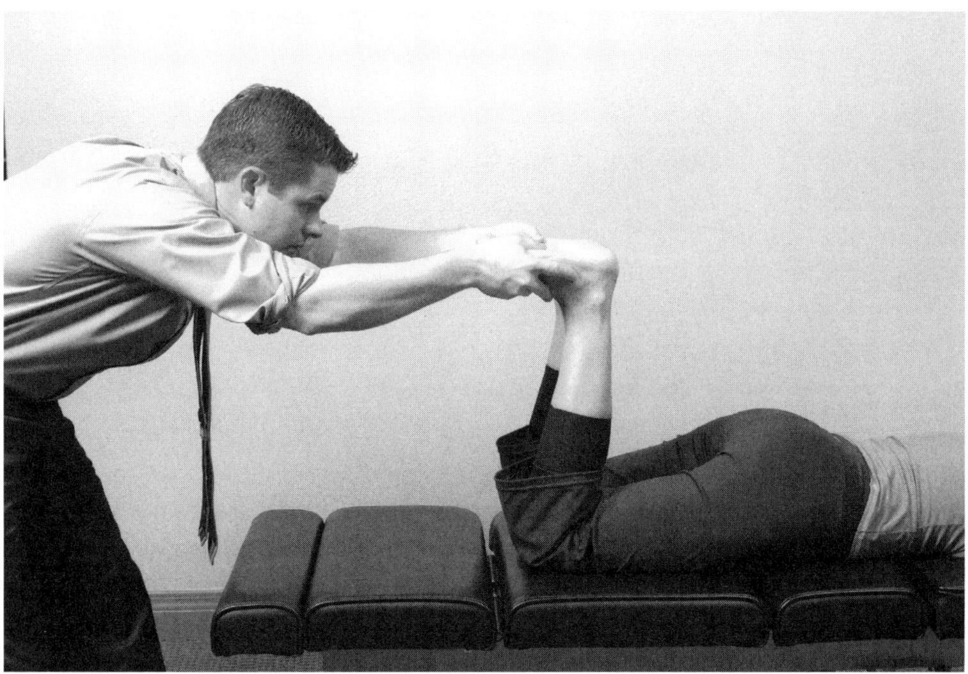

Fig. 15-5 Prone knee flexion. The long leg shortens in relation to the opposite leg when the knees are flexed 90 degrees.

Treatment

Muscle Energy Technique: The supine patient contracts his gluteal and hamstring muscles into resistance provided by the therapist. This is held for 5", followed by a stretch into posterior rotation for 5". This is repeated five times into end-range (Fig. 15-6).

Mobilization/Manipulation: With the patient in sidelying with the involved side up, the clinician flexes the involved hip until end-range is reached. He contacts the ischial tuberosity and drives anterior and superior, rotating the innominate posteriorly (Fig. 15-7). This is done repetitively as a mobilization. A manipulation must be more specific and is comprised of many more steps to ensure safety and specificity. The reader is urged to learn this skill hands-on.

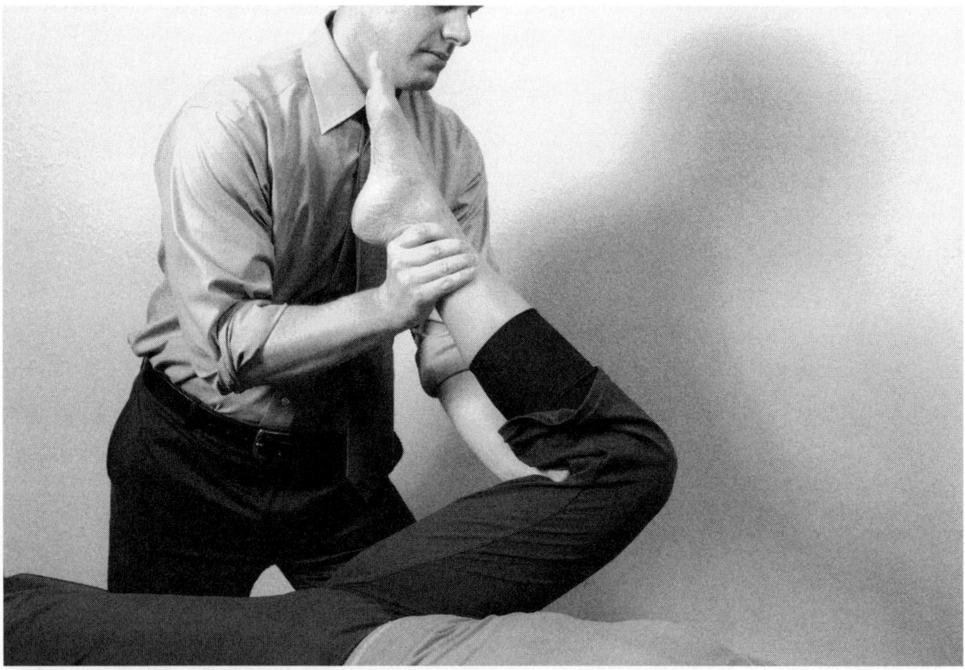

Fig. 15-6 MET for AS/Anterior Innominate: Have the patient push her thigh into the therapist's hand, followed by stretching into further hip flexion.

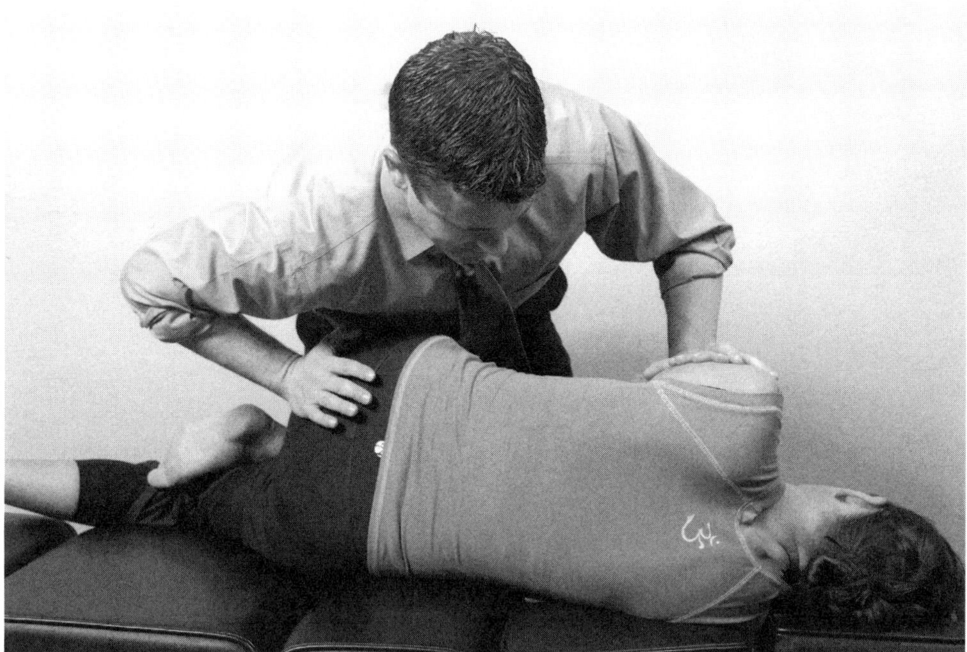

Fig. 15-7 Mobilization of AS/Anterior Innominate: Contact the ischial tuberosity and drive superior and anterior.

POSTERIOR INNOMINATE ROTATION/PI INNOMINATE

Diagnosis

There are several methods to confirm this diagnosis. In standing, the ASIS on the affected side is superior and the PSIS is inferior. The PSIS on the affected side moves before the opposite PSIS during the standing forward flexion test. In the long-sitting test, the affected leg is shorter in extension but lengthens on long-sitting. Lastly, the affected leg presents as shorter than the opposite leg in prone.

Treatment

Muscle Energy Technique: The supine patient pushes his thigh upwards into the clinician's hand. This is maintained for 5", followed by a stretch into anterior rotation for 5". This is repeated five times into end-range (Fig. 15-8). This

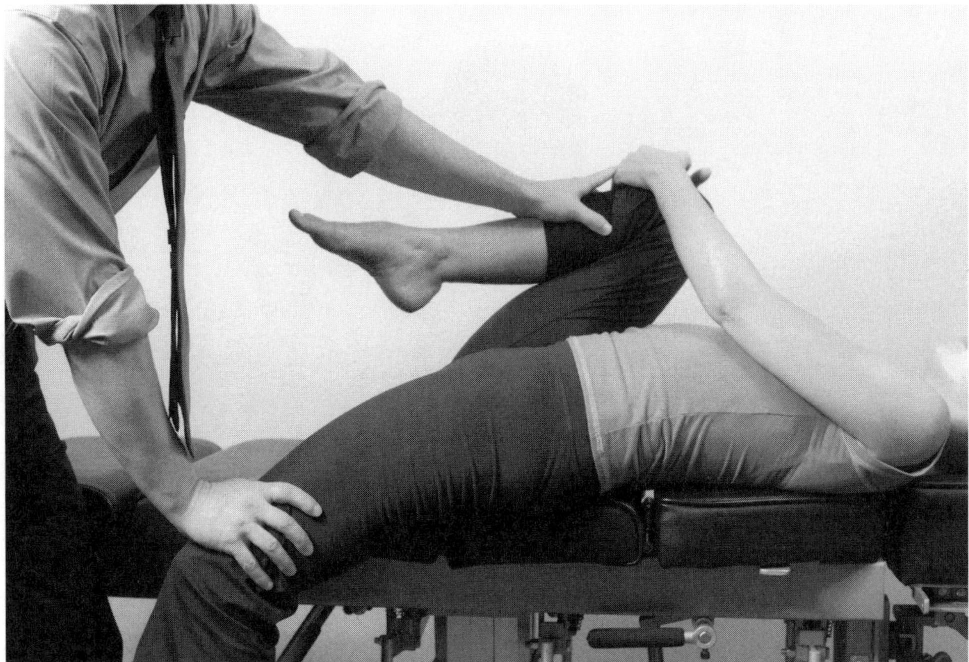

Fig. 15-8 MET for the PI/Posterior Innominate: Have the patient contract the thigh into the therapist's hand. When the patient relaxes, stretch the thigh into further extension. Repeat 5 times.

technique can be applied in sidelying as well. In both positions, the patient must maintain hip flexion on the opposite side by pulling the knee to the chest.

Mobilization/Manipulation: With the patient in sidelying (involved side up), the clinician flexes the hip until movement is perceived at the sacroiliac joint. He contacts the PSIS and drives anterior and superior, rotating the innominate anteriorly. This is done repetitively as a mobilization. A manipulation must be more specific and is comprised of several more steps to ensure safety and specificity. The reader is urged to learn this skill hands-on.

POSITIVE AND NEGATIVE DERIFIELD LISTINGS

The positive and negative Derifield listings are two versions of the posterior innominate described in the Thompson technique. The positive Derifield is basically a posterior innominate rotation about an axis located through the acetabulum. It is found through prone leg length examination. The involved leg is short when the knee is straight but lengthens when the knees are flexed. Correction is performed on a drop table with anterior and superior-directed pressure on the PSIS.

The negative Derifield is more rare than the positive Derifield. It involves posterior rotation around the pubic symphysis. Diagnosis is performed through the prone leg length check; this time the short leg stays the same length (in comparison to the long leg) or shortens upon knee flexion. Combined with this diagnostic method, the patient must also have tenderness to palpation of multiple points. These include the ipsilateral gastrocnemius, medial knee, ischial tuberosity, sacroiliac joint, pubic tubercle, and the contralateral erector spinae, psoas and 2nd rib interspace anteriorly. Correction is a two-part adjustment performed on a special drop table; it consists of pressure to push the innominate superiorly followed by thrusts to push it posteriorly. When the patient presents with myofascial problems involving these regions be sure to look for this pattern. Once again, this is another example how pelvic dysfunction is involved in reflexive patterns.

BILATERAL ANTERIOR INNOMINATE ROTATION

Bilateral anterior innominate rotation is rarely evaluated for, although it is a part of the common pattern/lower crossed syndrome. One of the few authors to place importance on this listing is physical therapist Richard DonTigny, who points to the structure of the pelvis as the primary reason for the resultant anterior rotation. In his writings[155] he suggests this misalignment is the primary cause of insidious-onset low back pain. Treatment is accomplished with traditional methods as described previously. In addition, DonTigny suggests tractioning the leg with the hip flexed 30 degrees. This rotates the pelvis posteriorly and actually causes a functional shortening after treatment. This is applied bilaterally.

OUTFLARE/IN INNOMINATE

Diagnosis

The standing forward flexion test indicates the side of involvement. Palpation demonstrates the PSIS on the affected side is displaced medially compared with the opposite PSIS. The gluteal appears wider on this side as well. Look for the foot on the affected side to be turned outwards.

Treatment

Muscle Energy Technique: The patient is supine. Bring the knee across the patient's midline until the point of resistance. Then have him push his knee laterally into the clinician's hand. Hold for 5", then stretch the hip further medially. Repeat five times (Fig. 15-9).

Mobilization/Manipulation: The patient is prone. Stand on the side opposite the affected side while contacting the medial aspect of the ischial tuberosity.

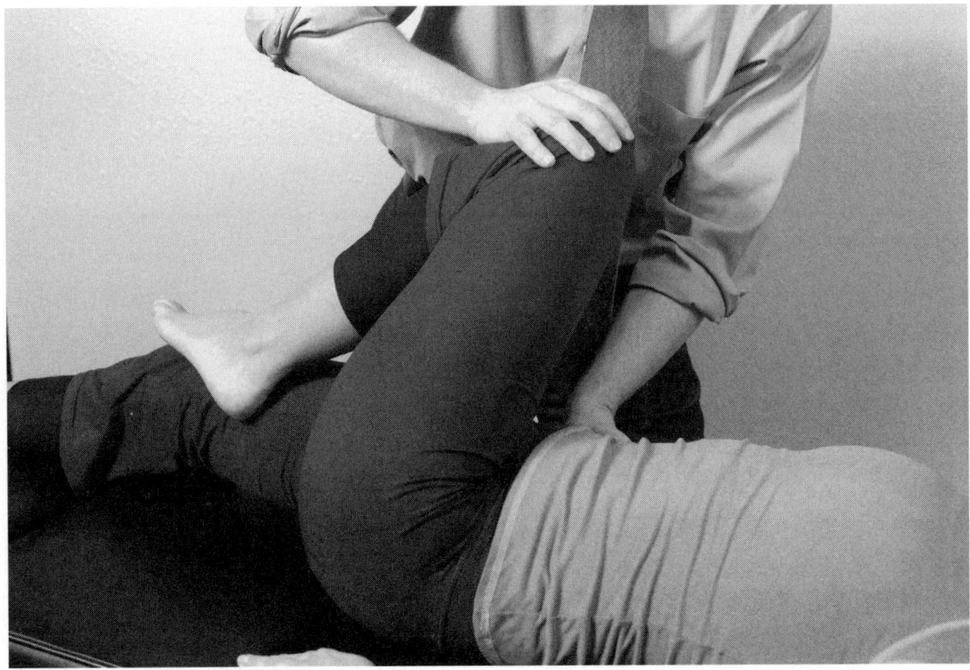

Fig. 15-9 MET for Outflare/IN Innominate: Bring the patient's knee across her body and then have her push the thigh into resistance. Upon relaxation, stretch the hip further across the body.

Mobilize by pushing laterally and anteriorly. Manipulation can be performed with a drop table or in the side posture position.

INFLARE/ER INNOMINATE

Diagnosis

The standing forward flexion test indicates the side of involvement. Palpation demonstrates the PSIS on the affected side is displaced laterally compared with the opposite PSIS. The gluteal appears more narrow on this side as well. In addition, look for the foot on the affected side to be turned medially.

Treatment

Muscle Energy Technique: The patient is supine. Put the hip into the "figure 4" position. Next, push the knee towards the table until the point of resistance. Then have him push his knee superiorly into resistance. Hold for 5", then stretch the hip further downwards. Repeat five times (Fig. 15-10).

Mobilization/Manipulation: The patient is prone. Stand on the affected side and contact the lateral aspect of the PSIS. Mobilize by pushing medially. Manipulation can be performed with a drop table or in the side posture position.

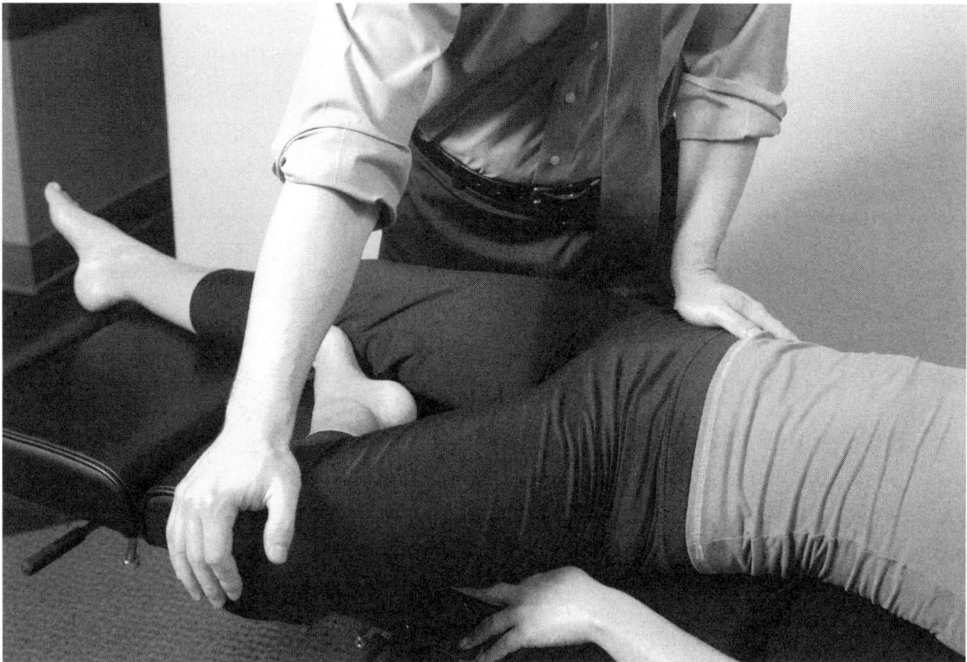

Fig. 15-10 MET for Inflare/ER Innominate: Have the patient in the figure-4 position. Have her push her knee into resistance. Upon relaxation, stretch the hip further towards the floor.

UPSLIP

Diagnosis

The standing forward flexion test is positive on the side of involvement. Observation and palpation reveal superior displacement of the ASIS and PSIS on the same side. This leg will be short in supine and prone. Additionally, there will be no change during the long-sitting test.

Treatment:

Manipulation: The patient is supine with the legs extended. Grasp the affected leg just above the ankle (or proximal to the knee if there is knee pathology) and rotate the hip slightly internally. Have the patient cough three times. On the third cough, quickly traction the extremity inferiorly.

Myofascial Release—Leg Pull: This technique is exceptionally gentle and should be used when high velocity techniques are contraindicated. In addition to being effective at correcting an innominate upslip, this procedure is touted as a great method to release myofascial restrictions throughout the entire lower extremity and lumbar spine. To perform this maneuver, begin by taking the supine patient's extremity and applying gentle traction (Fig. 15-11). As the tissue releases, slowly externally rotate and abduct the hip. Take it to the point of restriction and wait until the tissue gives way once more. Remain here until maximal external rotation and abduction are achieved through repetitive tissue releases. From here, bring the extremity across the patient's body while adding internal rotation. Give a gentle traction with the free hand on the pelvis. Again, wait for the tissue to release and then pursue increased motion. Follow this until maximum range of motion is reached (Fig. 15-12).

PUBIC DYSFUNCTION

Pubic dysfunction typically occurs secondary to the other misalignments of the pelvic girdle. As with the other regions of the pelvis, there are specific diagnostic techniques to determine subtle movement or structural dysfunction here. The reader is welcomed to choose one of these approaches to learn these techniques in greater detail, as they are not taught in this text. Instead, the approach to pubic dysfunction in this text is to simplify things as much as possible. The pubic shotgun technique is just the answer.

As the name implies, the "pubic shotgun" is a technique designed to treat any and all forms of pubic dysfunction with a single (yet far-reaching approach). It begins by having the supine patient flex his hips and knees. The clinician stands alongside the patient and makes contact with the outside of his knees with her hands. Next, she has him push his knees into her hands at least three times, holding for three seconds each time. After he is finished with the third contraction, she places her hands on the inside aspect of his knees and asks him to squeeze his knees together. Again, he performs three contractions of three seconds duration. During the third contraction the therapist pulls the knees apart with a quick but light force. This separation, along with the adductor contraction, is intended to separate the pubic bones. This separation allows them to fit together properly.

THE SACRUM

The sacrum may be listed in almost any possible direction. Despite this hypothetical "freedom" of motion, both the chiropractic and osteopathic literature agree that the most common finding is that of a unilateral anterior malposition of the sacral base. In the chiropractic literature, this finding is termed an

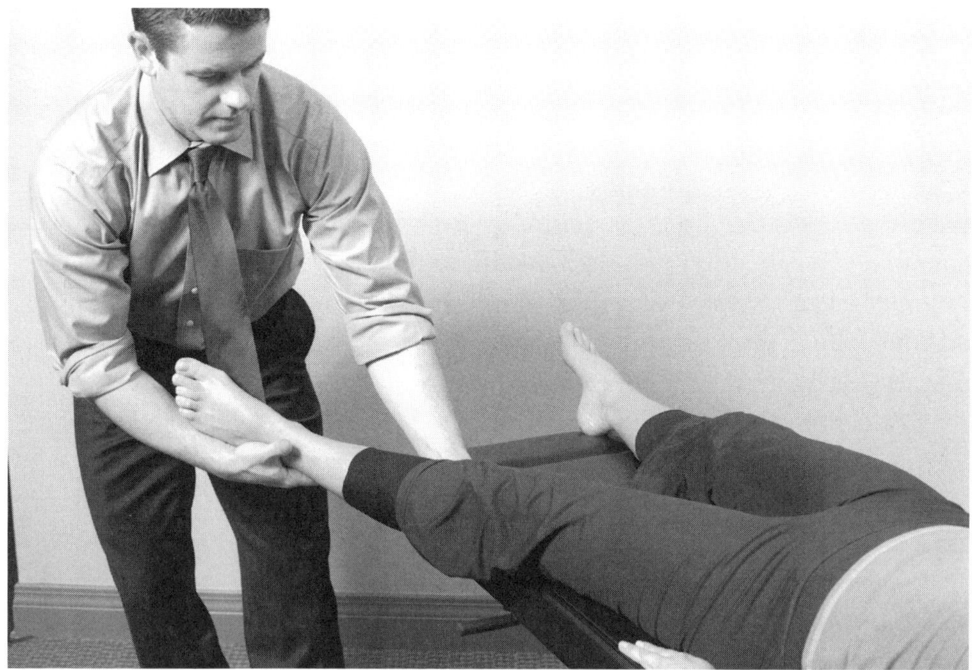

Fig. 15-11 Myofascial release leg pull. Begin with a gentle traction force.

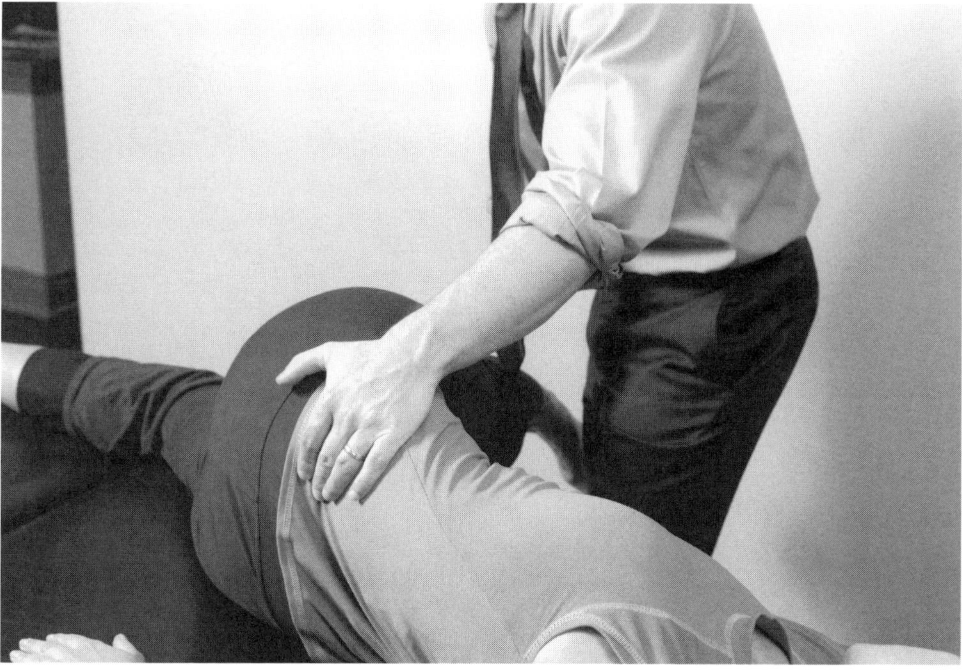

Fig. 15-12 Last phase of the myofascial release leg pull.

anterior-inferior (AI) sacrum. In the osteopathic literature, this is termed a left-on-left or right-on-right sacral torsion. Oftentimes, this is in response to a PI ilium on the same side. Other times it is due to trauma.

An effective way of detecting an A-I sacrum in addition to standard palpation is followed in the Thompson protocol. In this instance, the patient is prone and the clinician stabilizes the sacrum by applying a posterior-to-anterior pressure to it. The patient is then asked to raise the extended lower extremity as high as possible. Pain and/or restriction on one side indicates an A-I sacrum on that side (Fig. 15-13). Inability to raise either leg at least 4" indicates a base posterior sacrum (analogous to a counternutated sacrum).

Correction of an A-I sacrum via Thompson protocol utilizes a drop table. However, similar results may be obtained through mobilization/manipulation in a side-posture position. Have the patient lie involved side down. Contact the contralateral sacral apex and drive anterior and superior. This pulls the sacral base posteriorly.

Correction of a base posterior sacrum can be performed in side posture as well. This time it does not matter which side is down. Contact the S2 tubercle and thrust anterior and inferior (Fig. 15-14). Another way to correct a base posterior sacrum is by contacting the sacral base with the patient prone. Apply an anteriorly-directed mobilization in this position.

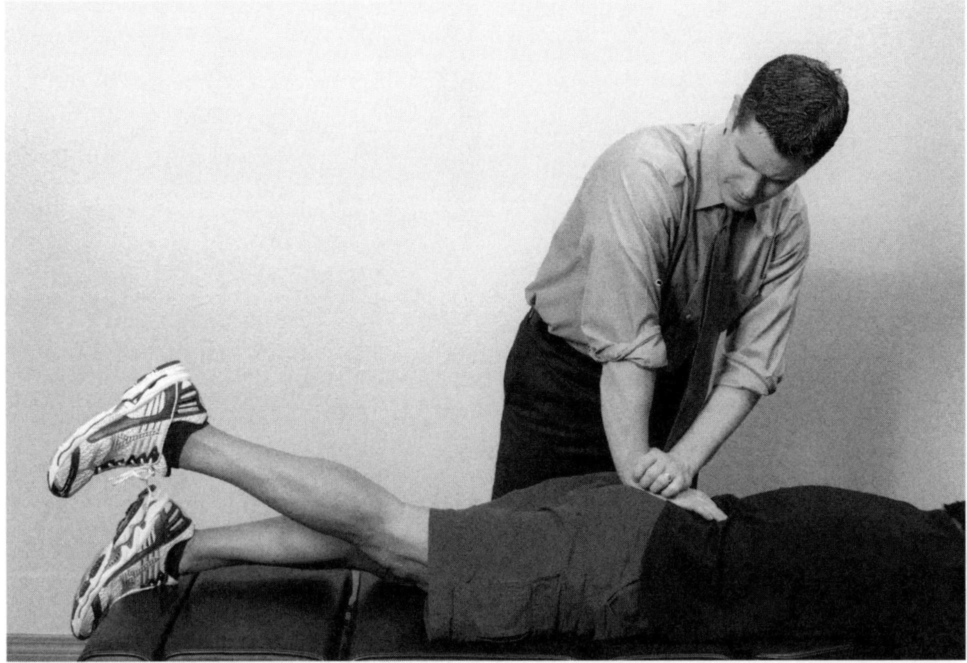

Fig. 15-13 Prone leg extension demonstrating limited motion.

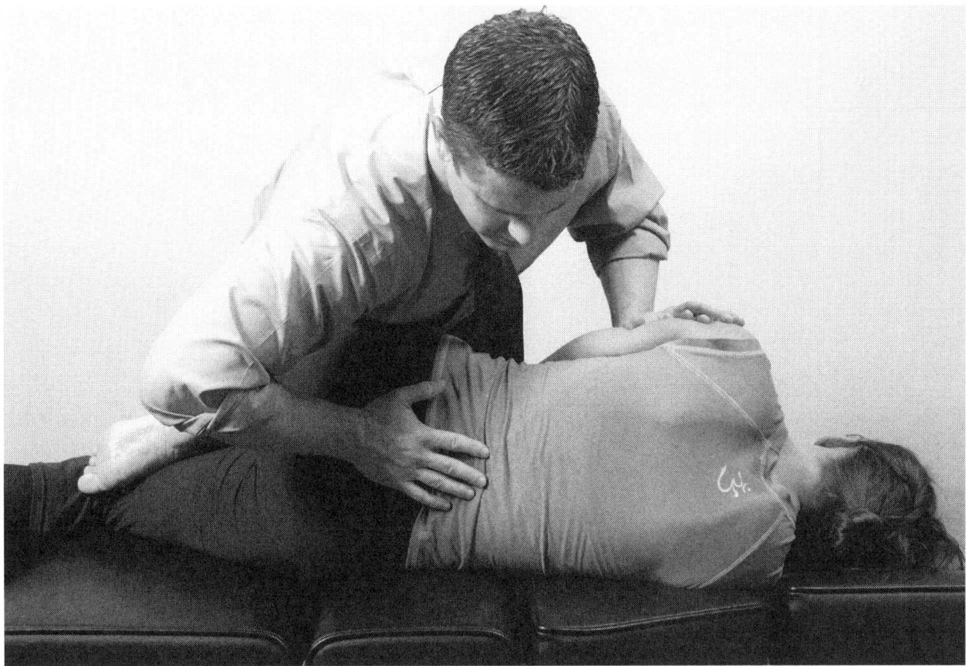

Fig. 15-14 Adjustment of a posterior sacral base in the side posture position.

Strain-counterstrain gives the practitioner another simple method to evaluate sacral malposition. The practitioner starts by palpating the border of the sacrum for tender points. When found, he applies an anterior pressure on the opposite side of the sacrum in order to lift (and take tension off) the tender area. Treatment can begin in this position if desired. Or, the clinician can use this knowledge of the sacrum's malposition and then mobilize/manipulate it into the opposite direction. For further information on in-depth sacral analysis, the reader is urged to consult the osteopathic literature, SOT or applied kinesiology.

THE COCCYX

The coccyx plays a more important role in the health of the individual than most people realize. Not only is it the final attachment point for the meninges (filum terminale), but it is also the seat for the ganglion impar. This ganglion gives rise to the nervi erigentes, which controls parasympathetic function to the lower colon and urogenital systems. Given these neurological connections it is no wonder why a 65-year-old woman can remember falling on her tailbone 45 years ago as if it was yesterday! It is also no surprise why correcting coccygeal dysfunction has such widespread benefit.

The first clue to coccygeal dysfunction comes from the patient's history. Whether or not the patient remembers falling on her tailbone initially is not important. What is important is her reporting that it hurts to sit on a *hard* surface, though on a soft surface she is fine. This always indicates coccygeal dysfunction. Once this is ascertained, ask them about falls directly on the tailbone. Sure enough, they will remember. If a fall is ruled out, remember that childbirth often results in similar problems.

From a chiropractic standpoint, the coccyx is normally considered to subluxate anteriorly. This may be combined with laterality as well. Correction can be through the rectum but only as a last resort. An adjustment taught by Gonstead is especially helpful. It consists of tractioning the skin from the tip of the coccyx superiorly and then thrusting superiorly, using the opposite hand to drive the contact hand upwards (Fig. 15-15).

The strain-counterstrain approach described by Jones is also helpful. The prone patient is palpated for a tender point one and three-quarter inches inferior and one-fourth inch medial to the lower edge of the PSIS. The position of ease is accomplished by raising the hip into extension and then adducting it so that it is above the opposite leg. This position is held for 90 seconds.[178]

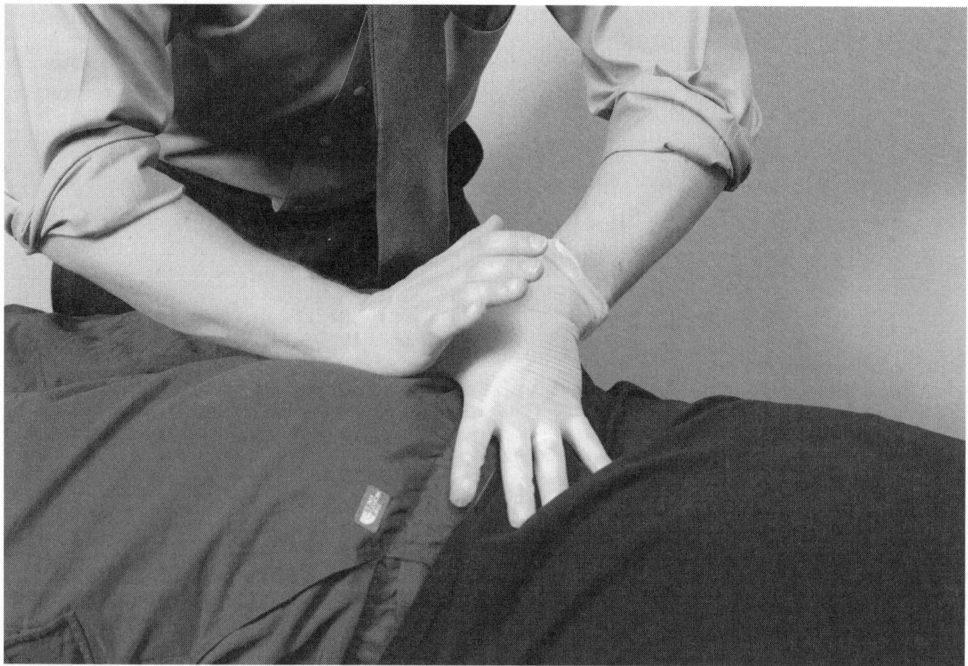

Fig. 15-15 Coccyx adjustment.

Another non-invasive technique is proposed by Upledger.[70] He suggests having the supine patient extend the flexed thigh into the clinician. This recruits the gluteus maximus, which pulls the coccyx posteriorly.

THE PELVIC LIGAMENTS

In Chapter 3 the importance of the pelvic ligaments was discussed in detail. To summarize, Logan Basic, Dvorak and Dvorak's work, and Gillet's work were introduced, and their perspectives on the pelvic ligaments was discussed. Logan Basic technique is more complex than these other two approaches and is not presented here. The other two techniques are fairly simple and are described below.

Spondylogenic Reflexes. Dvorak and Dvorak detail the neurological connections between points along the sacrospinous and sacrotuberous ligaments and different levels of the cervical and thoracic spine.[42] Furthermore, they describe how treatment of these ligaments can benefit dysfunction in these regions of the spine. This begins with finding a tender point alongside the spine. Next, add pressure to the prone patient's sacrospinous/sacrotuberous ligaments (especially where they intersect). Change the vector of pressure (which is generally superior, posterior and lateral to some degree) while monitoring for a drop in tenderness in the spine (Fig. 15-16). When the vector associated with a maximal drop in spinal tenderness is found, maintain this pressure until both regions relax. There may even be a change in the patient's breathing pattern to signify a change in autonomic function.[14]

Henri Gillet. Recall from Chapter 3 that Dr. Gillet and his colleagues find pelvic ligament dysfunction is involved in several different spinal fixation complexes—each of which affects other areas throughout the spine.[179] To aid in the treatment of these complexes, these authors suggest specific stretching techniques. To stretch the sacrospinous and sacrotuberous ligaments, the seated patient brings his knee to his chest. To stretch the posterior sacroiliac ligaments, the seated patient brings his knee across his body and in front of the opposite knee. The anterior sacroiliac ligaments are stretched by the therapist. She sits behind the seated patient and pulls his knees laterally, abducting his hips. The authors report that these gentle moves are often as effective as traditional manipulative techniques; immediate improvement in other regions of the spine is noted when ligamentous stretching is indicated. Please see *Motion Palpation and Chiropractic Technic* for further information on these complexes.

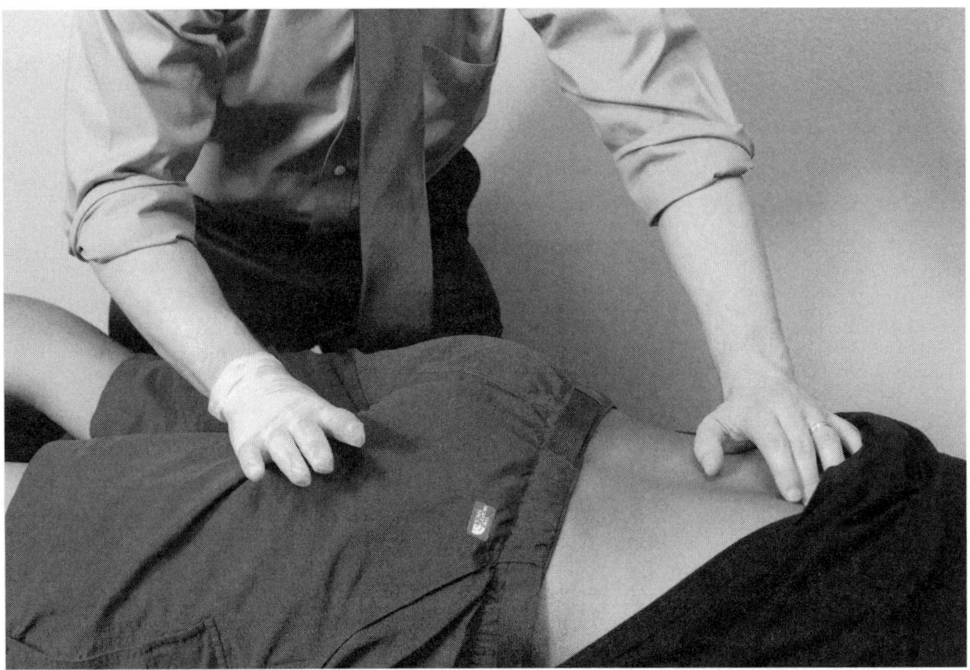

Fig. 15-16 Monitor the spine for a drop in tenderness while pressing the junction of the sacrotuberous and sacrospinous ligaments posteriorly, superiorly, and laterally.

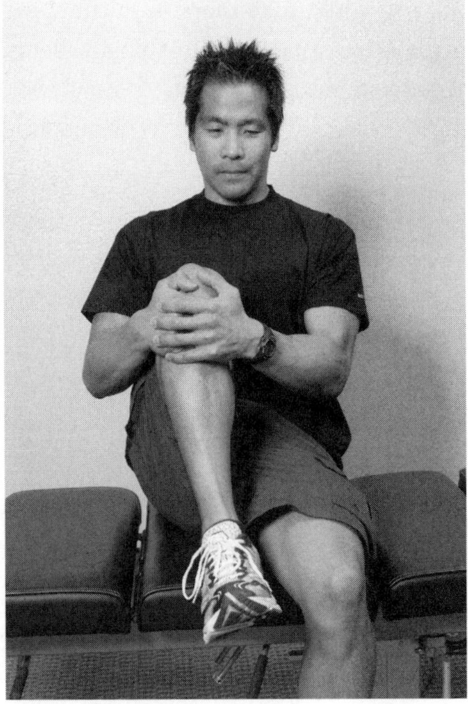

Fig. 15-17 Sacrospinous and sacrotuberous ligament stretch.

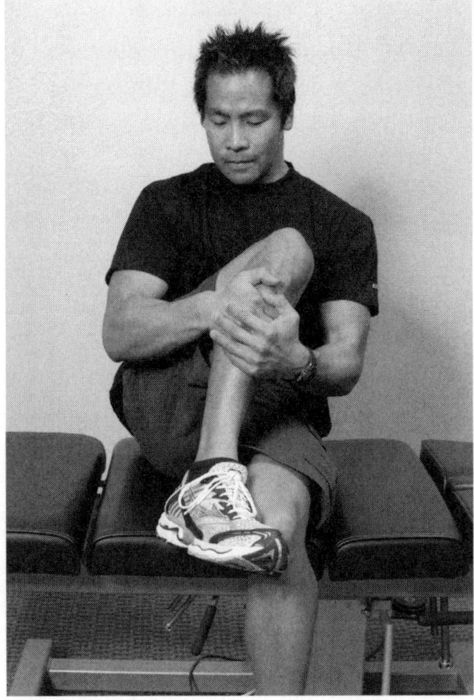

Fig. 15-18 Posterior sacroiliac ligament stretch.

CATEGORY I PELVIS

It is essential that the reader is familiar with the Category I pelvis. Briefly stated, this is a form of pelvic dysfunction described in Sacro Occipital Technique as a torsion of the pelvis without osseous misalignment at the sacroiliac joint.[14] This torsion has global repercussions, as the malalignment interferes with the flow of CSF and creates asymmetrical tension on the dura mater. In fact, as Walther points out, patients presenting with a CAT I pelvis oftentimes complain of neck pain when turning the head, as when backing up the car. Besides this, he notes, there seems to be a cause-and-effect relationship between this form of pelvic dysfunction and thoracic outlet syndrome. So powerful is the correction of the malalignment that it often negates orthopedic tests previously positive for TOS.

Presented below is the applied kinesiology approach to CAT I pelvic assessment and treatment. The author finds this method is quicker and easier to learn than the original methods described in SOT.

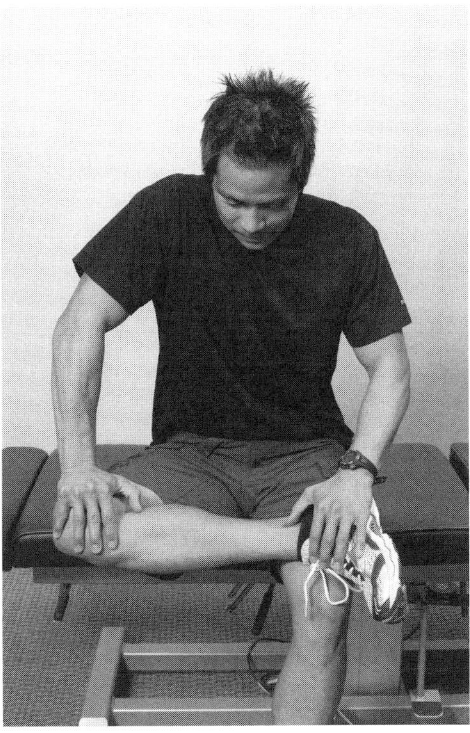

Fig. 15-19 Anterior sacroiliac ligament stretch.

Diagnosis

Assessment begins by finding a strong indicator muscle, such as the hamstrings or piriformis (Fig. 15-20 and 15-21). Then have the patient therapy localize (touch) both sacroiliac joints. This will cause the muscle to go weak if the patient has a Category I pelvis. Then touch both hands to the same sacroiliac joint. Only one side will cause weakness. This indicates the positive side.

Now, the practitioner will find what direction the pelvis is misaligned in by gently pressing on the PSIS and opposite ischial tuberosity and then testing the indicator muscle. This is repeated by pressing on the opposite PSIS and ischial tuberosity (Fig. 15-22). One of these will cause weakening. The pelvis is misaligned in the direction the clinician's pressure caused the pelvis to rebound towards. In other words, if the patient's hamstring became inhibited when the therapist pushed posterior-anterior on the right PSIS and left ischial tuberosity, then the patient has a posteriorly rotated right pelvis and anteriorly rotated left pelvis.

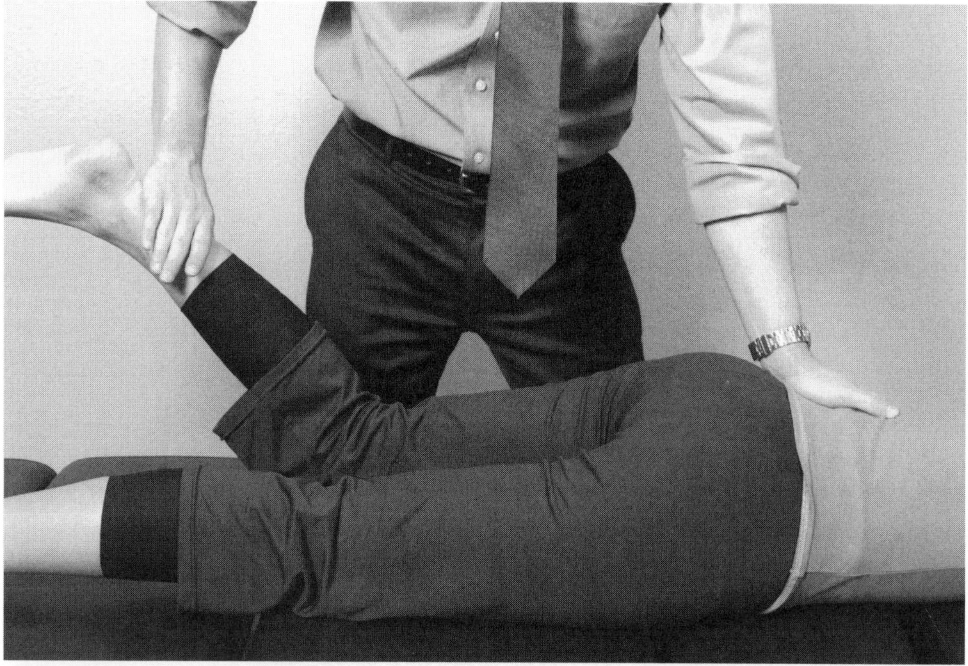

Fig. 15-20 Muscle testing the hamstrings. The applied kinesiology muscle test is not a traditional strength test. Instead, it is more gentle and is an evaluation of the patient's ability to recruit the muscle when asked to "hold." A positive test is a muscle which cannot immediately lock when gentle resistance is applied.

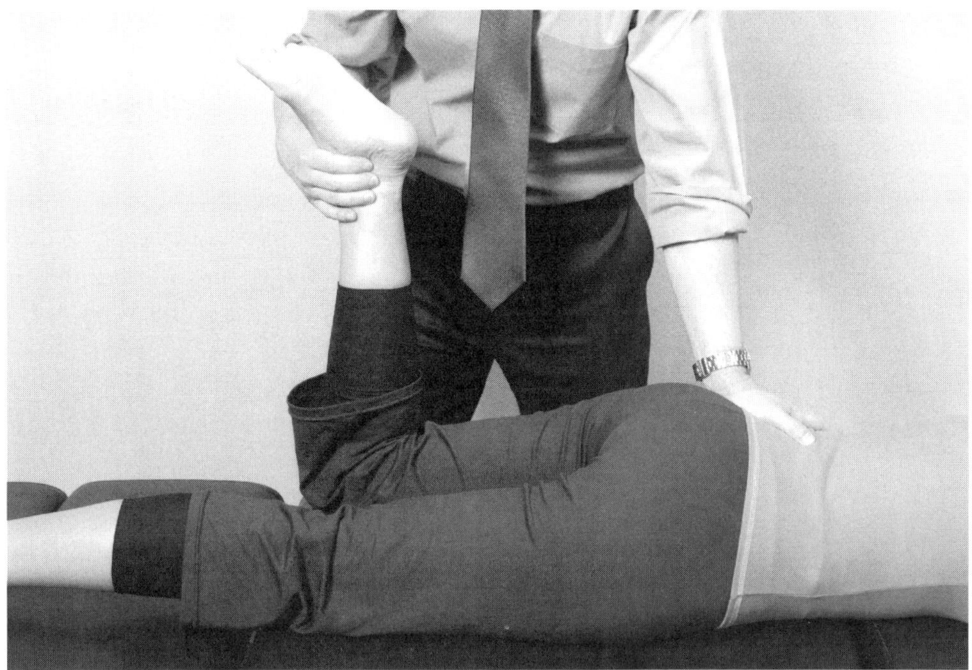

Fig. 15-21 Muscle testing the piriformis.

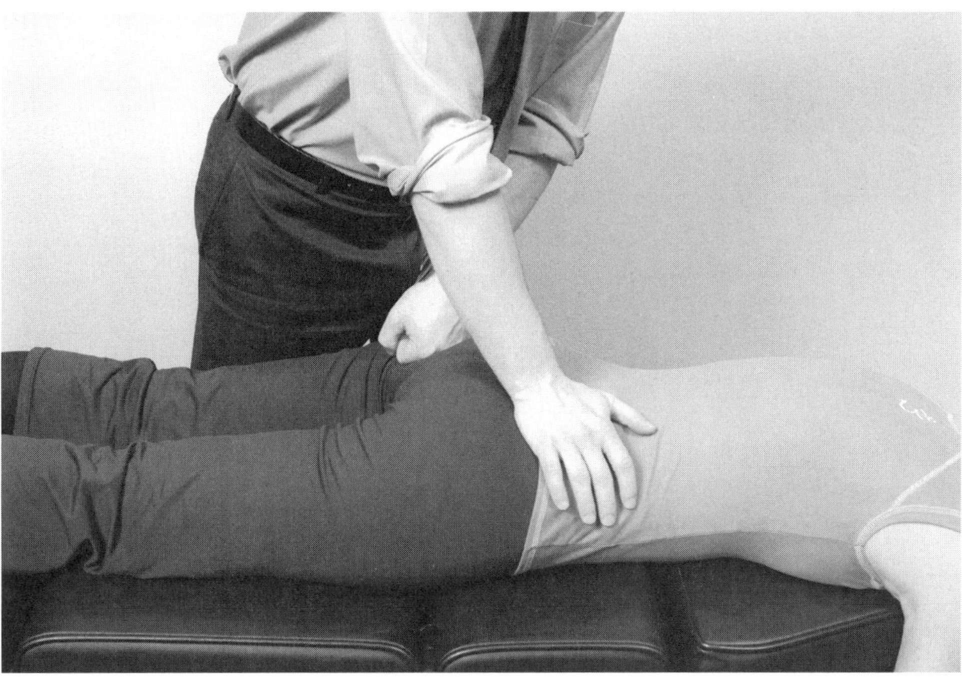

Fig. 15-22 Challenging the pelvis. Push posterior-anterior on the PSIS and opposite ischial tuberosity and then re-test the indicator muscle.

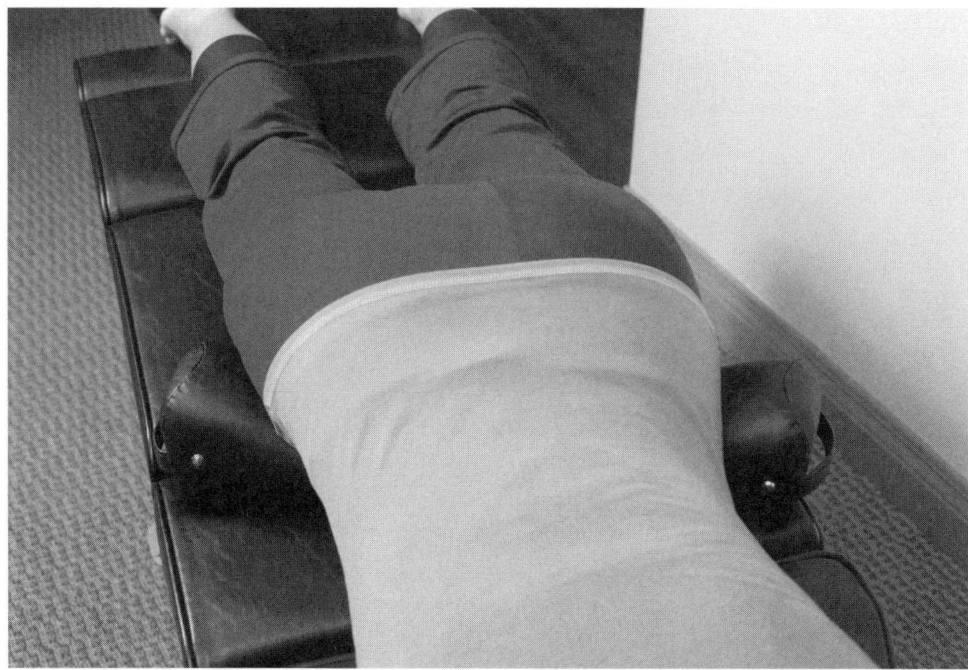

Fig. 15-23 Blocking the patient with a CAT I pelvis, right posterior and left anterior.

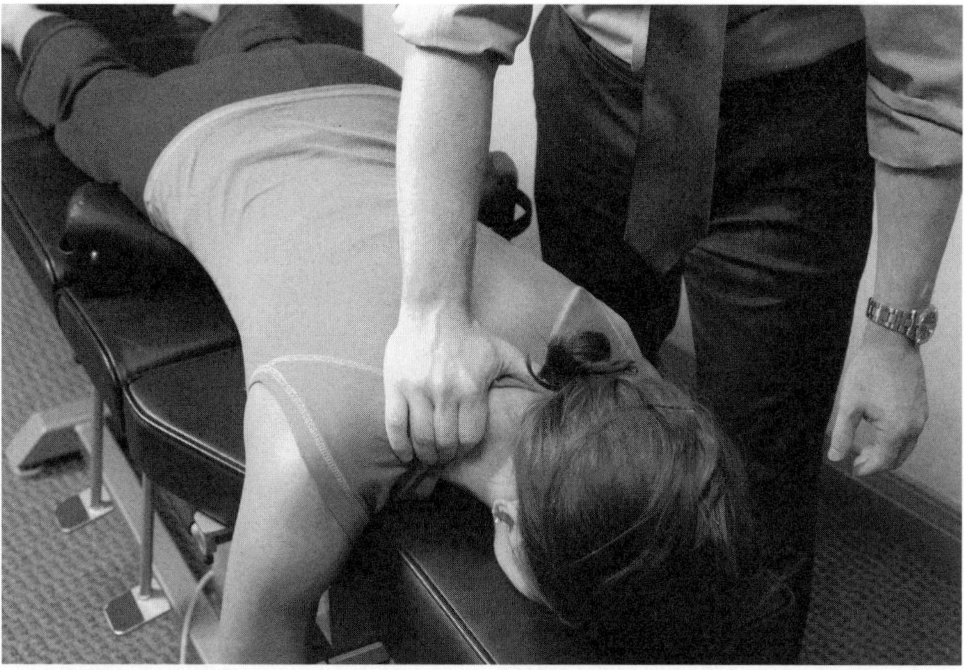

Fig. 15-24 The patient with CAT I pelvic dysfunction will have tenderness of the first rib on one side. This tenderness will diminish with appropriate therapy and can be used as a way to monitor the efficacy of treatment.

Treatment

To treat the patient, DeJarnette blocks are used (but shoes or towel rolls may be substituted as well). With the patient prone, the blocks are placed under the patient's ASIS and lesser trochanter so that the weight of the body causes a corrective rotation at the pelvis. For the example described above, put the blocks under the right lesser trochanter and the left ASIS (Fig. 15-23). Have the blocks/shoes facing one another, and leave the patient on them for 2-10'. The practitioner can monitor the patient's response by feeling the first rib (Fig. 15-24). On one side the patient with a CAT I pelvis will have tenderness that diminishes when he is placed on the blocks in the proper position. After several minutes, this tenderness will drop even further.

POSTURE OF THE PELVIS

The pelvis most often falls into an anterior tilt posture. This stresses the lumbosacral articulation, the lumbar spine, the sacroiliac joints, the pubic symphysis and the hip joints. The various structural malalignments described previously also place undue stress on the pelvis while adding asymmetrical stress to the rest of the body. Consider this in all patients, as the pelvis is not only the foundation of the spine, but it also has myofascial and neurological connections capable of influencing the entire body. This makes manual correction of structural/functional pelvic asymmetry a priority. It should also be noted that when correction does not hold, the practitioner must look at true functional shortcomings (small hemipelvis, short leg syndrome) as potential aggravating factors needing correction.

MOVEMENT PATTERNS

The pelvis tends to fall into the lower crossed pattern just as one would expect. This involves an anterior pelvic tilt due to hypertonicity of the erector spinae and iliopsoas along with inhibition of the lower abdominals and hip extensors. This imbalance affects numerous movement patterns of the spine, pelvis, and lower extremity. Most notable is the excessive anterior tilt during arising from sitting as diagnosed and treated by Alexander. Of course, this one motion is not the only time dysfunctional pelvic motor control negatively affects the body. After all, the pelvis and "core" musculature are the foundation from which lower extremity and spinal motion are anchored upon. To be sure, any aberrant pelvic motion or instability will result in problems throughout the kinetic chain.

A frequent casualty of pelvic muscle imbalance is incompetence of the abdominal and pelvic floor muscles. This compromises the stability of the lumbar spine provided by the abdominal cavity. This allows the lumbar spine and abdominal viscera to translate anteriorly, thereby bringing the person's center of gravity further forward in the process. Along with loss of core strength is the loss of optimal force closure normally providing pelvic stability. This allows for excessive sacroiliac motion, creating or maintaining local problems.

Pelvic floor dysfunction adds to the problems described above by compromising abdominal cavity pressure and lessening force closure of the pelvis. This creates pelvic instability and the eventual onset of symptoms. In fact, O'Sullivan and Beales found that patients with sacroiliac joint dysfunction, particularly those with a positive active straight leg raise test, had improper breathing patterns as well as poorly functioning pelvic floor muscles.[180] Retraining both areas led to improved functional ability in these areas, and more importantly led to a negative active straight leg raise test and the elimination of symptoms. Weak pelvic floor muscles will also invite visceral problems such as incontinence. Exercising these muscles while also removing the cause of their inhibition will benefit the patient on all fronts.

ENERGY-BASED THERAPIES

Auricular Acupressure. Gently squeeze the point corresponding to the pelvis with two fingers. Hold for 5 seconds, then relax 5 seconds. Increase the amount of pressure with each cycle for a total time of one minute (6 cycles). Do this initially on the ear on the involved side only; treat the opposite ear as well if the patient does not improve.

Reflexology. Begin by massaging the entire foot. Walk up the foot with the thumbs along the five zones. Treat both the plantar and dorsal surfaces. Work the toes as well. Spend extra time on the medial border of the foot corresponding with the spine. Also, work on areas associated with different organs needing an extra "boost." Following this long warm-up, massage the area on the foot corresponding with the pelvis.

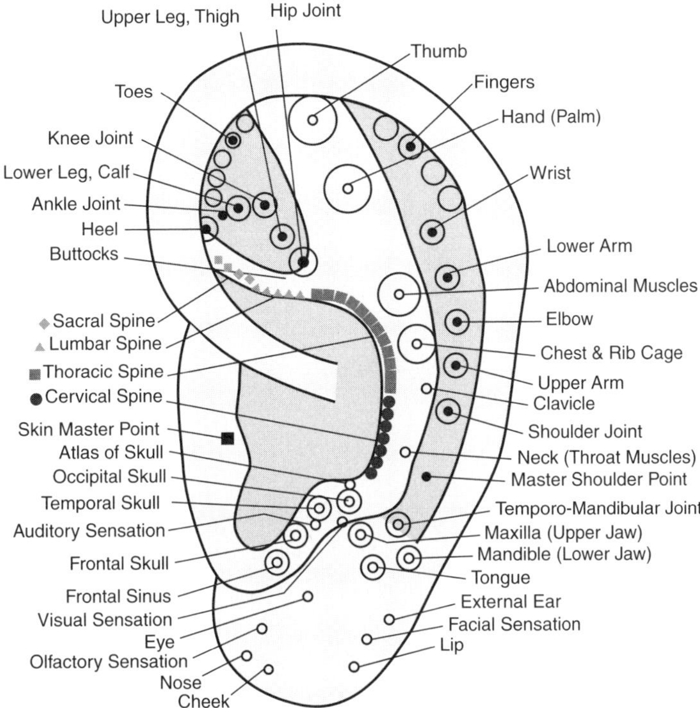

Fig. 15-25

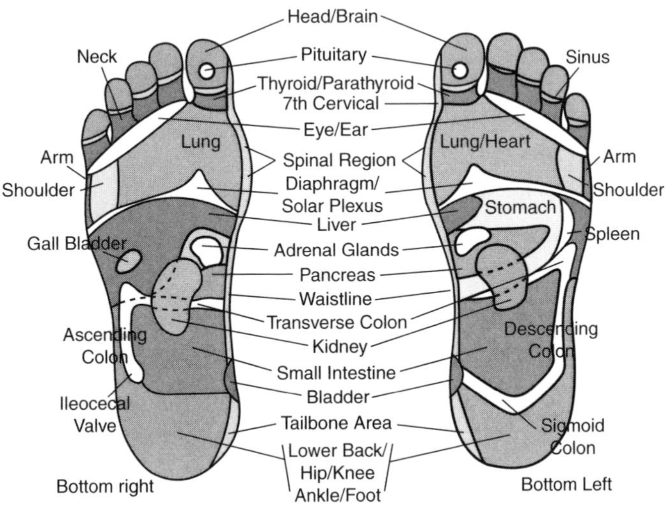

Fig. 15-26

THE HIGH-YIELD SCAN

Perform a scan of the other high-yield elements of the body including:

- Gait
- Posture
- Sit-to-Stand
- Miniature Squat
- Respiration
- Romberg Test
- Fukuda's Test
- Upper Cervical Spine
- Middle and Lower Cervical Spine
- TMJ
- Feet
- Stress Screen

EVALUATION AND TREATMENT OF THE SECONDARY FACTORS

Please see the corresponding section in Ch. 14, the Lumbar Spine for ways to reduce stress on the pelvic girdle. In addition to these factors, also address the following habits:

Sitting. The way a person sits can also influence the condition of his pelvic girdle. For instance, many people tend to cross their legs when they sit. Moreover, many are predisposed to crossing their legs in a particular pattern. This causes patterns of strain and compression in the hip and pelvic girdle. Encourage the patient to avoid this way of sitting.

Standing. Individuals frequently stand more on one leg than the other. Look for this in the clinic, and ask the patient to note any preferences at home. Encourage him to make a conscious effort to stand with his weight evenly distributed so that aberrant stress is not borne by the pelvic girdle secondary to this habit.

16 The Hip

EXAMINATION AND TREATMENT OF THE PRIMARY FACTORS

Iliopsoas. Palpate the muscle for hypertonicity, fascial adhesions, tenderness, and trigger points. Utilize soft tissue techniques including myofascial release, sustained pressure, and strumming to address the findings (Fig. 16-1). Post-isometric relaxation and strain/counterstrain are also useful in reducing tone (Fig. 16-2 to 16-4).

The iliopsoas is facilitated as part of the common pattern. This alters hip, pelvic, and lumbar spine mechanics. It also refers pain to the low back. This point is missed by many clinicians, as the patient does not complain of pain anteriorly. In fact, most people are astonished to have pain upon palpation, although the rapid improvement after massaging this muscle is a welcomed surprise.

Expect the iliopsoas to compress the hip joint and to keep the femur in a flexed position. This stresses the joint itself while greatly altering the gait mechanism. Contracture will even tension the shoulder girdle and can be involved in upper quarter complaints. In short, dysfunction in this muscle wreaks havoc on the body. Remember to examine it in all patients with hip, lumbopelvic, or lower quarter complaints. For more information on the iliopsoas please consult Liz Koch's The Psoas Book, an entire text dedicated to this muscle. Besides providing wonderful treatment options for psoas dysfunction, Koch discusses how emotions (especially fear) influence this muscle.

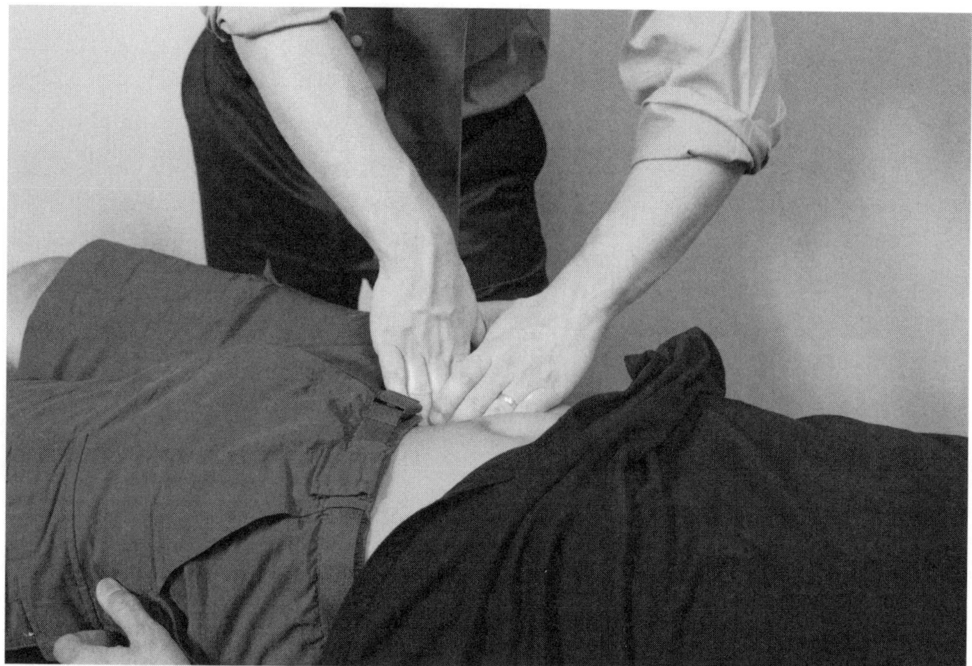

Fig. 16-1 The clinician can apply MFR, sustained pressure, strumming and ischemic compression in this position.

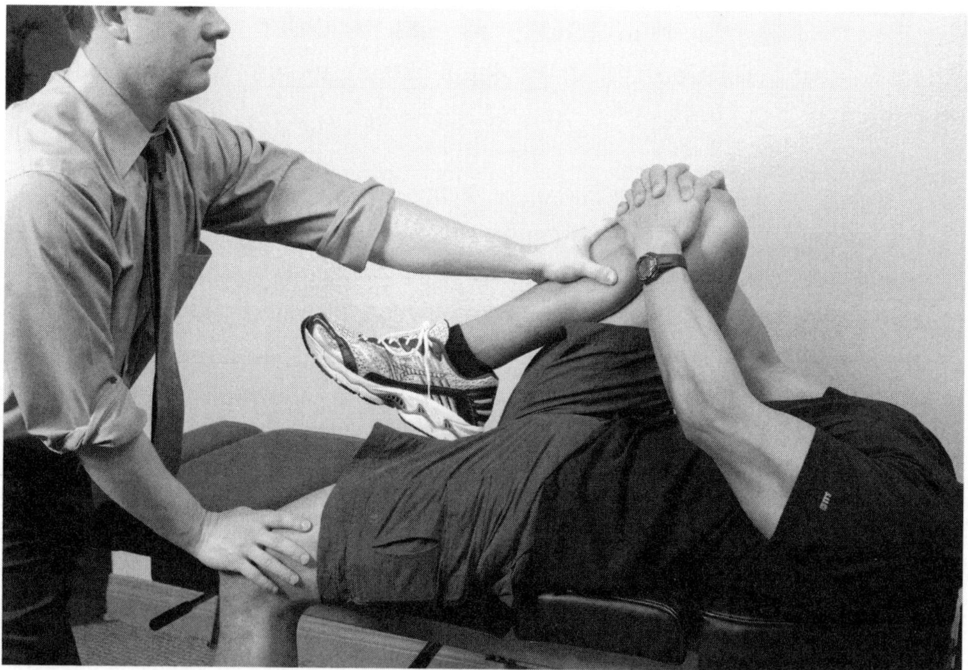

Fig. 16-2 Post-isometric relaxation stretching of the iliopsoas. The patient is in the Thomas test position with the affected leg hanging off the table. Have the patient gently flex the hip into resistance. Upon relaxation, take the hip into further extension. If the hip is externally rotated due to iliopsoas contracture, prevent further external rotation during the maneuver.

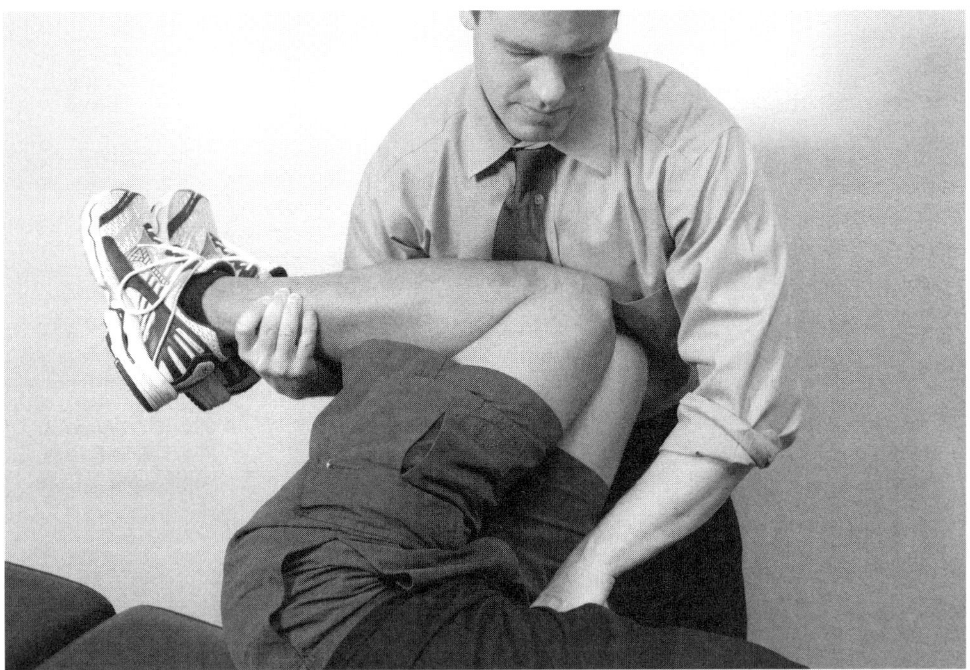

Fig. 16-3 Strain-counterstrain of the psoas. There are multiple tender points along the anterior surface of the psoas. One frequently involved is found two inches lateral and slightly inferior to the umbilicus. The position of ease involves flexing the hips 90 degrees, bringing the knees 60 degrees towards the ipsilateral side, and raising the feet to impart contralateral sidebending.[164]

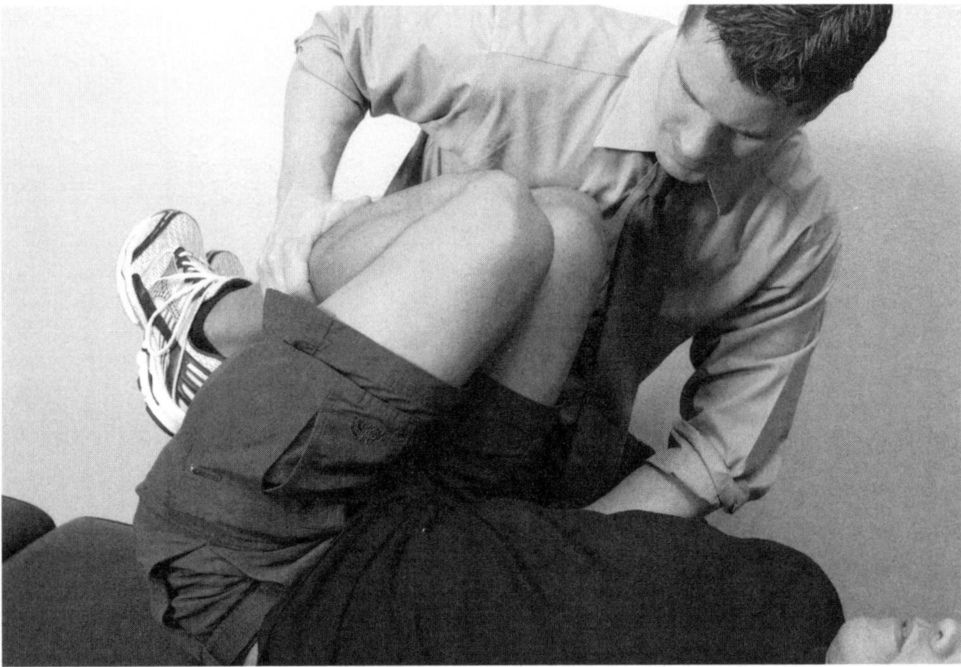

Fig. 16-4 Strain-counterstrain of the iliacus. Find the tender point just medial to the ASIS. Find the position of ease by flexing the hips, bringing them out to the ipsilateral side, and then laterally flexing to the ipsi- or contralateral side.

Hip Adductors. Palpate these muscles for hypertonicity, fascial adhesions, tenderness, and trigger points. Utilize soft tissue techniques including myofascial release, sustained pressure, strumming and ischemic compression to address the findings. Post-isometric relaxation is also useful in reducing tone and increasing flexibility (Fig. 16-5).

The adductors are facilitated as part of the common pattern. This causes weight bearing on the supero-lateral surface of the acetabulum, leading to hip pain and eventually osteoarthritis. At the knee, this posturing results in genu valgus. Local problems including groin strains are precipitated and/or perpetuated by this hypertonicity as well.

Tensor Fascia Lata. Palpate the muscle for hypertonicity, fascial adhesions, tenderness, and trigger points. Utilize soft tissue techniques including myofascial release, sustained pressure, strumming and ischemic compression to address the findings. Post-isometric relaxation is useful in reducing tone and increasing flexibility.

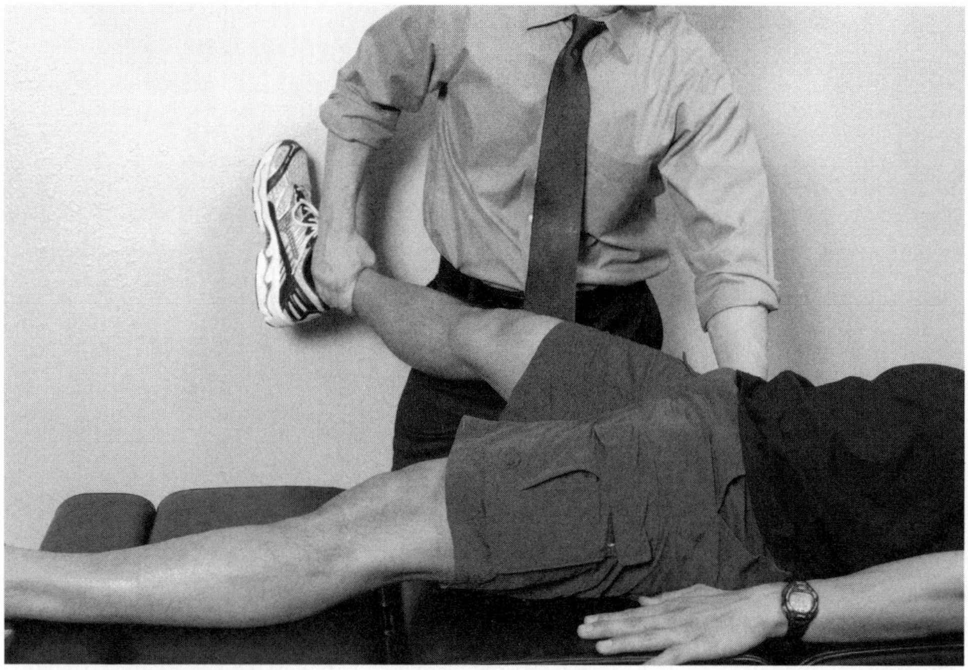

Fig. 16-5 PIR stretching of the hip adductors. Stretch the hip further into abduction following the patient's contraction into adduction.

The TFL is facilitated as part of the common pattern. This helps to further flex and internally rotate the femur, thereby stressing the hip and knee. TFL facilitation also tensions and changes the tracking of the iliotibial band. This contributes to problems including trochanteric bursitis, iliotibial band friction syndrome, patellofemoral syndrome, and sacroiliac joint dysfunction. Worthy of note is Schamberger's observation that the left ITB becomes strongly facilitated in all cases of sacroiliac malalignment no matter what the malposition. This signifies a form of neurological influence rather than tightening due to mechanical shortening or stretching.

Hip Abductors. Palpate theses muscles for hypertonicity, fascial adhesions, tenderness, and trigger points. Utilize soft tissue techniques including myofascial release, sustained pressure, strumming and ischemic compression to address the findings. Strain/counterstrain is also useful in reducing tone (Fig. 16-6).

The hip abductors are inhibited as part of the common pattern. This leads to coxa vara and weight bearing on the superior-lateral surface of the acetabulum. Expect tender

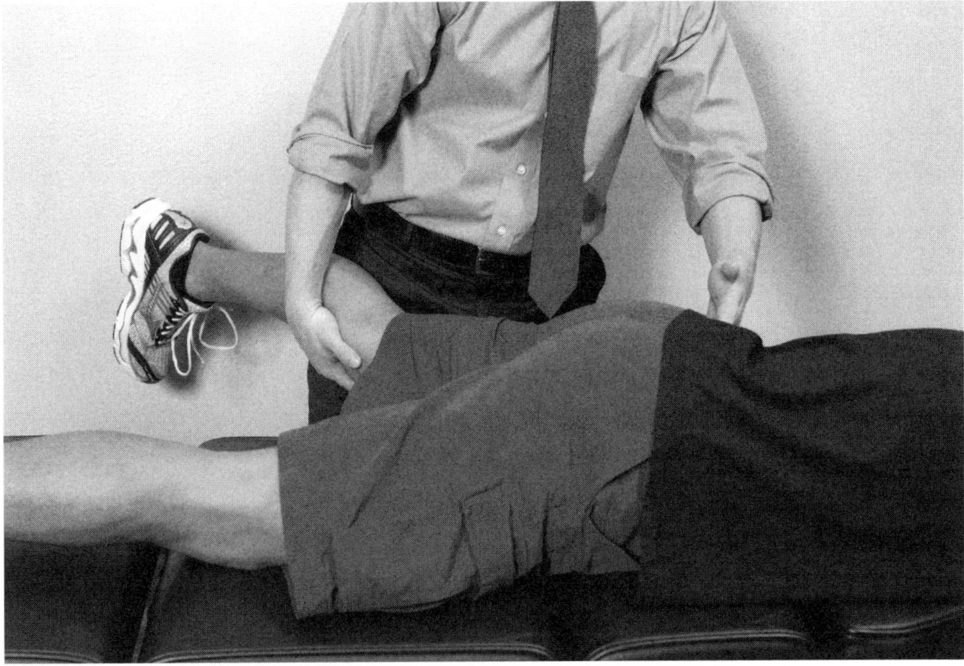

Fig. 16-6 Strain-counterstrain of the gluteus minimus. The position of ease is marked hip abduction combined with slight flexion or extension and internal or external rotation.

points in these muscles to cause/perpetuate hip and low back pain syndromes. Trigger points in the gluteus medius refer to the low back, sacroiliac region, and buttock. Trigger points in the gluteus minimus have a wider referral pattern, spreading from the buttock down the posterolateral thigh and leg. Travell and Simon[68] refer to the gluteus minimus's referral pattern as a form of "pseudo-sciatica."

Piriformis. Palpate the muscle for hypertonicity, fascial adhesions, tenderness, and trigger points. Utilize soft tissue techniques including myofascial release, sustained pressure, strumming and ischemic compression to address the findings. Post-isometric relaxation and strain/counterstrain are also useful in reducing tone (Fig. 16-7 and 16-8).

The piriformis is infamous for causing a variety of problems, including sciatic nerve entrapment, hip dysfunction, and sacroiliac dysfunction. Trigger points in this muscle can even refer down the lower extremity, mimicking sciatica symptoms. The manual therapist must be aware of the piriformis' role in each of these cases and treat it

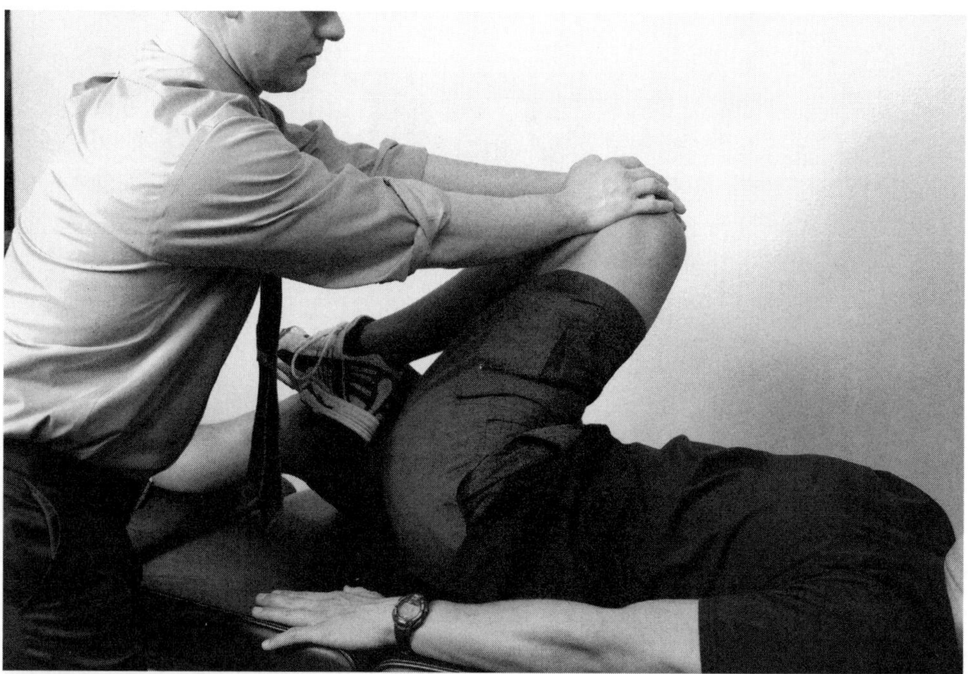

Fig. 16-7 Post-isometric relaxation stretching of the piriformis. Grasp the supine patient's knee, bringing the hip into adduction, flexion, and internal rotation. Have him gently contract into hip abduction, extension, and external rotation. Upon relaxation, take the hip into further adduction, flexion, and internal rotation.

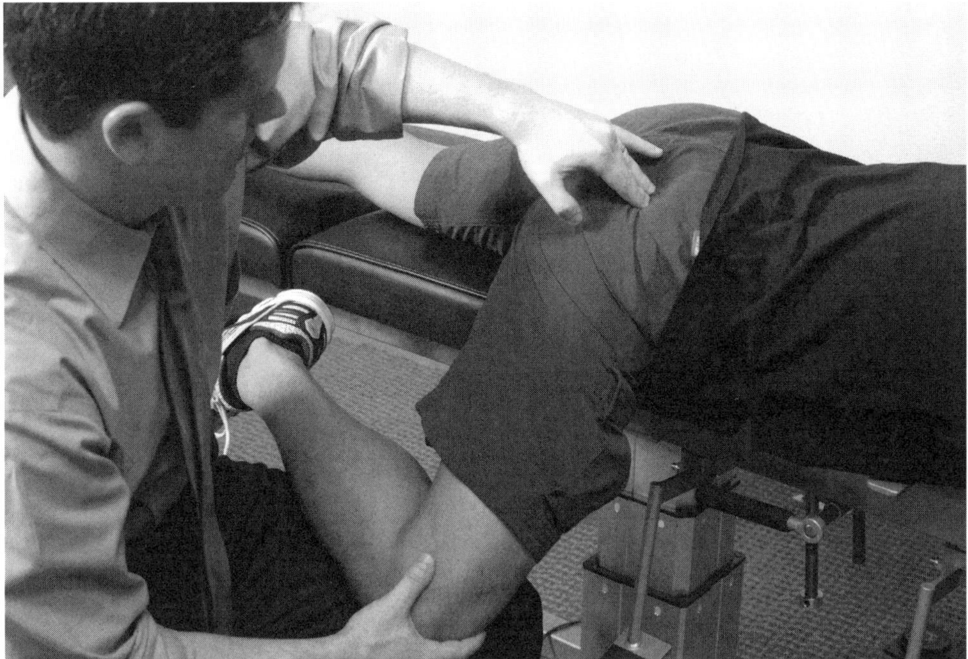

Fig. 16-8 Strain-counterstrain of the piriformis. Find the tender point in the belly of the muscle. The position of ease involves hip flexion, abduction, and external rotation.

accordingly to achieve a successful outcome. Besides this, he must find the cause of piriformis dysfunction. This can occur with sacroiliac problems or segmental dysfunction at L4/5. It may also be due to over-stretching of the muscle secondary to excessive hip internal rotation.

Upledger adds that the piriformis can negatively affect the craniosacral system due to its attachment on the sacrum. This is just one more reason to address this important muscle.

Gluteus Maximus. Palpate the muscle for hypertonicity, fascial adhesions, tenderness, and trigger points. Utilize soft tissue techniques including myofascial release, sustained pressure, strumming and ischemic compression to address the findings. Post-isometric relaxation is useful in reducing tone and improving flexibility (Fig. 16-9).

The gluteus maximus is inhibited as part of the common pattern. This allows for increased pelvic anterior rotation, hip flexion, and hip internal rotation. Hypertonicity in the muscle can also result in low back pain; Walther suggests treating it with

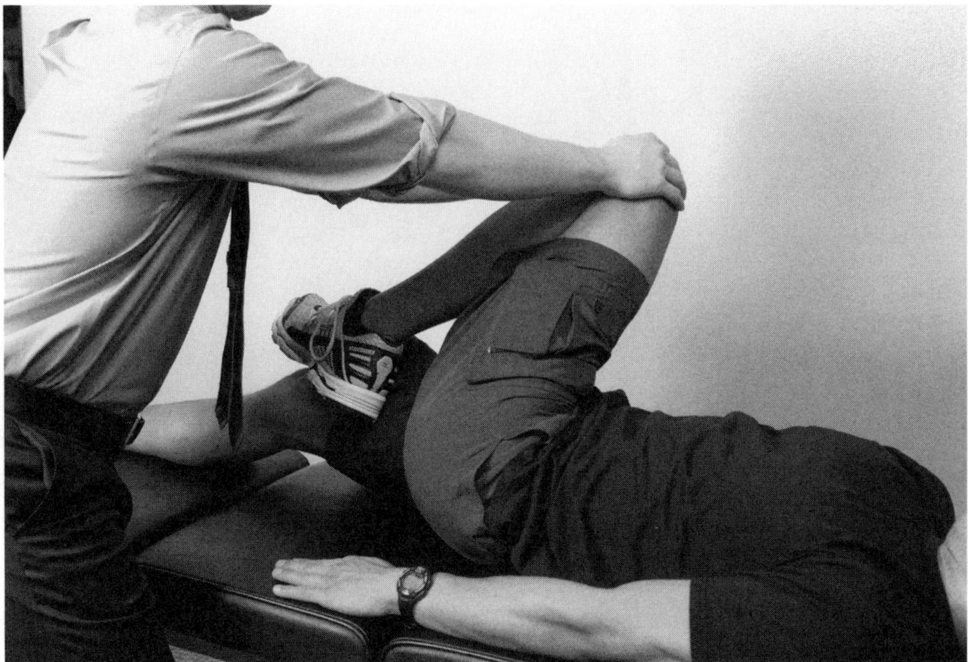

Fig. 16-9 Post-isometric relaxation stretching of the gluteus maximus. Have the supine patient gently extend and slightly externally rotate the hip into resistance. Follow this by stretching the hip into flexion and slight internal rotation.

strain/counterstrain in conjunction with specific treatment of the iliolumbar ligament. As with the piriformis, Upledger believes the gluteus maximus influences the craniosacral system due to its origination on the sacrum.

MUSCLE STRENGTH

Evaluate the strength of the hip muscles with traditional methods. Make sure to assess both the ability to initiate a contraction as well as sheer strength. Most often, what we perceive as weakness is more a matter of inhibition. This will follow the common pattern and/or be due to local or segmental dysfunction. Treating the causative factor restores normal strength in these cases. In cases of true muscle weakness, such as those involving muscle atrophy, remedial strengthening is indicated. This is done with traditional strengthening techniques. Remember to begin strength training with light weight, having the patient focus mostly on muscle contraction and recruitment of the target muscle. Then, as strength and control improve, advance the patient into weight-bearing, functional exercises to maximally challenge the weak muscle.

FEMORAL HEAD MOBILITY

The femoral head most often subluxates anteriorly, though this is not an absolute. Consequently, the manual therapist must assess all planes of motion to determine the restricted plane(s), and deliver appropriate therapy. Utilize conventional methods of joint examination to find capsular restrictions. When one encounters capsular restrictions during testing, the examination technique is quickly turned into a therapy. It is wise to remember that capsular tightness is a common finding in the hip joint. When present it will restrict internal rotation, extension, and adduction.

HIP POSTURE

Examine the posture of the hip with two different goals in mind. First, look at the position of the femur in relation to the acetabulum. From the common pattern, we can expect it to be flexed, internally rotated, and adducted in the majority of individuals. However, there are patients with differing presentations, so do not blindly assume this posture is present.

The second thing to assess is the position of the pelvis. This is important because the pelvis' position helps determine the position of the femoral head. It also changes the demands placed on the femur. For instance, an anteriorly tilted pelvis necessitates the femur flex more than average during normal gait. A posteriorly-rotated hemipelvis forces extra extension during normal gait. Either malposition places added strain on a joint complex best utilized at mid-range and not end-range. Expect these malpositions to alter demands on local muscle groups and distant joints in addition to just affecting the coxafemoral joint.

SEGMENTAL DYSFUNCTION

Dysfunction of the thoracolumbar junction and the L2 and L3 levels may directly cause referred pain in the hip. Dysfunction in L3-S1 causes hip problems as well by changing muscular recruitment patterns.

MOVEMENT PATTERNS

The hip follows the lower crossed pattern as one might expect. The manual therapist has many different ways to examine for this. General observation is the most basic method. Look for the patient to display excessive hip flexion/internal rotation/adduction during gait; this is made much worse with squatting, rising from sitting or ascending stairs.

Improper muscle recruitment patterns often go hand-in-hand with this pattern. A technique described by Greenman is useful in assessing these by palpating specific muscles during the initiation of motion. The first of these is used to test the recruitment pattern used in hip extension. Extension should begin with hamstring contraction, followed by contraction of the gluteus maximus, contralateral lower lumbar erector spinae, and ipsilateral lower erector spinae. A common dysfunctional firing pattern involves early firing of the hamstrings and erector spinae muscles.[5]

Hip abduction is assessed with muscle palpation in a similar manner. One should feel the muscles fire in the following sequence: gluteus medius, tensor fascia lata, quadratus lumborum, and erector spinae. A dysfunctional pattern often involves early contraction of the tensor fascia lata or quadratus lumborum.[5]

Treatment for these faulty movement patterns begins by teaching the patient to recruit inhibited muscles during activities of daily living. In combination with this, he should be taught to hold the pelvis and hips in the proper position during normal activities. Special emphasis should be placed on ascending/descending stairs, bicycling, and arising from sitting.

A great aid to helping the patient recruit inhibited muscles is by having him practice the hip extension and abduction tests. He can be shown how to palpate the hip muscles just as the clinician did and taught how to recruit these muscles in the proper fashion. This will help him turn these muscles on in more functional situations where he needs these muscles to fire.

Last, but certainly not least, the clinician must assess the entire gait mechanism. Remember from Chapter 4 that the kinetic chain connects virtually all bodyparts during gait; this means the therapist must include the entire locomotor system in his assessment. Please see Chapters 4 and 6 for specific details on the biomechanics of gait as well as available therapies.

ENERGY-BASED TECHNIQUES

Auricular Acupressure. Gently squeeze the point corresponding to the hip with two fingers. Hold for 5 seconds, then relax 5 seconds. Increase the amount of pressure with each cycle for a total time of one minute (6 cycles). Do this initially on the ear on the involved side only; treat the opposite ear as well if the patient does not improve.

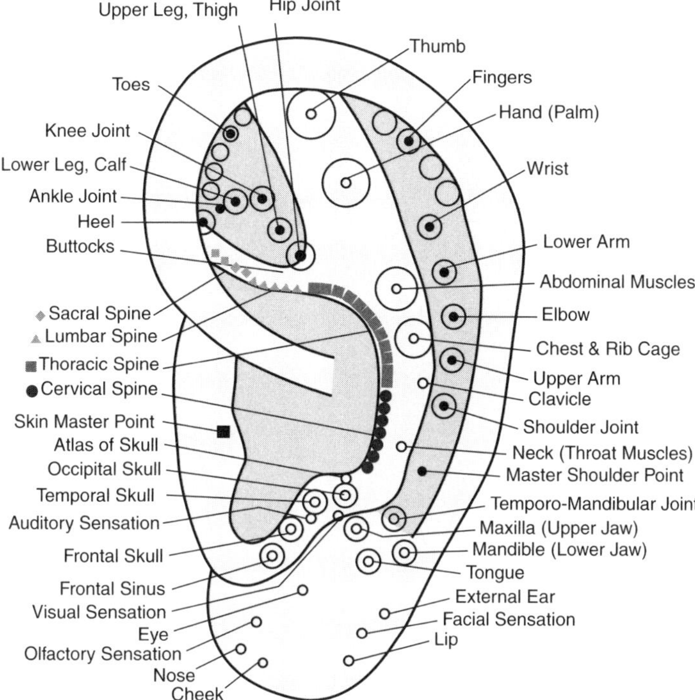

Fig. 16-10

Reflexology. Begin by massaging the entire foot. Walk up the foot with the thumbs along the five zones. Treat both the plantar and dorsal surfaces. Work the toes as well. Spend extra time on the medial border of the foot corresponding with the spine. Also, work on areas associated with different organs needing an extra "boost." Following this long warm-up, massage the area on the foot corresponding to the hip.

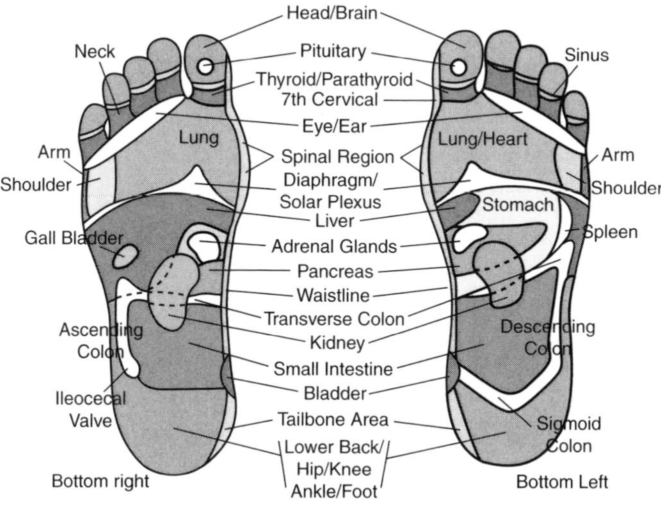

Fig. 16-11

EVALUATION OF HIGH-YIELD REGIONS

Perform a scan of the high-yield elements of the body including:

- Gait
- Posture
- Sit-to-Stand
- Miniature Squat
- Respiration
- Romberg Test
- Fukuda's Test
- Upper Cervical Spine
- Middle Cervical Spine
- TMJ
- Pelvis
- Feet
- Stress Screen

EVALUATION AND TREATMENT OF THE SECONDARY FACTORS

Sleeping. Lying on the affected hip usually aggravates the patient's symptoms, so it is advised to have him sleep on the opposite side. Besides this, instruct him to place a pillow between the knees to prevent excessive adduction that will occur if the knee falls onto the bed.

If circumstances (such as bilateral hip pain) necessitate the patient sleep on the affected leg it is best to unweight the hip. This is accomplished by placing pillows under the lumbar spine and ribcage so the greater trochanter does not take all of the person's weight. It can also be helpful to put small pillows under the ilium to further unweight the greater trochanter.

Standing. Please see corresponding section in Chapter 15, The Pelvis.

Sitting. Please see corresponding section in Chapter 15, The Pelvis.

17 The Knee

EVALUATION AND TREATMENT OF THE PRIMARY FACTORS

Quadriceps. Palpate these muscles for hypertonicity, fascial adhesions, tenderness, and trigger points. Utilize soft tissue techniques including myofascial release, sustained pressure, strumming and ischemic compression to address the findings. Post-isometric relaxation is also useful in reducing tone and improving flexibility (Fig. 17-1).

> *The quadriceps is inhibited as part of the common pattern. This affects the tibiofemoral joint, the patellofemoral joint, and the quadriceps muscle itself. Pathology in each often ensues. Soft tissue work applied to the quadriceps is beneficial in its ability to reduce localized pain and improve muscle activation if dysfunction is present.*

Hamstrings. Palpate these muscles for hypertonicity, fascial adhesions, tenderness, and trigger points. Utilize soft tissue techniques including myofascial release, sustained pressure, strumming and ischemic compression to address the findings. Post-isometric relaxation is also useful in reducing tone and improving flexibility (Fig. 17-2).

> *The hamstrings are facilitated as part of the common pattern. They neurologically "overpower" the quadriceps and lead to further quadriceps inhibition. With the prolonged facilitation the hamstrings are under it is no wonder these muscles are strained over and over again in many people. Quite frankly, the demand placed on them is just too high.*

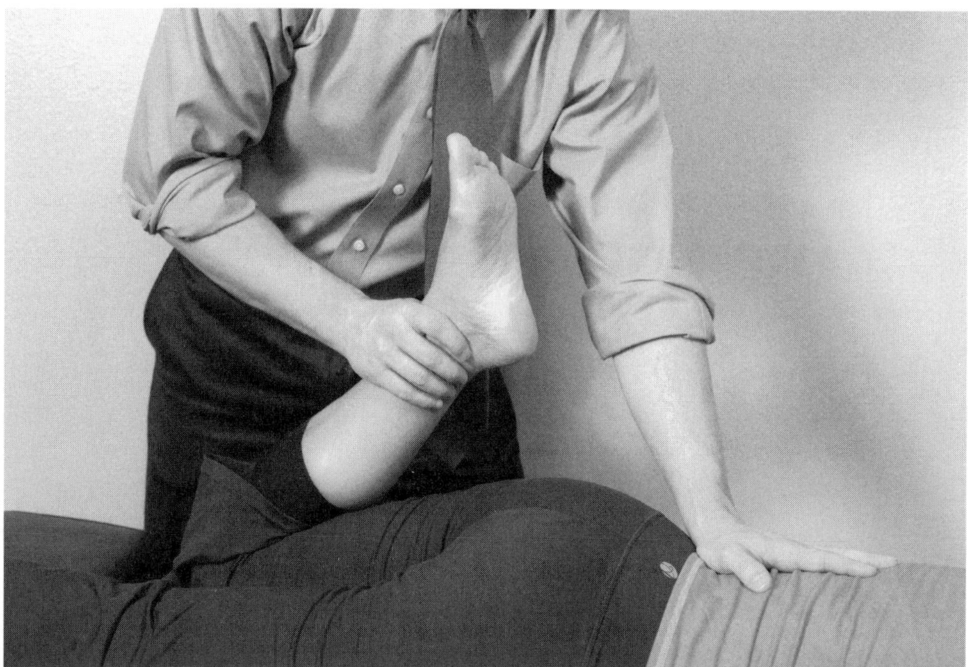

Fig. 17-1 PIR of the quadriceps. Have the patient extend her leg against resistance followed by a stretch into knee flexion. To stretch the rectus femoris do the same and also have the patient flex the hip into resistance; stretch it into extension upon relaxation.

Another problem involving the hamstrings is sciatic nerve impingement, typically following a muscle strain. This is believed to be caused by scarring-down of the nerve during the healing process. Suffice it to say, without direct treatment this problem may not resolve itself and the patient is left with a constant pain in the hamstring area. Do not confuse this with muscle pain. Use adverse neural tension tests to differentiate neural from muscle dysfunction. A quick way to do this is by adding dorsiflexion to a straight-leg raise test; if pain worsens in the belly of the hamstring, neural entrapment is indicated. Adding cervical flexion, hip internal rotation and adduction are other ways the clinician can bias this test towards neural compression.

Iliotibial Band. Palpate the muscle for hypertonicity, fascial adhesions, tenderness, and trigger points. Utilize soft tissue techniques including myofascial release, sustained pressure, strumming and ischemic compression to address the findings.

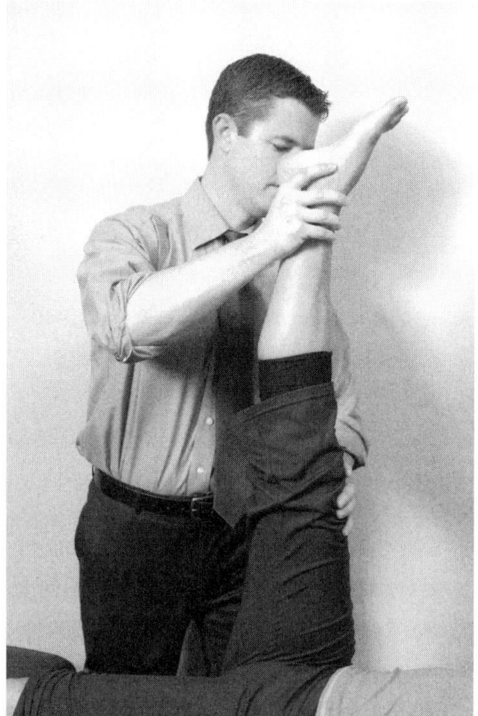

Fig. 17-2 PIR of the hamstrings. Have the supine patient flex the knee and extend the hip into resistance. Upon relaxation, stretch the patient into knee extension and hip flexion.

The ITB is notorious for being contracted. This causes localized pain where it passes over the lateral femoral epicondyle. It also causes lateral patellar tracking by way of increased lateral retinacular tension. Localized treatment is often beneficial in the short-term to help normalize patellar tracking. Successful long-term management must address the causes of ITB contracture.

Popliteus. Palpate the muscle for hypertonicity, fascial adhesions, tenderness, and trigger points. Utilize soft tissue techniques including myofascial release, sustained pressure, strumming and ischemic compression to address the findings. Post-isometric relaxation stretching is also useful in reducing tone and improving flexibility (Fig. 17-3).

The popliteus is the forgotten knee muscle due to its location. However, it has the power to influence joint mechanics and cause pain. Time spent addressing dysfunction here is well-worth it.

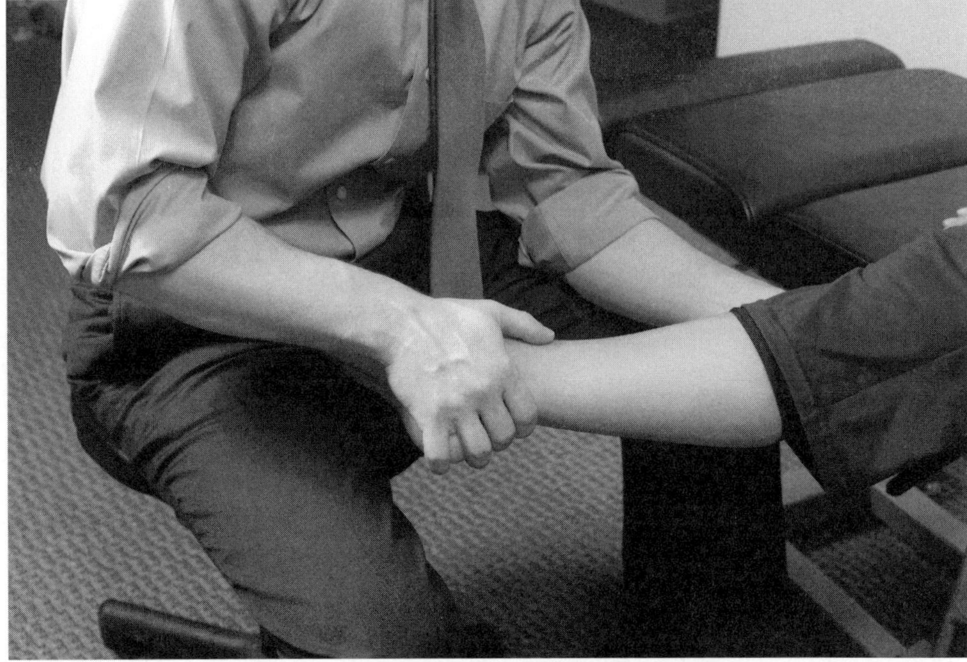

Fig. 17-3 PIR of the popliteus. The patient internally rotates and flexes the leg against resistance. Upon relaxation, stretch the leg into further external rotation and extension.

MUSCLE STRENGTH

Evaluate knee strength with traditional methods. Make sure to assess both the ability to initiate a contraction as well as sheer strength. Most often, what we perceive as weakness is more a matter of inhibition. This will follow the common pattern and/or be due to local or segmental dysfunction. Treating the causative factor restores normal strength in these cases. In cases of true muscle weakness, such as those involving muscle atrophy, remedial strengthening is indicated. This is done with traditional strengthening techniques. It is advisable to use closed-chain exercises over open-chain ones when the patient's condition allows. The miniature squat and the sensorimotor retraining exercises (from Chapter 6) are ideal in this regard; they are functional, utilize closed-chain principles, and strengthen weak/inhibited muscles such as the quadriceps and hip extensors.

The miniature squat is especially versatile in that it can be utilized by patients on both ends of the rehab spectrum. Persons with only subtle knee weakness can squat deeply to work the quadriceps, and even place more weight on the affected side to challenge the limits of his/her strength (Fig. 17-4). At the same time, the patient with acute knee pain can perform the exercise by squatting only a minimal amount (Fig. 17-5). This limits stress on the knee as well as the load on the quads. The patient can also be taught to focus on quadriceps recruitment in this position if that is the clinician's goal.

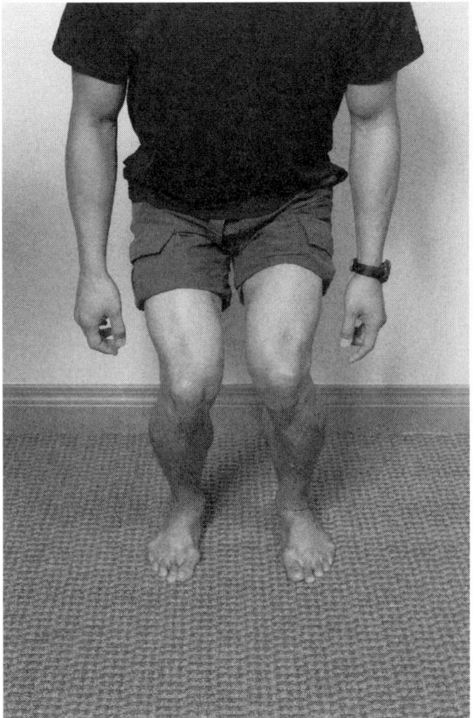

Fig. 17-4 Deep miniature squat.

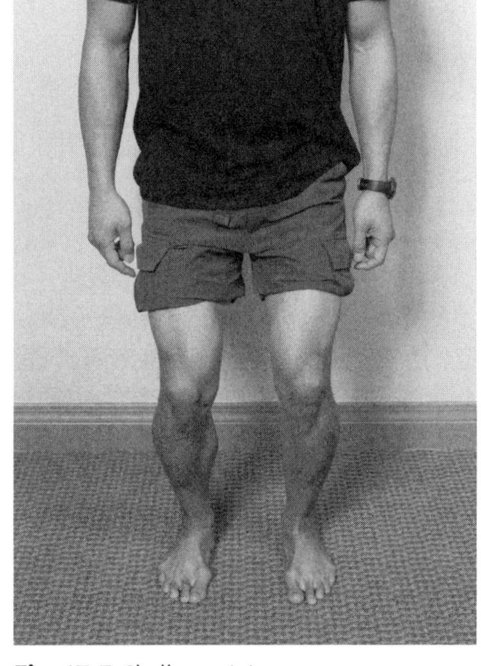

Fig. 17-5 Shallow miniature squat.

Regardless of where the patient is on the rehab spectrum, he needs to be taught to use impeccable form during the squat so that the knee and the rest of the kinetic chain are not stressed with this exercise. Starting from the ground-up, the clinician should make sure the foot, knee, hip, and pelvis stay in alignment and avoid falling into the miserable malalignment pattern (Fig. 17-6). From the top, the patient should be encouraged to utilize Alexandrian principles to optimize neuromuscular recruitment patterns. All of this ensures the patient will reap the greatest benefit from the miniature squat while not stressing the knee joint any further.

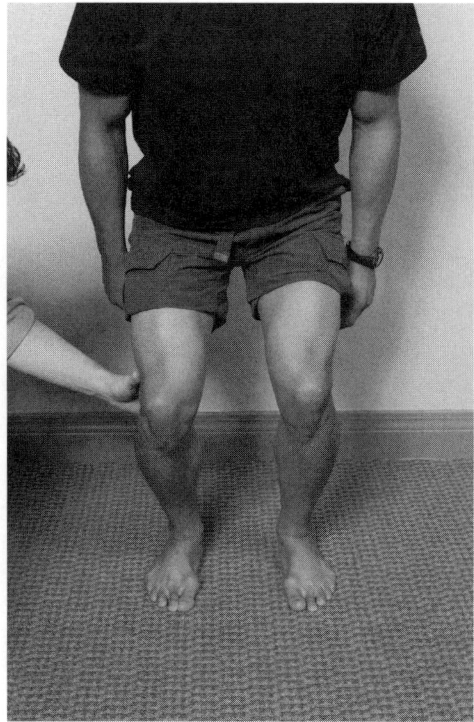

Fig. 17-6 Assuring proper patient form.

TIBIOFEMORAL JOINT MOBILITY

Assess the tibiofemoral joint's position and mobility using conventional methods. Most often, the tibia is found fixated posteriorly either unilaterally or bilaterally. Mobilize it accordingly (Fig. 17-7). It is a good idea to stay in a pain-free range of motion during treatment.

PATELLOFEMORAL JOINT MOBILITY

Assess the position and mobility of the patella. Oftentimes, it is malpositioned laterally and/or superiorly. Medially-directed patellar mobilization is frequently utilized (Fig. 17-8). This improves mobility and reduces pain at irritated joint surfaces.

Patellar taping is the best method to reduce patellofemoral symptoms immediately. Simply assess the patella's position, including its rotation, tilt, and medial-lateral position, and tape it accordingly. McConnell suggests that when this is done properly it will reduce pain by at least 50%.[181] Besides helping relieve pain, it also provides a stretch on contracted tissues (Fig. 17-9).

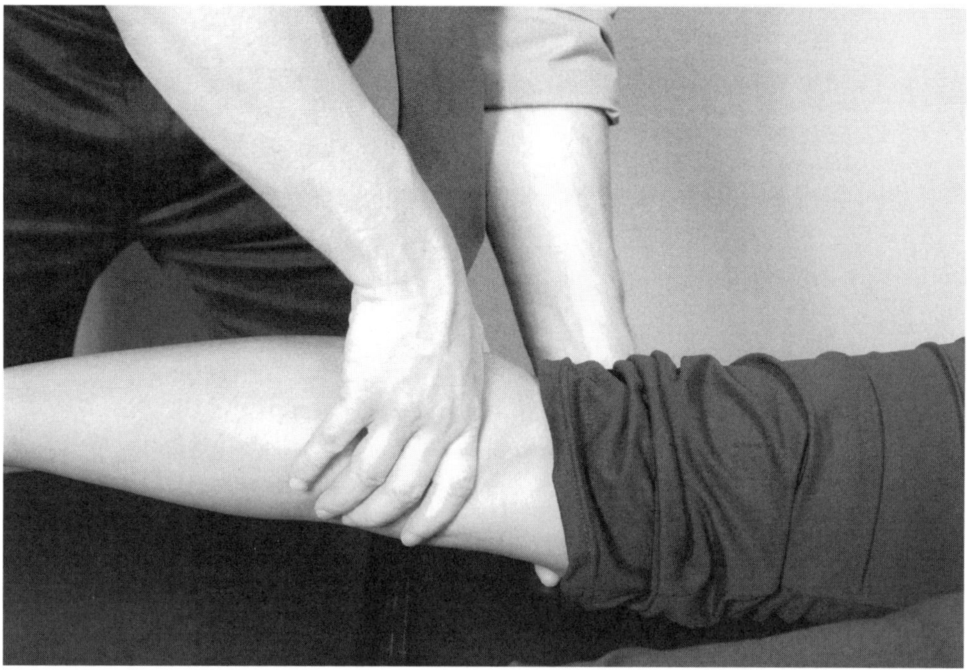

Fig. 17-7 Anterior mobilization of the tibia.

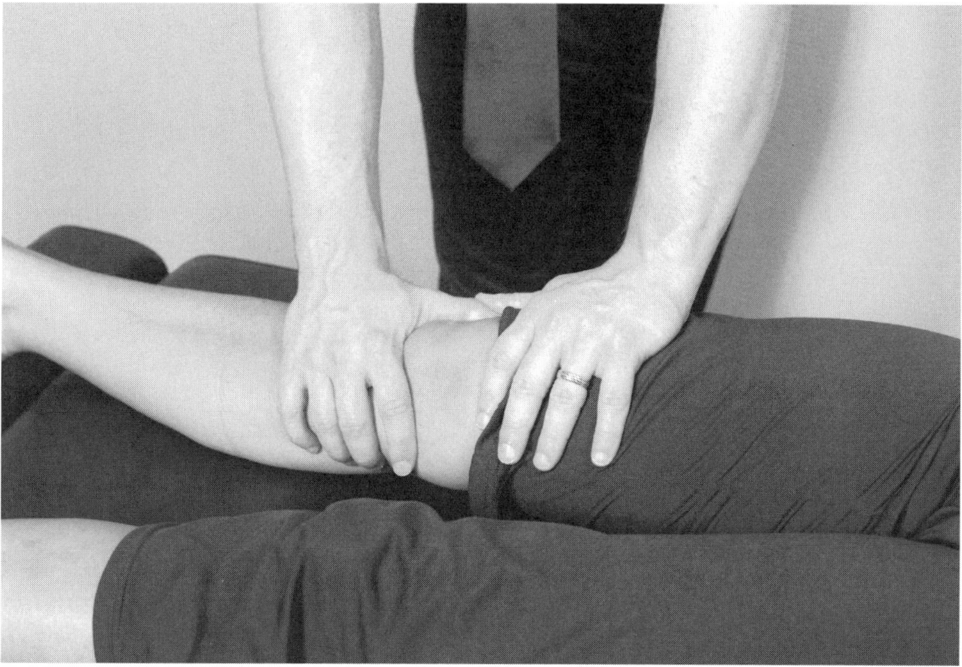

Fig. 17-8 Medial patellar mobilization.

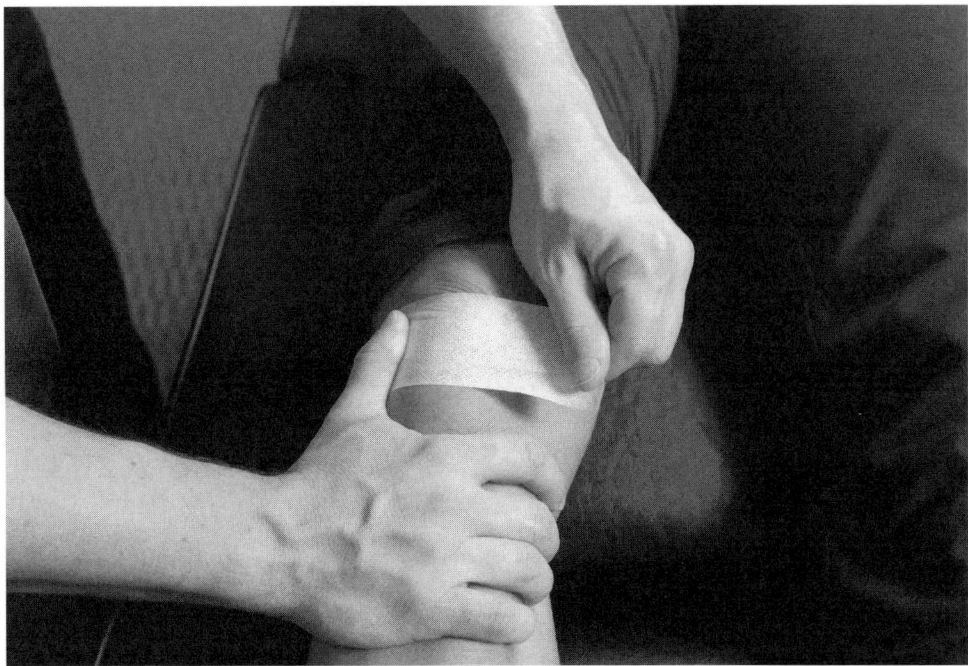

Fig. 17-9 Taping of the patella: Shown here is the taping technique for a laterally-displaced patella. The tape is applied to the lateral aspect of the patella and tractioned medially, thereby pulling the patella into a more medially-oriented position.

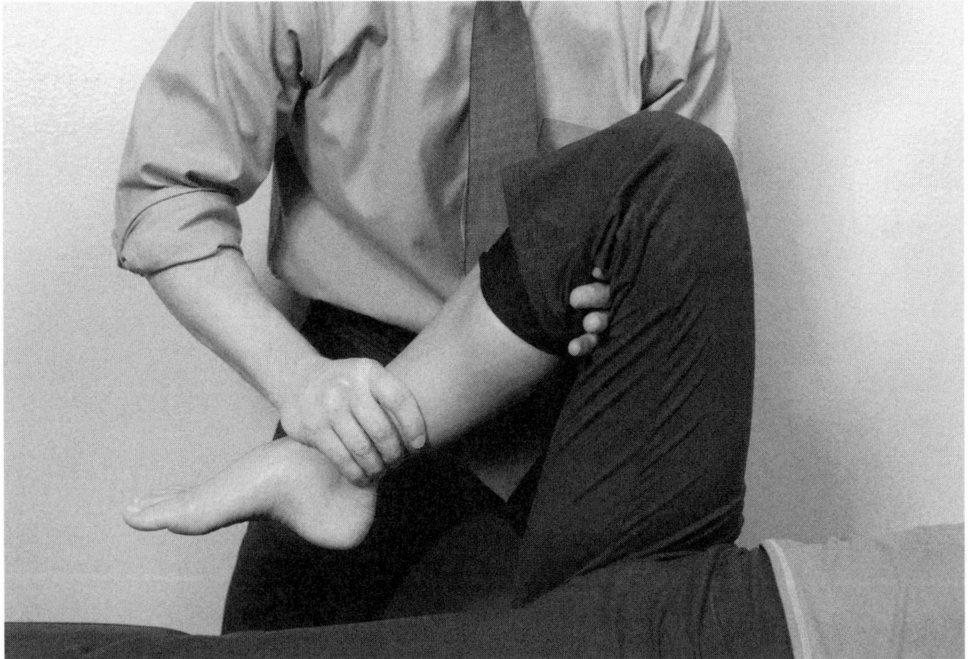

Fig. 17-10 Manipulation of a posterior fibular head.

PROXIMAL TIBIO-FIBULAR JOINT MOBILITY

Assess the position and mobility of the proximal fibula on the tibia. Most often it is stuck posterior and cannot move anteriorly. Correction can be through manipulation or mobilization (Fig. 17-10). Mulligan's MWM for the knee reinforces this, as the mobilization involves an anteriorly-directed force on the proximal fibula.

Expect fibular head involvement to occur with moderate-to-severe ankle sprains. As the distal fibula is pulled anterior and inferior, the proximal fibula goes inferior and posterior. This causes lateral knee pain difficult for the patient to localize. It may even be confused with ITB friction syndrome, which must be ruled out.

POSTURE OF THE LOWER EXTREMITY

Examine the posture of the lower extremity—from the foot all the way up to the pelvis. Look for the pattern of excessive pronation, genu valgus, hip internal rotation, hip adduction, hip flexion and anterior innominate rotation. This is present to some degree in most individuals. The opposing pattern occurs much less frequently, but be cognizant of it.

These patterns have great influence upon the knee. In fact, the knee is typically the "weak link in the chain." That is to say the knee often becomes symptomatic even though the real problem did not originate there. Instead, the real problem is what compromised the knee's structure and function in the first place.

It is still necessary to assess the knee's structure, such as the Q-angle. We just do not limit our treatment to it. We have to view the entire locomotor complex and determine what caused the problem in the first place. Is it the foot? Is it the hip? Is it the pelvis? Examine each joint to tell for sure.

SEGMENTAL DYSFUNCTION

Examine the L3 and L4 segments of the spine for signs and symptoms of dysfunction. Dysfunction here can refer pain to the knee joint itself. Or, it can indirectly cause knee problems by altering the function of muscles which control the joint. Please consult Chapter 14, The Lumbar Spine, for details on lumbar spine examination and treatment.

MOVEMENT PATTERNS

The movement patterns involving the knee go hand-in-hand with the "biomechanical avalanche" described previously. Fortunately, in this case we can use the nervous system to ease strain on the knee. This starts with teaching the patient to be cognizant of the knee's position when he/she is climbing stairs, arising from sitting, or standing up from a squat. Oftentimes in the case of the pronation pattern, the knee is tracking too far medially. Ideally, the patella should be directly above the 2nd toe (Fig. 17-11). This is good information to share with the patient; he or she can easily look down when climbing stairs or walking up an incline to make sure the patella isn't going too far medially. If it is, he can consciously correct the problem.

Higher up in the chain is the hip and pelvis. When these structures assume the common pattern (hip adduction, internal rotation, and anterior pelvic inclination), the knee can't help but suffer. Consequently, breaking up this pattern is especially beneficial. Hruska's Protonics brace is a good example of this point. As mentioned previously, it causes hamstring contraction, which rotates the pelvis posteriorly. This externally rotates the femur, thereby improving the alignment of the knee and patellofemoral joint. In many instances, this brace eliminates knee pain immediately.

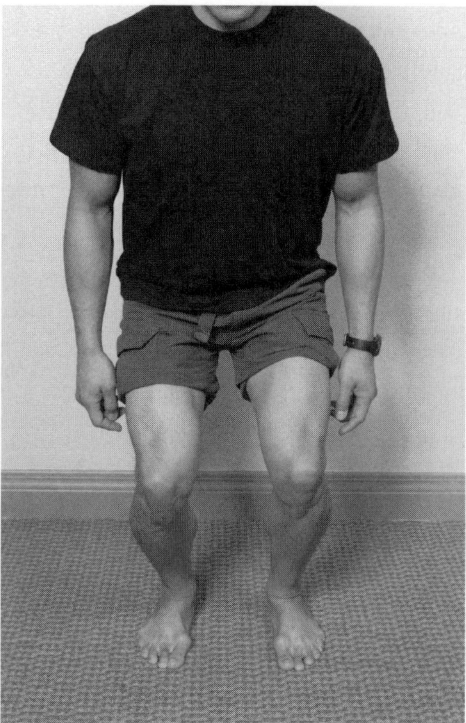

Fig. 17-11 Observation of the patella's position in relation to the foot. Ideally, the patella should track directly above the 2nd toe.

But what if you don't have the equipment? That's okay. The concept can still be utilized. Start by teaching the patient posterior pelvic tilt exercises. Progress the tilt exercises from supine to weight bearing and then have him maintain the tilt while performing a miniature squat. Oftentimes, the person with patellofemoral dysfunction will note increased pain-free range of motion while the posterior tilt is held. This is an excellent teaching tool for the patient. Encourage him to hold this position in the future while he squats, ascends stairs, or does anything else requiring knee flexion and extension.

The subject of posterior pelvic tilt exercises dovetails into the topics of core and hip strengthening, both of which are applicable to knee pain sufferers. That is because stabilizing the core and hip abductors/extensors is also important to minimize aberrant knee motion. It is also necessary for optimizing control of the knee in space. These techniques are presented in Chapters 6 and 16.

ENERGY-BASED TECHNIQUES

Auricular Acupressure. Gently squeeze the point corresponding to the knee with two fingers. Hold for 5 seconds, then relax 5 seconds. Increase the amount of pressure with each cycle for a total time of one minute (6 cycles). Do this initially on the ear on the involved side only; treat the opposite ear as well if the patient does not improve.

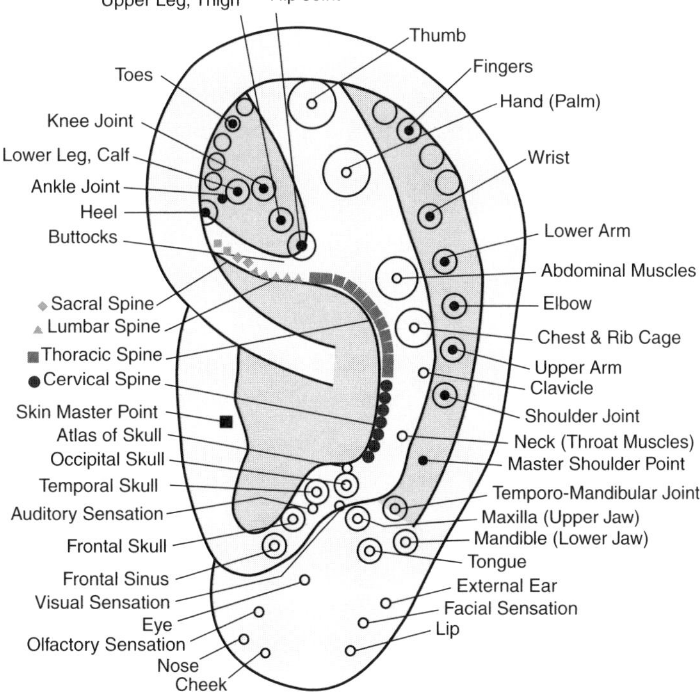

Fig. 17-12

Reflexology. Begin by massaging the entire foot. Walk up the foot with the thumbs along the five zones. Treat both the plantar and dorsal surfaces. Work the toes as well. Spend extra time on the medial border of the foot corresponding with the spine. Also, work on areas associated with different organs needing an extra "boost." Following this long warm-up, massage the area on the foot corresponding to the knee.

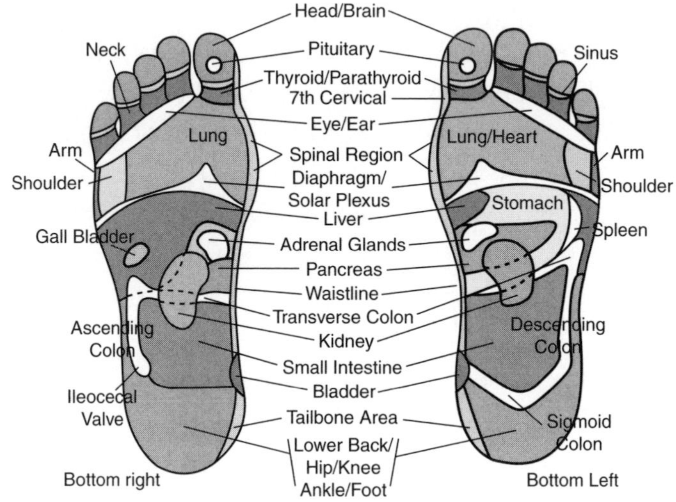

Fig. 17-13

THE HIGH-YIELD SCAN

Perform a scan of the high-yield elements of the body including:

- Gait
- Posture
- Sit-to-Stand
- Miniature Squat
- Respiration
- Romberg Test
- Fukuda's Test
- Upper Cervical Spine
- Middle Cervical Spine
- TMJ

- Pelvis
- Feet
- Stress Screen

EVALUATION AND TREATMENT OF THE SECONDARY FACTORS

Repetitive Motions. Intervention is similar to what was discussed in the movement patterns section. However, for this topic, the clinician focuses on things that can be altered outside the patient's body. This includes anything that reduces demands placed on the knee. Examples include advising the patient to avoid climbing stairs or squatting due to excessive pressure on the posterior surface of the patella. Likewise, if he or she is exercising, this needs to be discussed. Exercising on the Stairmaster should be substituted with something else. Other exercises should be modified. Take the stationary bike, leg press, and knee extension machines, for instance. Forcing the knee to start in extreme flexion places great pressure on the patellofemoral joint. In these instances, teaching the patient to modify these exercises by working closer to full extension automatically reduces strain.

There are many other activities that can be harmful to the knee. The clinician should use her knowledge of biomechanics to assess and address all potentially harmful activities.

Foot Structure and Footwear. These are important topics for the knee pain sufferer, as each of them has a strong influence over the knee. Please see Chapter 18, The Foot and Ankle, for more information.

18 The Foot and Ankle

THE FOOT IS A HIGH-YIELD REGION OF THE BODY AND MUST BE EXAMINED ON every patient. The reason for this is that the foot affects the entire body's mechanical system, nervous system, movement pattern schema, and energetic system. Mechanically, we know it functions as the body's foundation. We also understand the chain reaction occurring with gait, and we are aware of the widespread pathological forces resulting from abnormal biomechanics. It is under the mechanical model where orthotics are usually prescribed.

Neurologically, the foot plays just as large a role in affecting the body. This is exemplified by two different approaches which treat the foot as a means to influence the entire body. The first is podiatrist Brian Rothbart's approach, which uses minimally-invasive, flexible orthotics to support the first ray. This stimulates the anti-gravity muscles throughout the body. The second approach is applied kinesiology, which makes use of several "gait reflexes." These reflex points on the feet are acupuncture points which correspond with different patterns of weakness in gait-related muscles. Through AK analysis and treatment, the clinician can correct faulty recruitment patterns involving muscle groups such as: the hip flexors and contralateral shoulder flexors, the hip abductors and contralateral shoulder abductors, the hip extensors and contralateral shoulder extensors, as well as several others.

Foot function affects the body's movement patterns through both mechanical and neurological means. This is because the gait pattern itself is primarily a reflex activity, requiring the reciprocal activation and inhibition of different muscle groups. Therefore, proper foot motion is vital to providing the central nervous system with the right information at the right time.

Energetically, the best example of the foot's influence over the body is by studying the field of reflexology. After all, reflexology practitioners can limit themselves to treating specific reflex points on the foot in order to address maladies throughout the entire person. This says it all.

EXAMINATION AND TREATMENT OF THE PRIMARY FACTORS

Ankle Plantarflexors. Palpate these muscles for hypertonicity, fascial adhesions, tenderness, and trigger points. Utilize soft tissue techniques including myofascial release, sustained pressure, strumming and ischemic compression to address the findings. Post-isometric relaxation is useful in reducing tone and improving flexibility (Fig. 18-1).

The plantarflexors become facilitated as part of the common pattern. This interferes with the gait pattern and promotes breakdown of the medial longitudinal arch. This facilitated state also promotes the formation of trigger points in the gastrocnemius and soleus. The clinician should be aware of the unique referral patterns of trigger

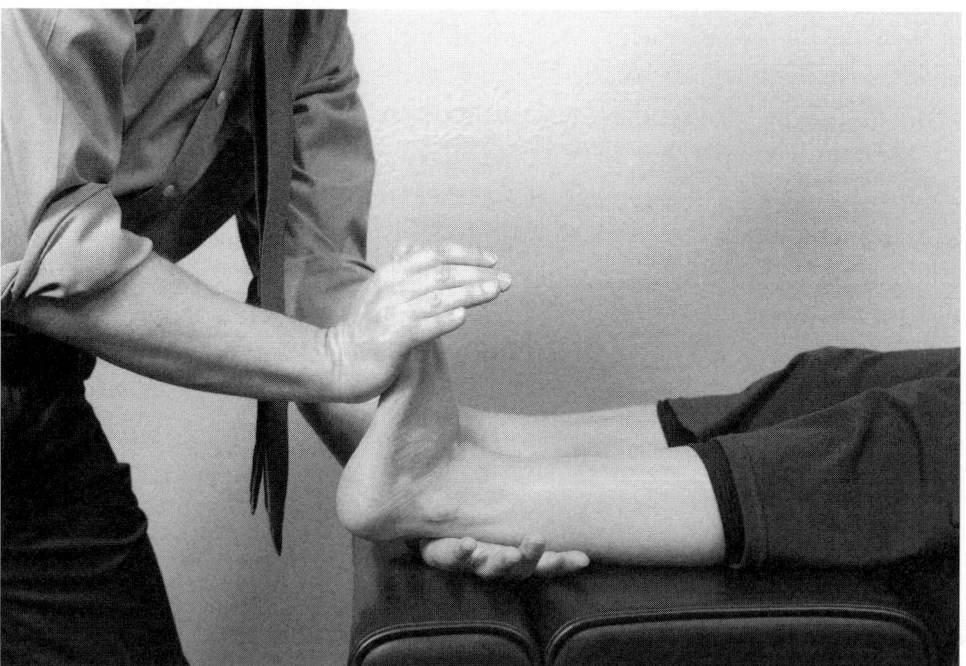

Fig. 18-1 PIR of the plantar flexors. Have the patient gently plantarflex into resistance. Upon relaxation, stretch her further into dorsiflexion. Do this with the knee flexed and extended so that the gastrocs and soleus are stretched.

points in these muscles. A trigger point in the medial gastroc may refer pain down the back of the leg to the heel. Trigger points in the soleus refer pain to the heel as well and even to the sacroiliac joint.[31]

Special conditions may also activate these muscles. One such case is the posterior ischium (or anterior innominate), which creates a tender point in the middle of the gastrocs. This tenderness disappears when the pelvic asymmetry is corrected. Another case is the negative Derifield (described in Chapter 15), in which there is notable tension/tenderness in the Achilles tendon ipsilateral to a posterior innominate rotation. Yet another example is associated with an atlas dural subluxation in SOT. In this case, a dural restriction causes impaired dorsiflexion at the ipsilateral ankle. Stressors such as those mentioned may activate the plantarflexors, thereby causing/perpetuating muscular and tendinous problems. The clinician is well-advised to correct these problems if present as well as any biomechanical issue from the ground-up in order to reduce added stress to these muscles.

Ankle Dorsiflexors. Palpate these muscles for hypertonicity, fascial adhesions, tenderness, and trigger points. Utilize soft tissue techniques including myofascial release, sustained pressure, strumming and ischemic compression to address the findings. Post-isometric relaxation is useful in reducing tone and increasing flexibility (Fig. 18-2).

The dorsiflexors are inhibited as part of the common pattern. To make matters worse, they are called upon to counter excessive pronation as the medial forefoot approaches the floor. This combination makes these muscles prone to overexertion injuries including shin splints and anterior compartment syndrome.

Ankle Invertors. Palpate these muscles for hypertonicity, fascial adhesions, tenderness, and trigger points. Utilize soft tissue techniques including myofascial release, sustained pressure, strumming and ischemic compression to address the findings. Post-isometric relaxation is useful in reducing tone and increasing flexibility (Fig. 18-3).

The ankle invertors become facilitated as part of the common pattern. In cases of extreme facilitation (i.e. traumatic brain injury, cerebral palsy), these muscles accentuate the arches of the foot and create a pes cavus deformity. In the average person, however, the effect of hypertonicity is just the opposite. By putting the forefoot and/or rearfoot in varus during the swing phase of gait, these muscles create excessive

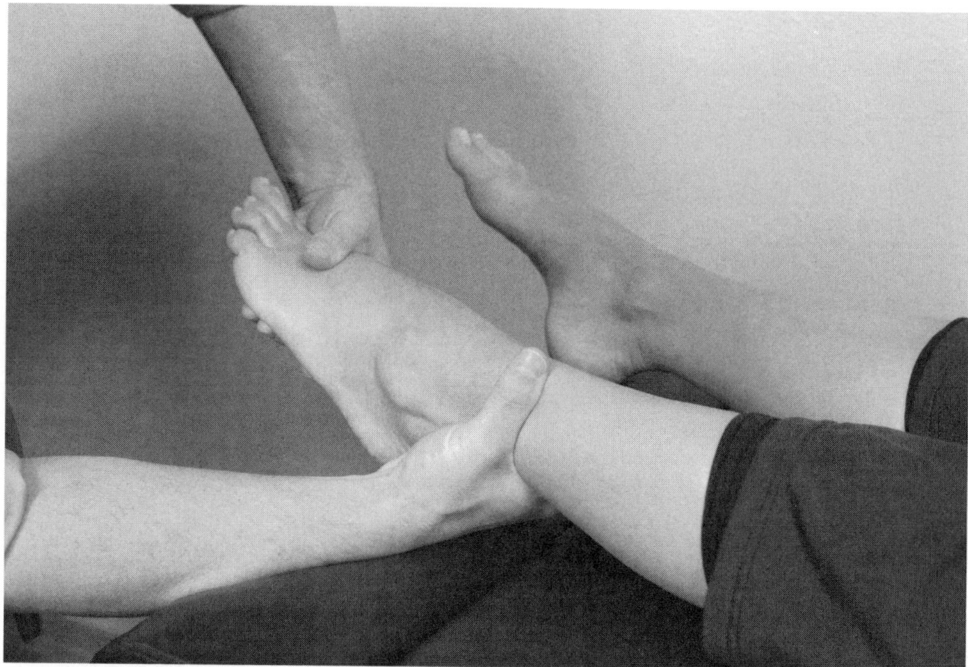

Fig. 18-2 PIR of the tibialis anterior. Have the patient dorsiflex and invert the foot into resistance. Upon relaxation, stretch her further into plantarflexion and eversion.

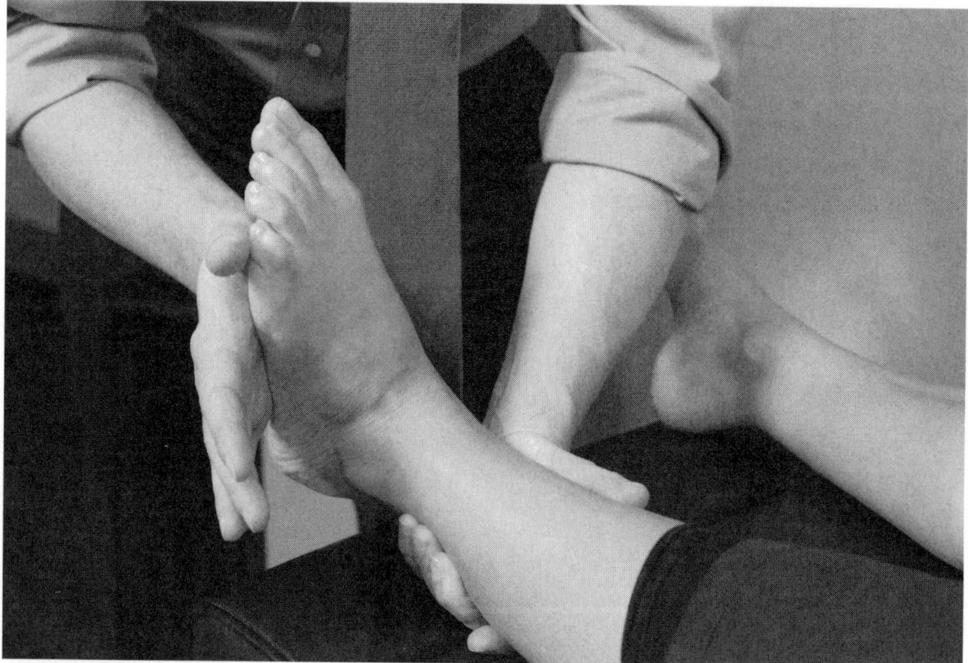

Fig. 18-3 PIR of the tibialis posterior. Have the patient gently plantarflex and invert the foot into resistance. Upon relaxation, stretch her further into dorsiflexion and eversion.

pronation by forcing the foot to pronate sharply during stance in order to form a rigid lever.

Excessive pronation (regardless of the cause) places added stress on the invertors. The tibialis posterior is especially vulnerable due to its many insertion points on the sole of the foot. It is quickly stretched with pronation and simultaneously asked to decelerate the rate of pronation through eccentric contraction. This sets the muscle up for problems including shin splints, tenosynovitis and sometimes even tendon rupture.

Ankle Evertors. Palpate these muscles for hypertonicity, fascial adhesions, tenderness, and trigger points. Utilize soft tissue techniques including myofascial release, sustained pressure, strumming and ischemic compression to address the findings. Post-isometric relaxation is useful in reducing tone and improving flexibility (Fig. 18-4).

The evertors should be closely evaluated in cases of ankle sprain as they are often strained. This will perpetuate many of the symptoms of the original injury and may alter the biomechanics of the foot. Most significant of these potential problems

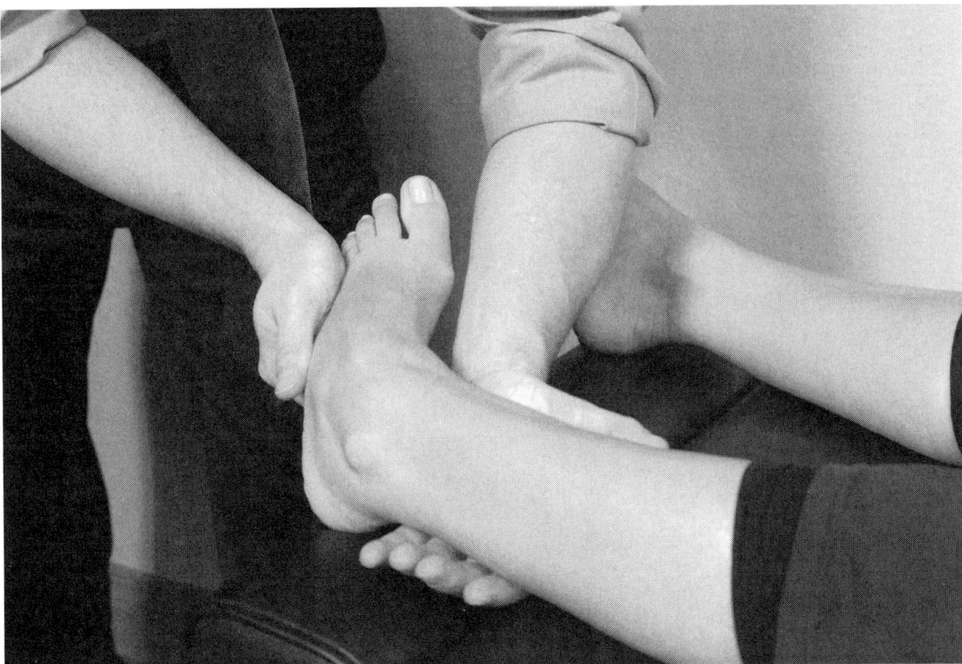

Fig. 18-4 PIR of the peroneus longus and brevis. Have the patient gently plantarflex and evert the foot against resistance. Upon relaxation, stretch the ankle further into dorsiflexion and inversion.

occurs if the peroneus longus is unable to contract fully; it plays an important role in stabilizing the first ray and everting the foot during gait. Without this function, the foot will not lock as it should and the person's bodyweight will pass over the lateral forefoot instead of over the first ray.

The Toe Muscles. Palpate these muscles for hypertonicity, fascial adhesions, tenderness, and trigger points. Utilize soft tissue techniques including myofascial release, sustained pressure, strumming and ischemic compression to address the findings (Fig. 18-5). Post-isometric relaxation is useful in reducing tone and improving flexibility (Fig. 18-6).

Of all the intrinsic and extrinsic muscles which control the toe, the most clinically significant ones are the abductor hallicus brevis and the flexor hallicus longus. The abductor hallicus is important because it can sometimes irritate the lateral plantar nerve, mimicking plantar fasciitis. The flexor hallicus longus is important as well; applied kinesiologists find that weakness of this muscle often contributes to tarsal tunnel syndrome. The toe flexors are clinically relevant as well because they have the propensity to become hypertonic and lead to a claw-toe deformity.

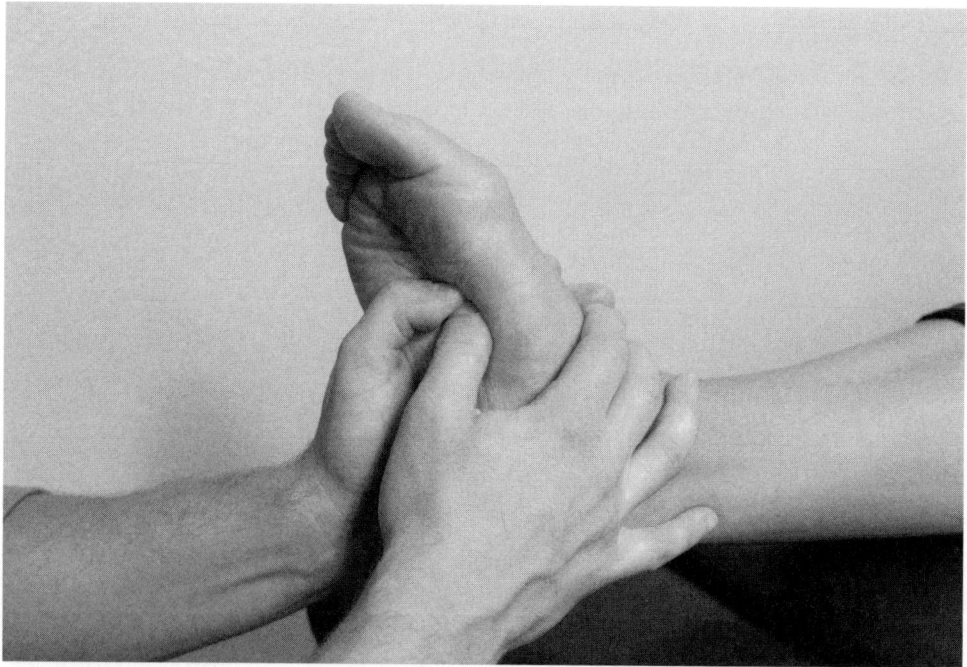

Fig. 18-5 The clinician can apply MFR, sustained pressure, strumming and ischemic compression in this position.

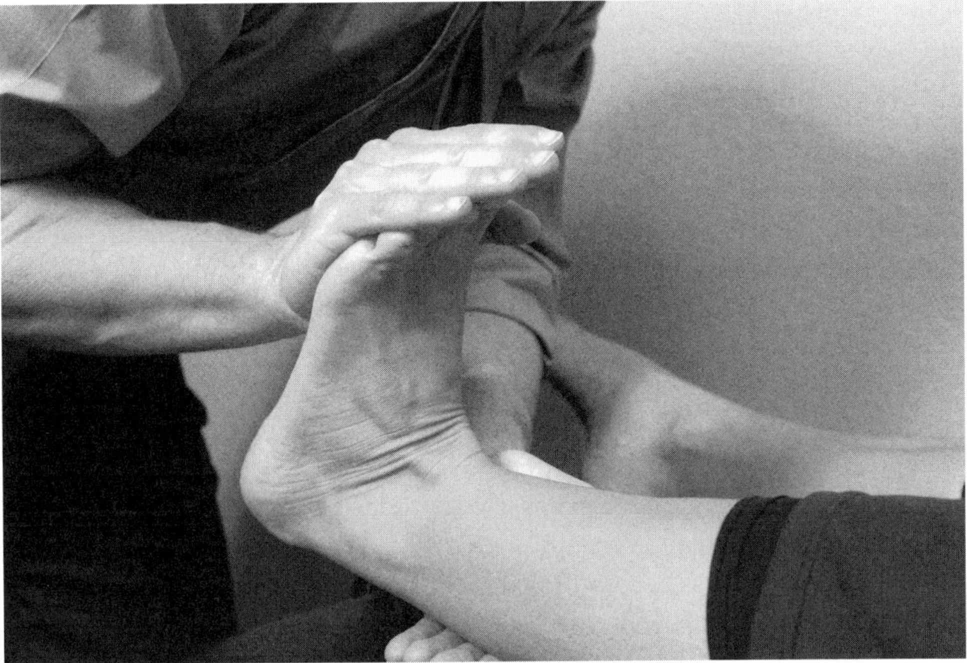

Fig. 18-6 PIR of the toe flexors. Have the patient gently flex the toes and plantarflex the ankle into resistance. Upon relaxation, stretch the toes further into extension and the ankle into dorsiflexion.

MUSCLE STRENGTH

Evaluate the strength of the foot and ankle muscles with traditional methods. Make sure to assess both their ability to initiate a contraction as well as their sheer strength. Most often, what we perceive as weakness is more a matter of inhibition. This will follow the common pattern and/or be due to local or segmental dysfunction. Treating the causative factor restores normal strength in these cases. In cases of true muscle weakness, such as those involving muscle atrophy, remedial strengthening is indicated. This is done with traditional strengthening techniques including resisted ankle inversion, eversion, plantarflexion and dorsiflexion. Occasionally strengthening of the toe flexors and extensors is indicated as well.

Proprioceptive exercises are also beneficial in strengthening the foot and ankle muscles. Simple exercises, such as single-leg standing and wobble board training recruit muscles at reflex speed. This is helpful in strengthening these muscles and improving coordination and balance. These exercises are presented in Chapter 6, Movement Pattern Considerations.

JOINT MOBILITY

Use conventional methods to assess foot and ankle motion. Treat restricted joint motion with standard mobilization and manipulation techniques (Fig's 18-7 to 18-12). Sometimes joint dysfunction does not resolve with standard techniques, and one can use Mulligan's mobilizations with movement for specific disorders. One of his most popular techniques for the foot and ankle is the lateral fibular repositioning MWM(Fig. 18-13). When indicated, this technique works wonders. Clinicians more interested in treating articular dysfunction related to abnormal foot posture are urged to follow Charrette's extremity adjusting protocol. This protocol addresses predictable subluxations of the feet which occur with excessive pronation and supination.

For 1st MTP dysfunction, the author has found Maitland's compression technique highly effective. This form of mobilization actually compresses the 1st MTP surfaces and reproduces joint pain (Fig. 18-14). This is believed to benefit the articular cartilage and is an excellent treatment for cases of metatarsophalangeal joint pain, metacarpophalangeal joint pain, and patellofemoral pain.

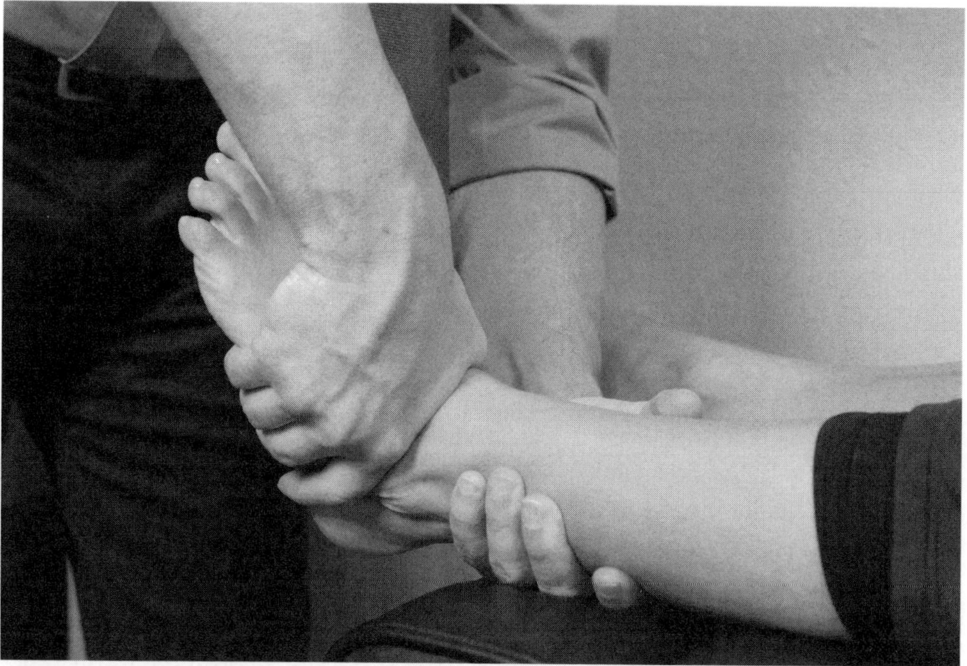

Fig. 18-7 Assessment of talocrural motion. Stabilize the posterior aspect of the distal tibia and fibula while assessing posterior motion of the talus. Reverse hand contacts to assess anterior talar motion. Restricted motion in either plane should be addressed with repetitive mobilization.

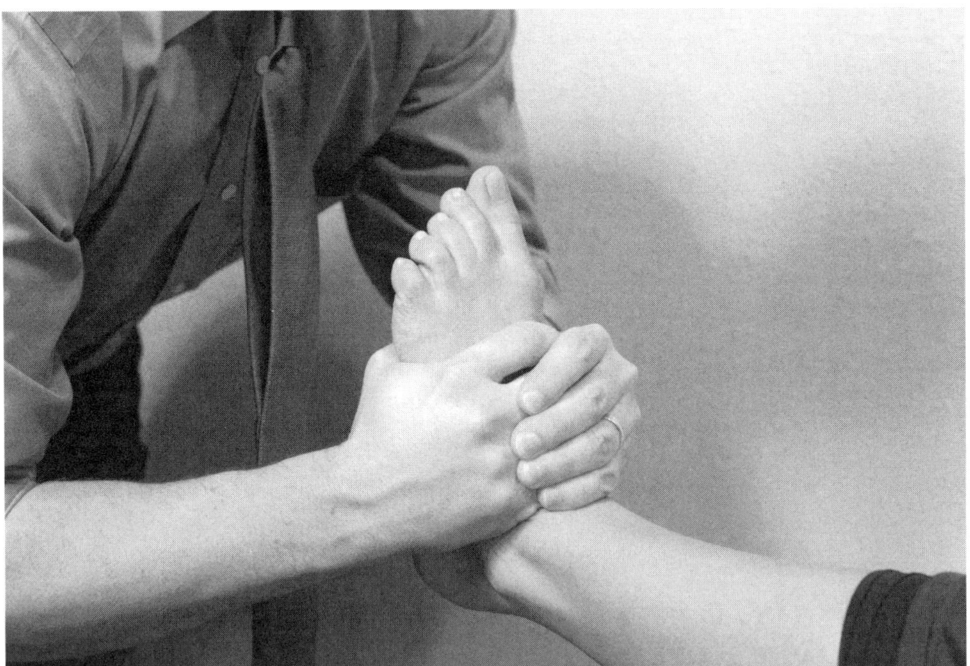

Fig. 18-8 Manipulation of the talocrural joint. The clinician grasps the anterior-superior aspect of the talus and applies gentle traction, taking the joint to end-range. He then applies a high-velocity, short amplitude traction inferior and posterior. This corrects the common anterior talus malposition.

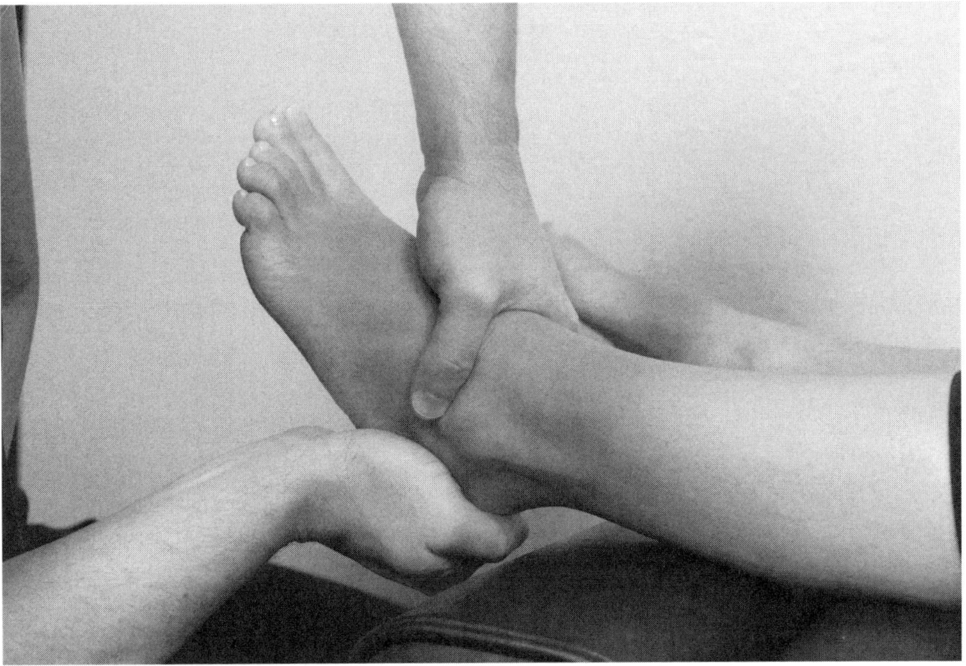

Fig. 18-9 Assessment of subtalar motion. Stabilize the talus while gliding the calcaneus medially and laterally. Restricted motion in either plane should be addressed with repetitive mobilization.

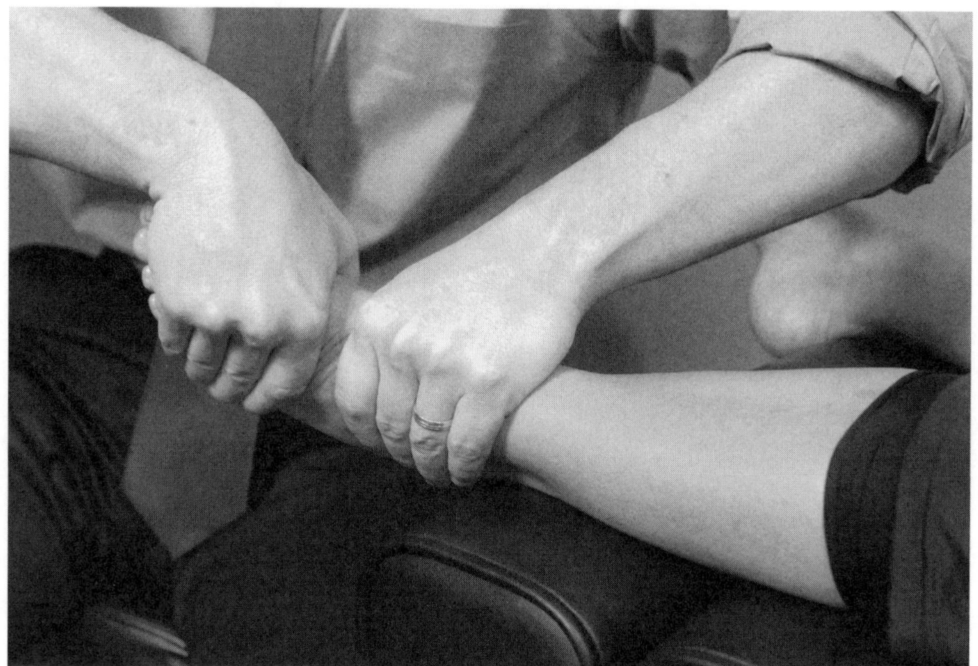

Fig. 18-10 Assessment of tarsal motion. The clinician can assess mobility at each joint in the foot by individually stabilizing one bone and moving its neighbor.

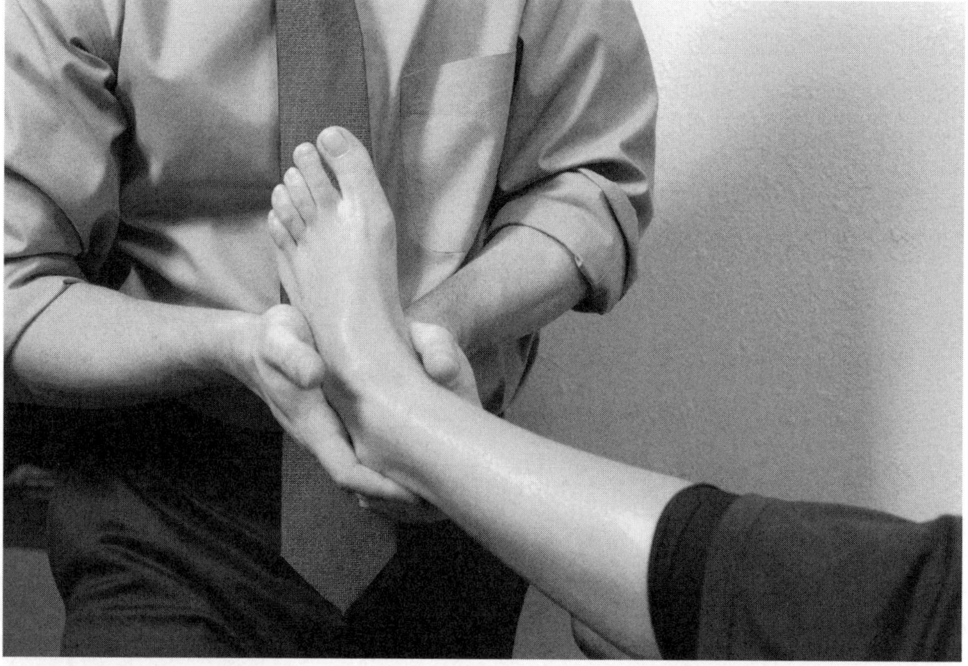

Fig. 18-11 Manipulation of the navicular bone. The navicular bone is typically displaced inferior and medial with a pronated foot posture. The clinician drives the navicular superior and lateral as a correction.

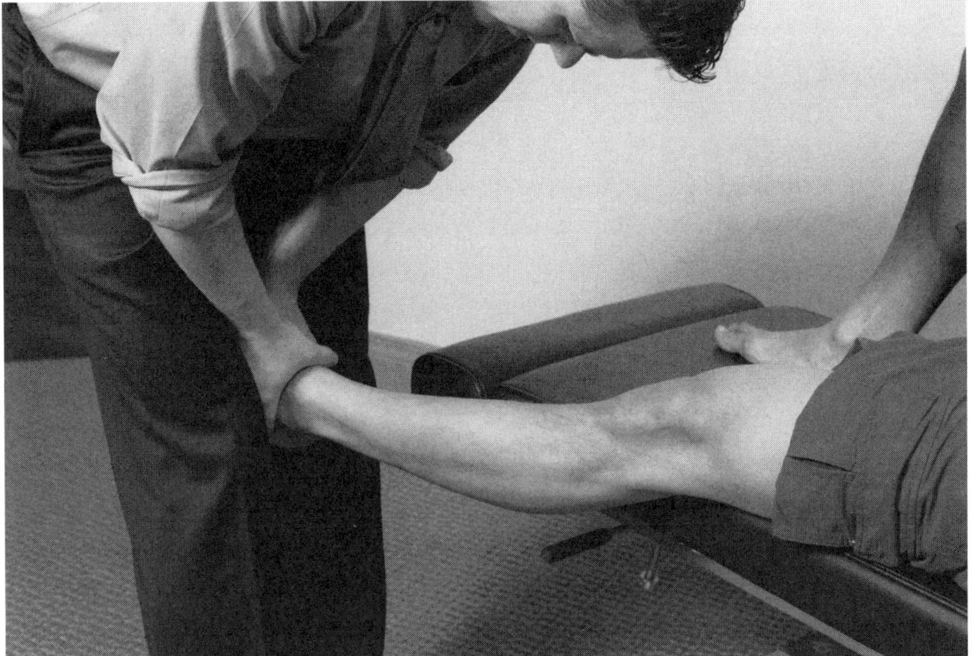

Fig. 18-12 Manipulation of the cuboid bone. The cuboid bone is typically displaced superiorly and laterally. The clinician corrects this malposition by driving it inferiorly and medially. This is achieved primarily by adducting the extending the clinician's knees.

FOOT POSTURE

The assessment of foot posture is really a biomechanical evaluation. To do this, one must examine the foot in non-weight bearing and in weight bearing. Needless to say, the clinician must have a thorough knowledge of biomechanics to properly perform and interpret these tests.

Beginning with the non-weight bearing examination, the clinician will first determine the patient's subtalar neutral position. This is achieved by palpating the medial and lateral aspects of the head of the talus with one hand while putting the foot into neutral dorsiflexion/plantarflexion with the other. From this position, the foot is alternately inverted and everted until a position is found where the head of the talus feels equally prominent medially and laterally. This is the patient's subtalar neutral position. Next, observe the relationship between the distal leg and the calcaneus. Note whether the calcaneus is in a varus or valgus position. Forefoot position is examined immediately afterwards while the foot is still in subtalar neutral. Again, note whether it is in a varus or valgus position.

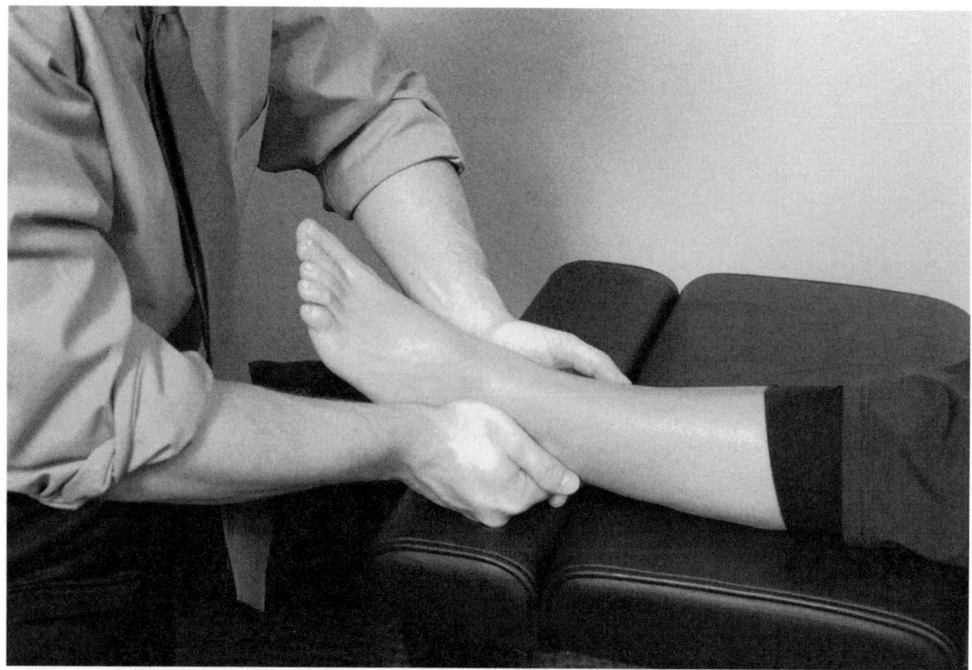

Fig. 18-13 Lateral fibular repositioning. Pre-test the patient by having her move her ankle in a direction which is painful or restricted. In the case of an ankle sprain, oftentimes inversion is both painful and limited. Then, apply a posteriorly-directed pressure on the lateral malleolus and have the patient repeat the movement. When indicated, the person's pain-free motion will increase instantaneously. This is then repeated 10 times and may be used throughout the day until symptoms improve. Mulligan also teaches a technique to tape the fibula posteriorly to mimic this technique.[182]

The static weight-bearing examination is performed next. Observe the general position of the foot from all sides. The clinician can determine if the person has a pes planus or pes cavus foot relatively easily. A useful adjunct to passive observation is by marking the navicular tubercle and then measuring the distance it drops when the patient goes from non-weight bearing to weight bearing (Fig. 18-15). It is acceptable for the navicular to drop by up to 3 mm. According to some authorities, a drop of 4–6 mm reflects a moderate indication for orthotics and a drop of 7mm or more signifies a high indication for orthotics.

Once a biomechanical evaluation is performed, there are two schools of thought in terms of treatment: orthotic recommendation and corrective training. Orthotic recommendation is by far the most popular choice. Orthotics are used to support the foot; most often this is to reduce excessive pronation.

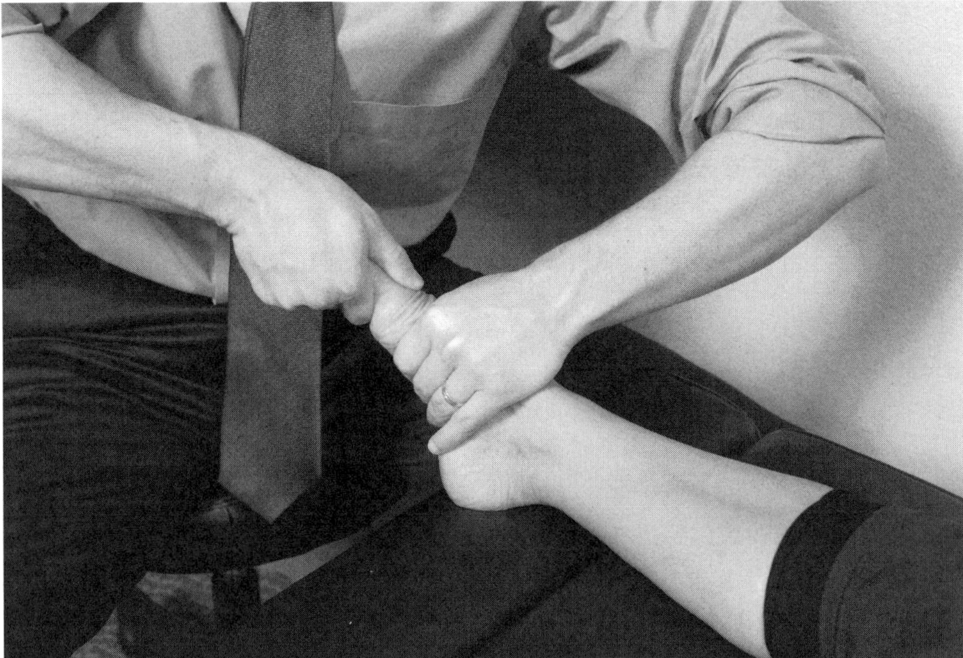

Fig. 18-14 First metatarsophalangeal dysfunction. Compress the joint surfaces to reproduce the patient's pain. Repeat this compressive force multiple times while also gliding the joint up and down.

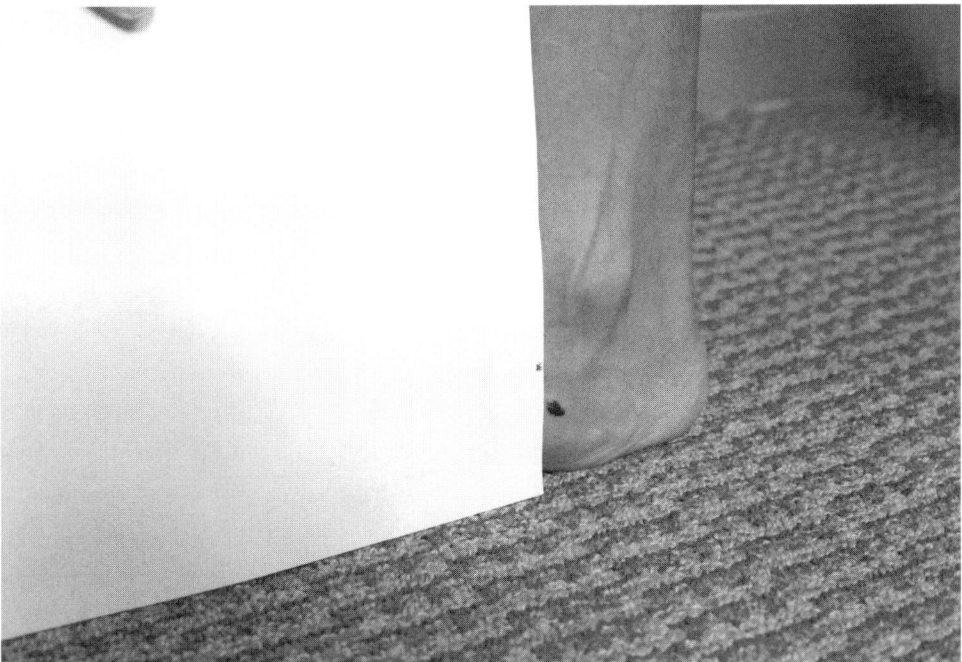

Fig. 18-15 Assessing navicular drop.

To many clinicians including podiatrists and manual therapists, orthotics are very helpful in managing patients with knee, hip, sacroiliac, and low back pain related to foot structure abnormality.

The other school of thought looks at foot structural abnormality as a potentially correctible condition. Treatment is carried out with adjustments and muscular re-education to support the arch of the foot. Some clinicians attest that proper therapy can improve foot structure and function, but the verdict is still out on whether or not this is effective. It is the author's speculation that therapies to naturally restore normal foot structure are more effective when the structural abnormality is due to the common pattern/lower crossed syndrome. On the other hand, a patient who has a pes planus foot structure due to systemic hypermobility is less likely to improve from such therapy and most likely needs orthotic support. On this note, it is wise for the clinician to screen her patients for hypermobility before making such important treatment recommendations.

MOVEMENT PATTERNS

There are several things the clinician can do to counter abnormal movement patterns. The most important one is to assess and correct any asymmetry in gait. This may involve the foot itself, or it may involve the knee, hip, pelvis, or spine. Remember, any asymmetry in these important joints will negatively impact the body. Sometimes, making the patient cognizant of the asymmetry is therapeutic in itself. He/she can then be taught to simply walk in a more symmetrical fashion, and this will reduce or eliminate the problem. Sherry Brourman's text, *Walk Yourself Well*, is a great resource on this topic. She describes many different abnormal gait patterns and lists ideas to help the patient correct each one. Please consult this book for further information.

Addressing neuromuscular recruitment patterns will once again fall under the common pattern. In this case, many of the techniques to address the lower crossed syndrome will again be very helpful. Treating asymmetries such as anterior pelvic tilt and genu valgus will inherently help the patient with excessive pronation. Beyond this, teaching the patient to activate his dorsiflexors and invertors during the stance phase will help reduce problems related to excessive pronation.

In addition to these options, the clinician should also assess where the patient bears the majority of his weight while standing. Many people tend to bear more weight on one side or the other. This may be due to neurological or structural asymmetry. Other times, the person bears too much weight either anteriorly or posteriorly (Fig. 18-16). Most often he bears too much weight anteriorly, thereby forcing contraction of the ankle and foot flexors and even stressing the plantar fascia. In this case, he should be taught to stand in a more symmetrical posture. This will reduce unnecessary strain on the structures mentioned.

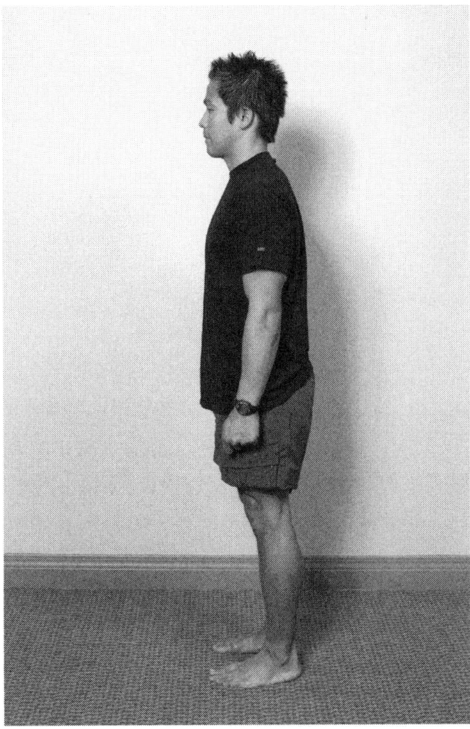

Fig. 18-16 Excessive weight bearing on the ball of the foot.

ENERGY-BASED TECHNIQUES

Auricular Acupressure. Gently squeeze the point corresponding to the foot and ankle with two fingers. Hold for 5 seconds, then relax 5 seconds. Increase the amount of pressure with each cycle for a total time of one minute (6 cycles). Do this initially on the ear on the involved side only; treat the opposite ear as well if the patient does not improve.

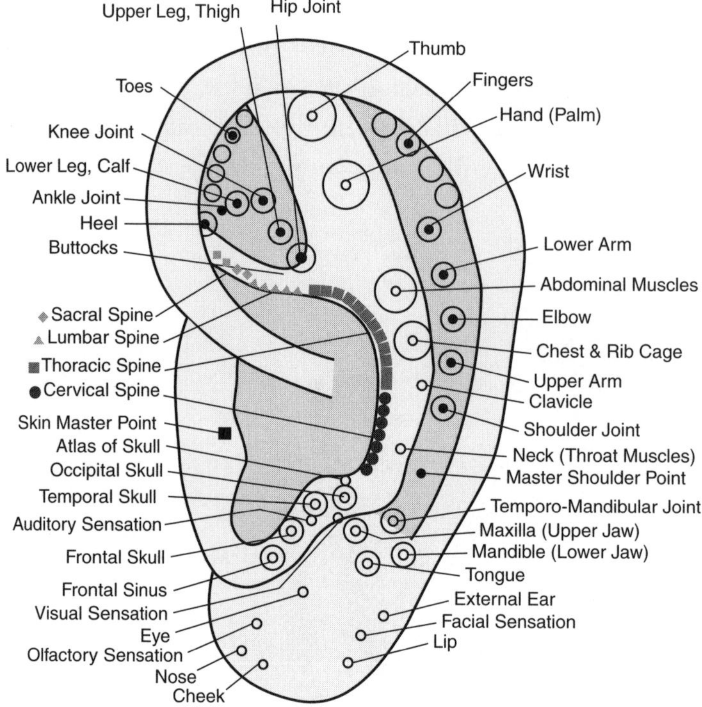

Fig. 18-17

Reflexology. Begin by massaging the entire foot. Walk up the foot with the thumbs along the five zones. Treat the plantar and dorsal surfaces. Work the toes as well. Spend extra time on the medial border of the foot corresponding with the spine. Also, work on areas associated with different organs needing an extra "boost." Following this long warm-up, massage the area on the foot corresponding to the foot and ankle.

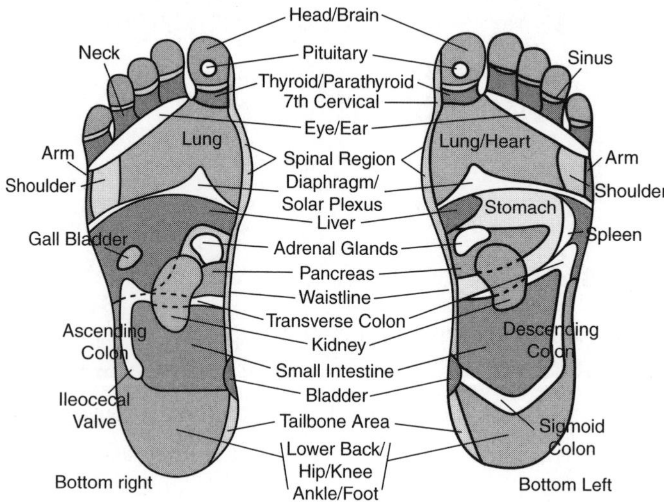

Fig. 18-18

HIGH-YIELD SCAN

Perform a scan of the other high-yield elements of the body including:

- Gait
- Posture
- Sit-to-Stand
- Miniature Squat
- Respiration
- Romberg Test
- Fukuda's Test
- Upper Cervical Spine
- Middle Cervical Spine
- TMJ
- Pelvis
- Stress Screen

EVALUATION AND TREATMENT OF THE SECONDARY FACTORS

Standing. Much can be gained from a therapeutic standpoint by modifying the stresses the foot is under when the person is standing. First, take note of where on the foot the person is bearing weight. Is it anterior, lateral, medial, or posterior? If so, advise him to change this habit so that weight is distributed more evenly.

Next, find out what surface he stands on all day. If his job requires that he stand on a concrete surface all day long, this will almost always cause problems. In this case, he should be urged to add inserts to attenuate as much shock as possible just to minimize this inherent stress. External changes, such as adding a foam mat to his work area is another modification the patient can take up with his boss. Again, any small change to reduce the repetitive compression will have positive results.

Footwear. Assess the patient's shoes. Are they right for his foot type? Are they supportive? Do they cushion the foot while standing and walking? What about signs of wear and tear? Is the heel counter firm and supportive or is it damaged and tilted in relation to the sole? What about the bottom of the shoe? Is the sole worn down on one side? Pronators often make initial contact on the lateral heel, and this area will be worn down relative to the medial side.

An equally-important footwear issue is the style of footwear the person utilizes. High heels, flip-flops and narrow-toed shoes each pose their own problems to the patient. High-heeled shoes throw the bodyweight forward, increasing lumbar lordosis, forward head posture, and greatly stressing the forefoot. Flip-flops provide almost no support to the foot while also demanding a degree of toe flexion to keep them on during the toe-off and swing phase of gait. This interrupts the normal recruitment patterns of gait, altering synergistic patterns throughout the body. Narrow-toed dress shoes are often responsible for causing pain at the MTP joints, as expected. They also alter gait mechanics due to the extended toe box.

19 The Shoulder

EVALUATION AND TREATMENT OF THE PRIMARY FACTORS

Subscapularis. Palpate the muscle for hypertonicity, fascial adhesions, tenderness, and trigger points. Utilize soft tissue techniques including myofascial release, sustained pressure, strumming and ischemic compression to address the findings (Fig. 19-1). Post-isometric relaxation is useful in reducing tone and improving flexibility (Fig. 19-2).

As part of the common pattern, the subscapularis is always in a hypertonic state. This alters glenohumeral mechanics, causing rotator cuff dysfunction. Besides this, it generates a great deal of pain on its own. This is normally not perceived in the axilla, but instead is felt in the lateral shoulder region. Additionally, myofascial trigger points present in the subscapularis will refer pain down the posterior arm and end up as a painful band around the wrist.[31] *Skillful treatment of this muscle often eliminates shoulder symptoms, negates positive orthopedic tests, and removes the signs of pseudoradiculopathy.*

Supraspinatus. Palpate the muscle for hypertonicity, fascial adhesions, tenderness, and trigger points. Utilize soft tissue techniques including myofascial release, sustained pressure, strumming and ischemic compression to address the findings (Fig. 19-3).

The supraspinatus is inhibited as part of the common pattern. Consequently, it is unable to perform the crucial task of depressing the humeral head and initiating

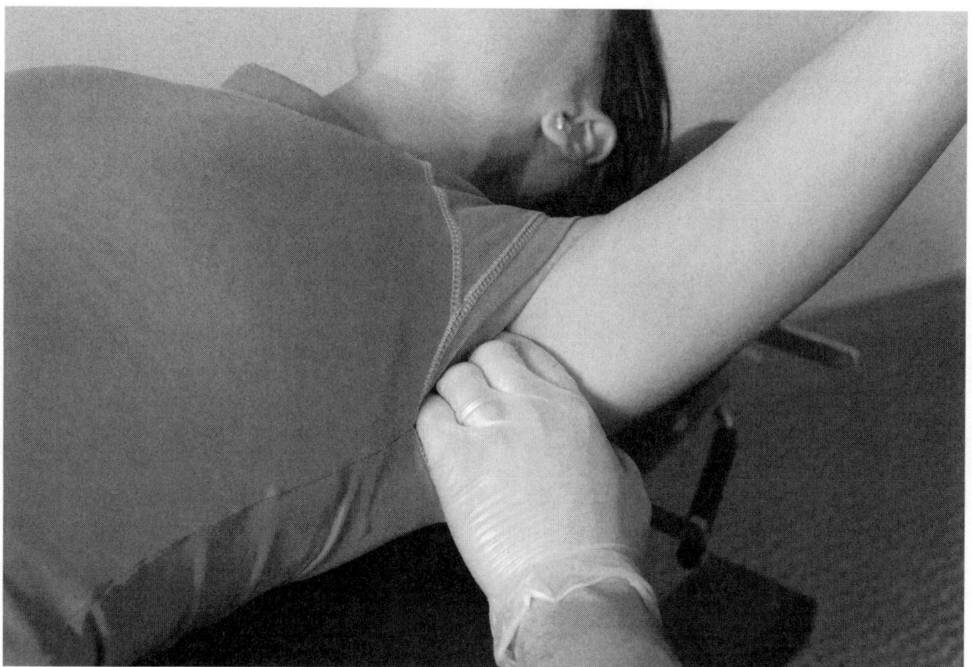

Fig. 19-1 The clinician can apply MFR, sustained pressure, strumming and ischemic compression in this position. Be sure to go far enough medially so that contact is made with the origin of the muscle. At the same time, do not go so far medially and superiorly that contact is made with the lower portion of the brachial plexus.

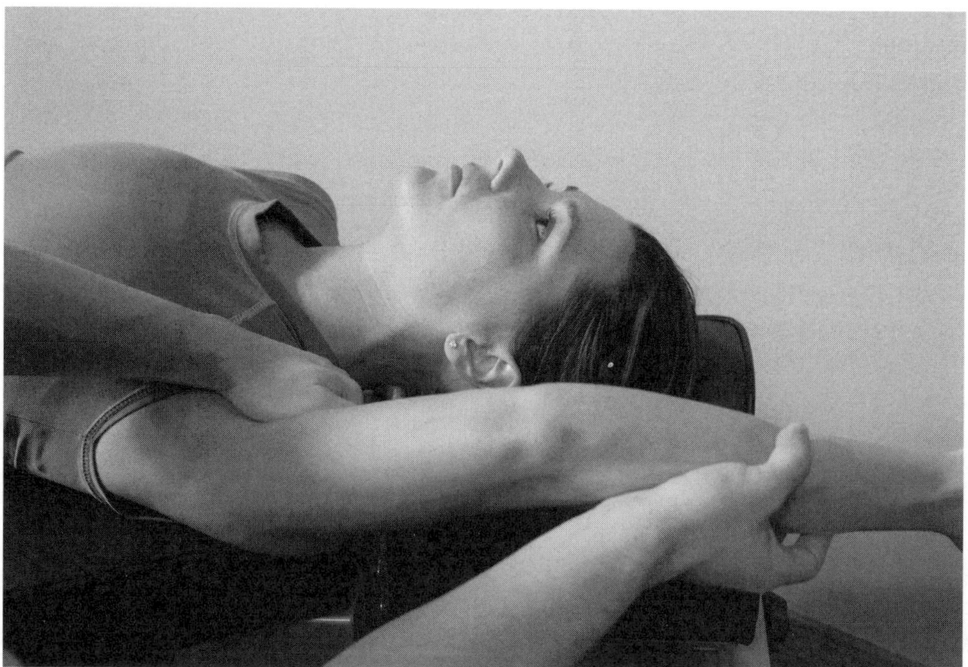

Fig. 19-2 PIR of the subscapularis. Stretch the patient into further external rotation, abduction, and flexion after the patient gently contracts into extension, adduction and internal rotation. Apply anterior-posterior pressure on the humeral head to prevent anterior translation.

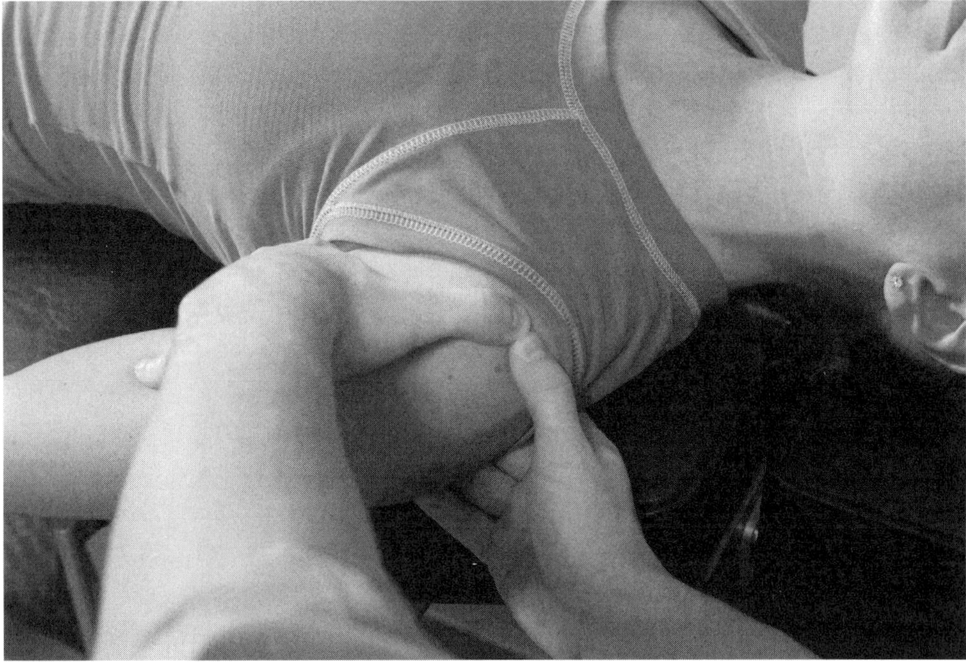

Fig. 19-3 Gentle friction massage applied to the supraspinatus tendon. This is intended to help reorganize collagen fibers and bring added circulation to this poorly vascularized tendon.

shoulder abduction. This leads to problems with the entire rotator cuff and causes impingement of the supraspinatus tendon. Manual therapy applied to this muscle reduces pain and increases strength right away.

Infraspinatus and Teres Minor. Palpate these muscles for hypertonicity, fascial adhesions, tenderness, and trigger points. Utilize soft tissue techniques including myofascial release, sustained pressure, strumming and ischemic compression to address the findings (Fig. 19-4).

These muscles are typically inhibited as part of the common pattern. This limits the external rotation strength they were designed to contribute to the rotator cuff complex. Expect trigger points in the infraspinatus to refer pain into the anterolateral shoulder and down the radial aspect of the arm and forearm. The teres minor will refer pain into the lateral shoulder and arm.

Teres Major. Palpate the muscle for hypertonicity, fascial adhesions, tenderness, and trigger points. Utilize soft tissue techniques including myofascial release, sustained pressure, strumming and ischemic compression to address the

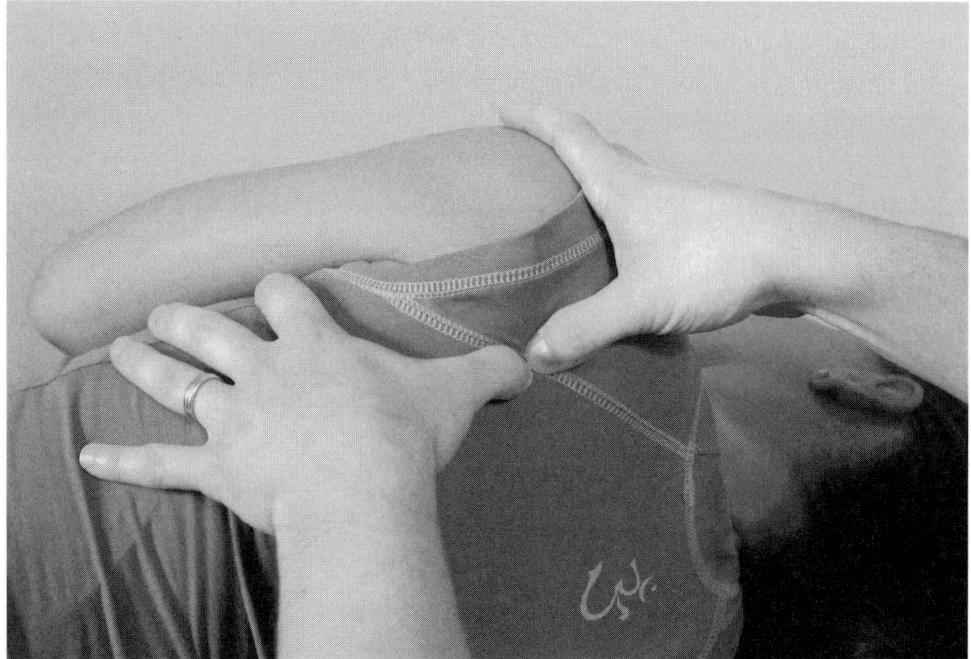

Fig. 19-4 The clinician can apply MFR, sustained pressure, strumming and ischemic compression in this position.

findings. Post-isometric relaxation is useful in reducing tone and improving flexibility (Fig. 19-5).

The teres major is facilitated as part of the common pattern. This adds to the pattern of humeral internal rotation, overpowering the inhibited external rotators. Trigger points in this muscle refer pain to the lateral shoulder, down the lateral arm, and into the dorsal forearm.[31]

Long Head of Biceps. Palpate the muscle for hypertonicity, fascial adhesions, tenderness, and trigger points. Utilize soft tissue techniques including myofascial release, sustained pressure, strumming and ischemic compression to address the findings (Fig. 19-6). Post-isometric relaxation is useful in reducing tone (Fig. 19-7).

The biceps is facilitated as part of the common pattern. This causes irritation of the tendon, resulting in well-localized anterior shoulder pain. Added to this stressor is poor posture, which causes impingement of the tendon when the arm is raised.

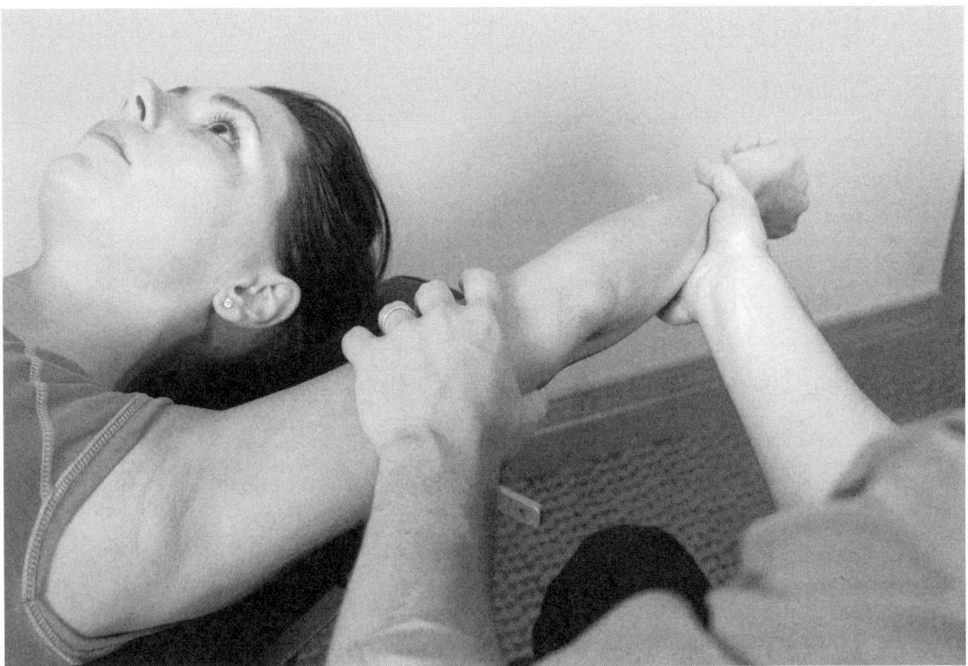

Fig. 19-5 PIR of the teres major. Stretch the patient further into flexion, abduction and external rotation after she gently contracts into extension, adduction and internal rotation.

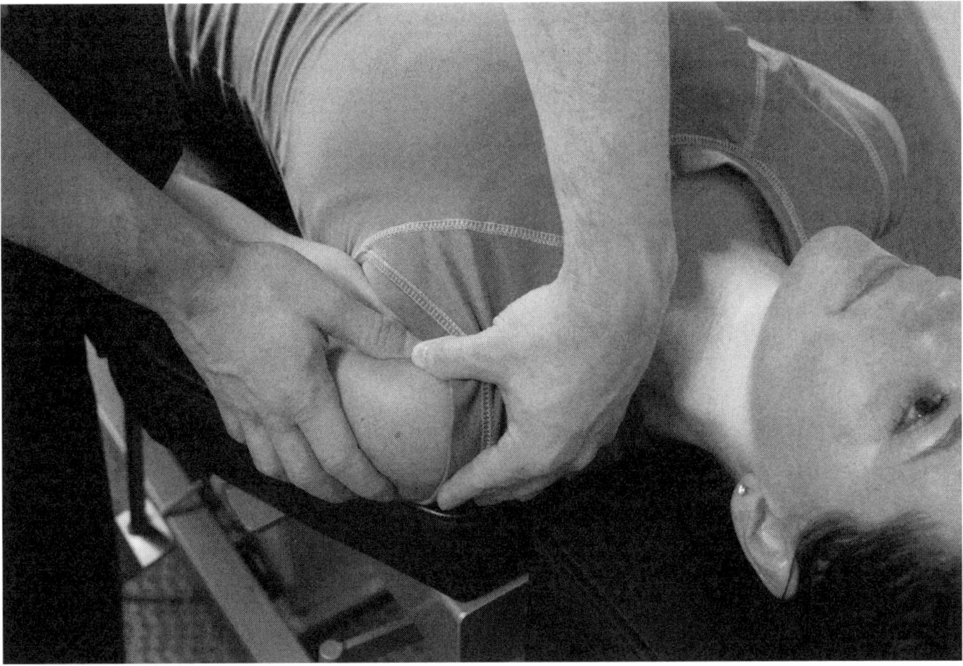

Fig. 19-6 The clinician can apply MFR, sustained pressure, strumming and ischemic compression in this position.

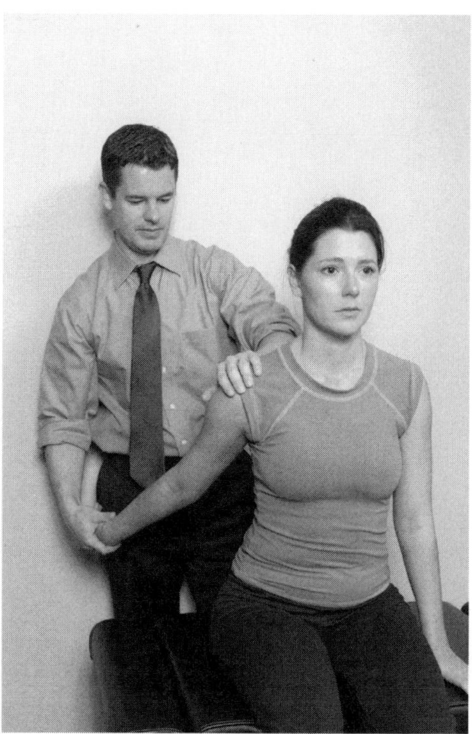

Fig. 19-7 PIR of the long head of the biceps. Stretch the patient further into extension, adduction, internal rotation and pronation after she gently contracts into flexion, abduction, external rotation and supination.

Deltoid. Palpate the muscle for hypertonicity, fascial adhesions, tenderness, and trigger points. Utilize soft tissue techniques including myofascial release, sustained pressure, strumming and ischemic compression to address the findings (Fig. 19-8).

Latissimus Dorsi. Palpate the muscle for hypertonicity, fascial adhesions, tenderness, and trigger points. Utilize soft tissue techniques including myofascial release, sustained pressure, strumming and ischemic compression to address the findings. Post-isometric relaxation is useful in reducing tone (Fig. 19-9).

The latissimus dorsi is facilitated as part of the common pattern. This adds to the pattern of humeral internal rotation, thereby overpowering the external rotators. It also helps depress the entire shoulder girdle. Look for trigger points in this muscle to

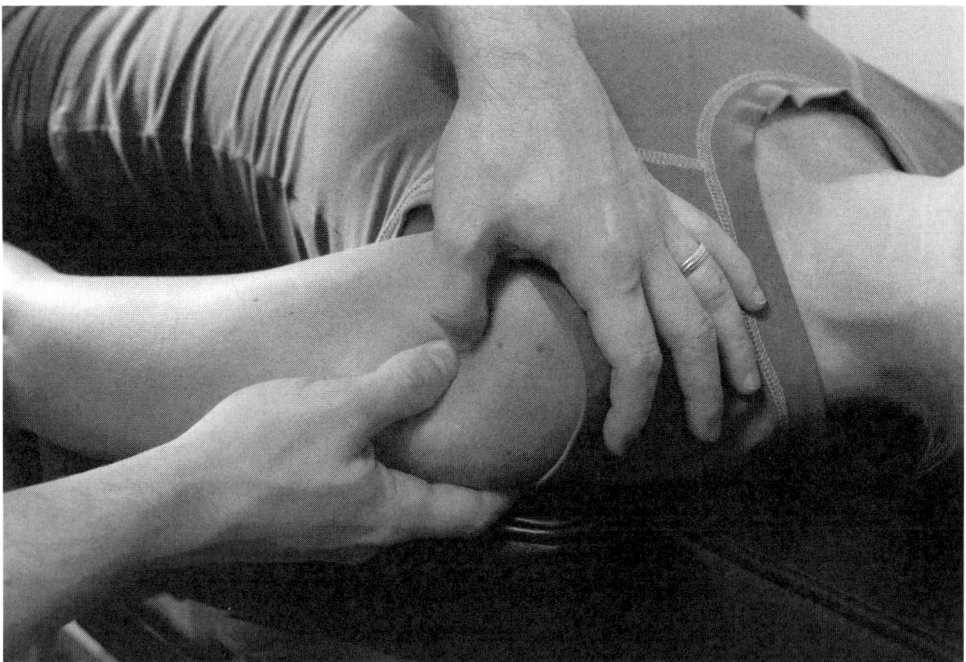

Fig. 19-8 The clinician can apply MFR, sustained pressure, strumming and ischemic compression in this position.

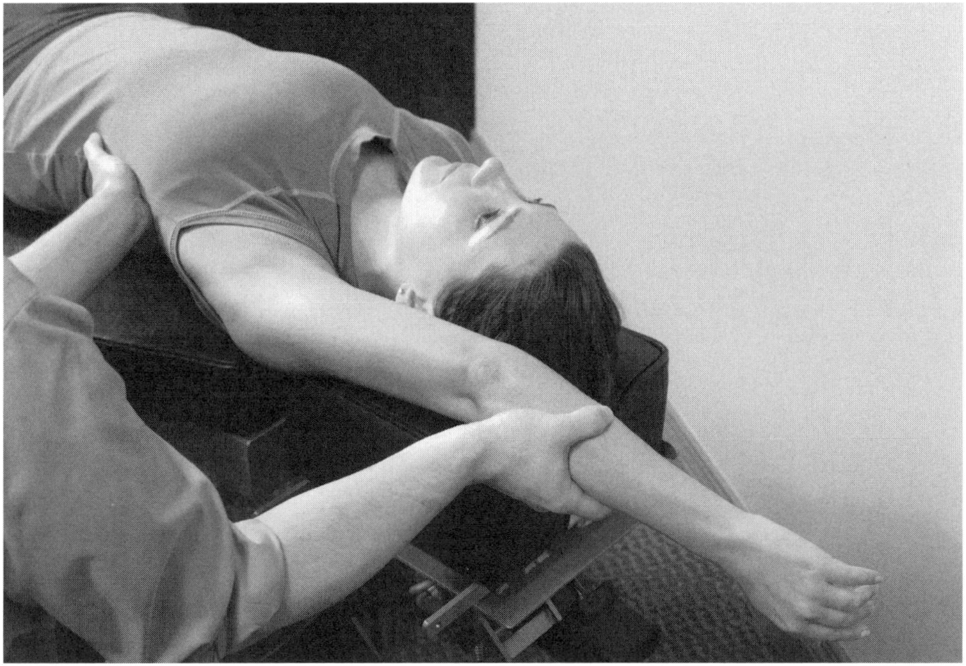

Fig. 19-9 PIR of the latissimus dorsi. Stretch the patient further into flexion, abduction and external rotation after she gently contracts into extension, adduction and internal rotation.

refer pain to the posterolateral ribcage and down the radial side of the arm, forearm and hand.

Subclavius. Palpate the muscle for hypertonicity, fascial adhesions, tenderness, and trigger points. Utilize soft tissue techniques including myofascial release, sustained pressure, strumming and ischemic compression to address the findings (Fig. 19-10).

The subclavius plays a role in two common disorders. In acromioclavicular dysfunction it is usually facilitated and develops trigger points. This results in increased pain in the region of the joint and alters joint mechanics even further. In other words, it makes a bad problem worse. The other disorder this muscle is involved in is costoclavicular thoracic outlet syndrome. In this instance, facilitation of the subclavius approximates the clavicle and rib cage, thereby reducing the space for neural and vascular structures.

Pectoralis Major and Minor. Palpate the muscle for hypertonicity, fascial adhesions, tenderness, and trigger points. Utilize soft tissue techniques including

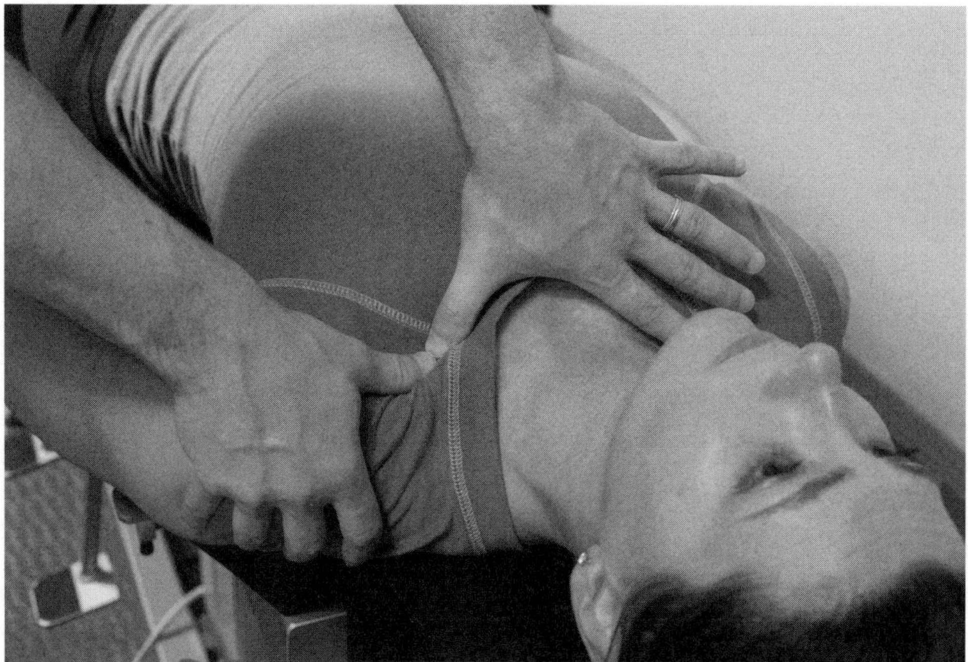

Fig. 19-10 The clinician can apply MFR, sustained pressure, strumming and ischemic compression in this position.

myofascial release, sustained pressure, strumming and ischemic compression to address the findings. Post-isometric relaxation is useful in reducing tone and improving flexibility (Fig. 19-11 and 19-12).

The pectoralis major and minor are facilitated as part of the common pattern. The pec major pulls the humerus into internal rotation, adduction, and extension. Trigger points in this muscle refer pain into the anterior chest, breast, and even into the ulnar aspect of the arm and hand. Travell reports that a particular trigger point on the right side will cause cardiac arrhythmia, and those on the left side may mimic ischemic heart disease.

The pec minor tilts the scapula forward, changing the biomechanics of the rotator cuff. Trigger points refer pain into the chest, anterior shoulder, and the ulnar aspect of the arm and hand. Trigger points on the left side may mimic angina.[31] *Hypertonicity in this muscle is also capable of causing a form of thoracic outlet syndrome*

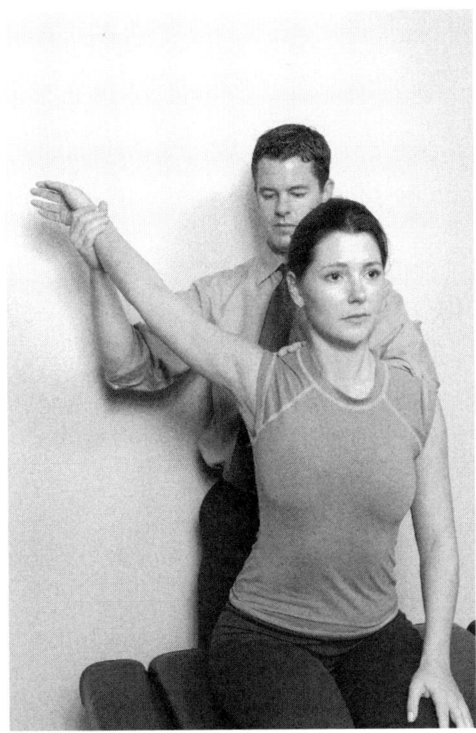

Fig. 19-11 PIR of the pectoralis major. Have the patient contract against resistance into extension and horizontal adduction. Upon relaxation, stretch the arm further into flexion and horizontal abduction.

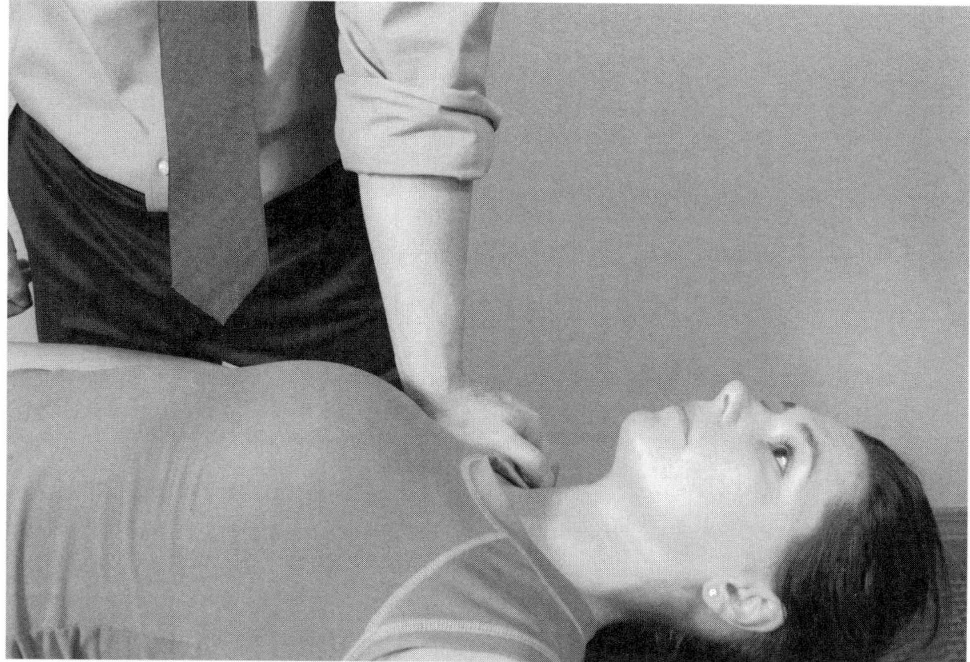

Fig. 19-12 PIR of the pectoralis minor. Have the patient contract against resistance into scapular protraction. Upon relaxation, stretch the scapula further into posterior tilting and retraction.

by compressing the brachial plexus and axillary artery between itself and the ribcage. Be certain to address the pec minor in any case suggestive of neurovascular compromise.

Rhomboids and Middle Trapezius. Palpate these muscles for hypertonicity, fascial adhesions, tenderness, and trigger points. Utilize soft tissue techniques including myofascial release, sustained pressure, strumming and ischemic compression to address the findings. Post-isometric relaxation is also useful in reducing tone and improving flexibility (Fig. 19-13).

These muscles are inhibited as part of the common pattern, allowing the scapulae to abduct. This adds to the common problem of scapular instability and fosters problems with the rotator cuff. Besides this, trigger points in these muscles fuel complaints of pain in the posterior ribcage.

MUSCLE STRENGTH

Evaluate the strength of the rotator cuff and scapular stabilizing muscles with traditional methods. Make sure to assess both their ability to initiate a contraction

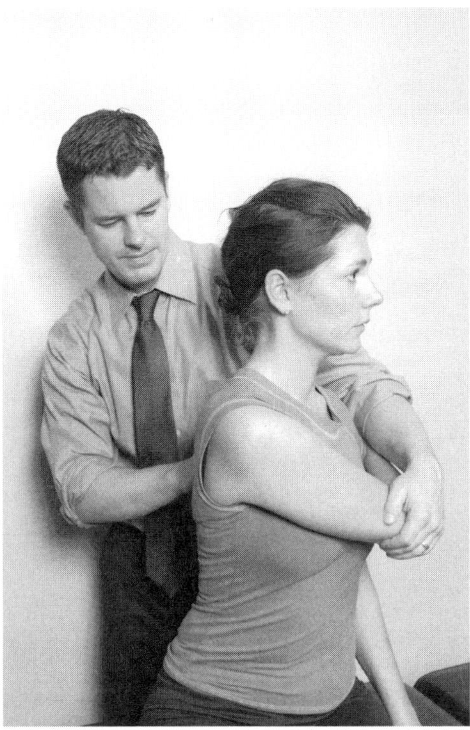

Fig. 19-13 PIR of the rhomboids and middle trapezius. Stretch the patient further into horizontal adduction after she gently contracts the scapular adductors.

as well as their sheer strength. Most often, what we perceive as weakness is more a matter of inhibition. This will follow the common pattern and/or be due to local or segmental dysfunction. Treating the causative factor restores normal strength in these cases. In cases of true muscle weakness, such as those involving muscle atrophy, remedial strengthening is indicated. This is done with traditional strengthening techniques.

GLENOHUMERAL JOINT MOBILITY

Assess mobility of the humeral head in all planes. Most often, one finds the humeral head held anteriorly while posterior motion is restricted. This is consistent with what is seen in the common pattern. Techniques including mobilization, manipulation, and Mulligan's mobilization with movement are useful in treatment (Fig's 19-14 through 19-16).

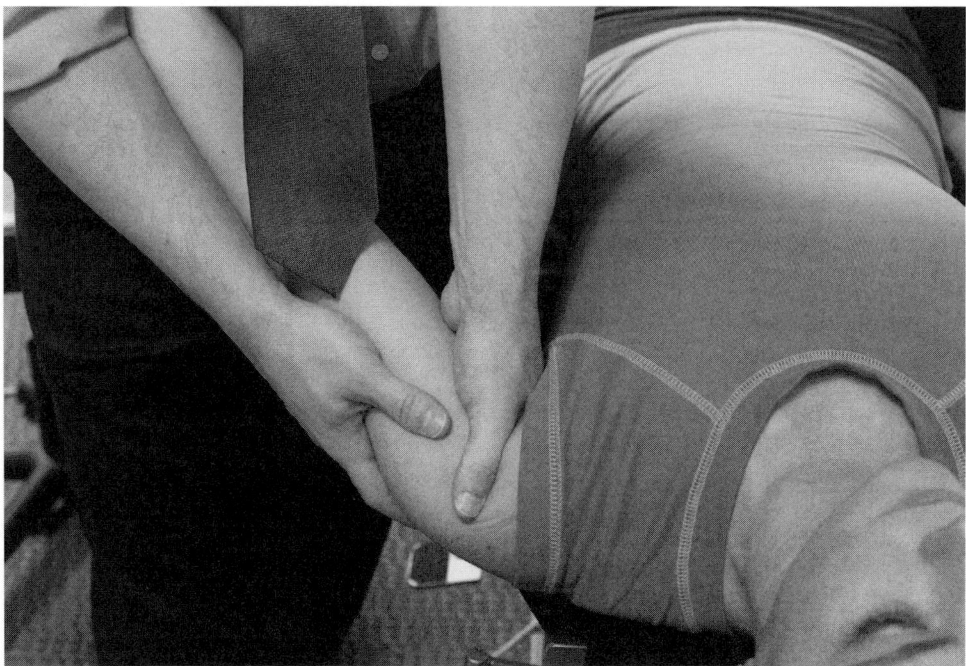

Fig. 19-14 Posterior mobilization of the humeral head while maintaining the arm in the loose-packed position during therapy: external rotation, flexion, and abduction.

ACROMIOCLAVICULAR JOINT MOBILITY

Assess the symmetry and mobility of the acromioclavicular joint using conventional methods. Most often, one finds the distal clavicle displaced superiorly. Use mobilization or manipulation to correct this finding (Fig. 19-17). The practitioner should also assess and treat the subclavius in cases of AC dysfunction. It often becomes hypertonic in these cases and makes the entire problem worse. It also adds to joint dysfunction by altering biomechanics. Treatment is presented in Figure 19-4.

STERNOCLAVICULAR JOINT MOBILITY

Assess the symmetry and mobility of the sternoclavicular joint with traditional methods. Most often, the proximal clavicle is displaced anteriorly. Use mobilization or manipulation to correct this finding (Fig. 19-18). Additionally, be sure to assess the structure of the cervicothoracic junction and ribcage. Asymmetry in these joints will certainly disrupt normal sternoclavicular joint function.

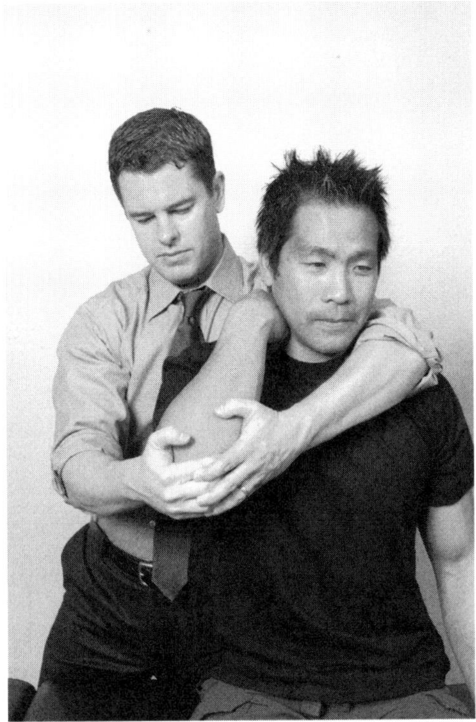

Fig. 19-15 Posterior manipulation of the shoulder. The arm is externally rotated and flexed when the impulse is delivered. Gentle pressure in this direction before the thrust should not cause pain.

SCAPULAR POSITION

Evaluate the position and general mobility of the scapula. In the structural assessment, look for signs of winging, anterior tilting, and abduction, all of which are components of the common pattern. When assessing mobility, move the scapula in all planes while feeling for restriction. Treatment for these asymmetries is through collective strengthening of the scapular stabilizers and corrective taping of the scapula. Strengthen the serratus anterior, rhomboids, and middle and lower trapezii as discussed previously. Corrective scapular taping is presented in Figure 19-19.

SEGMENTAL DYSFUNCTION

The C5 and C6 levels innervate the shoulder joint and the rotator cuff muscles. Dysfunction at either level may cause or contribute to shoulder symptoms via

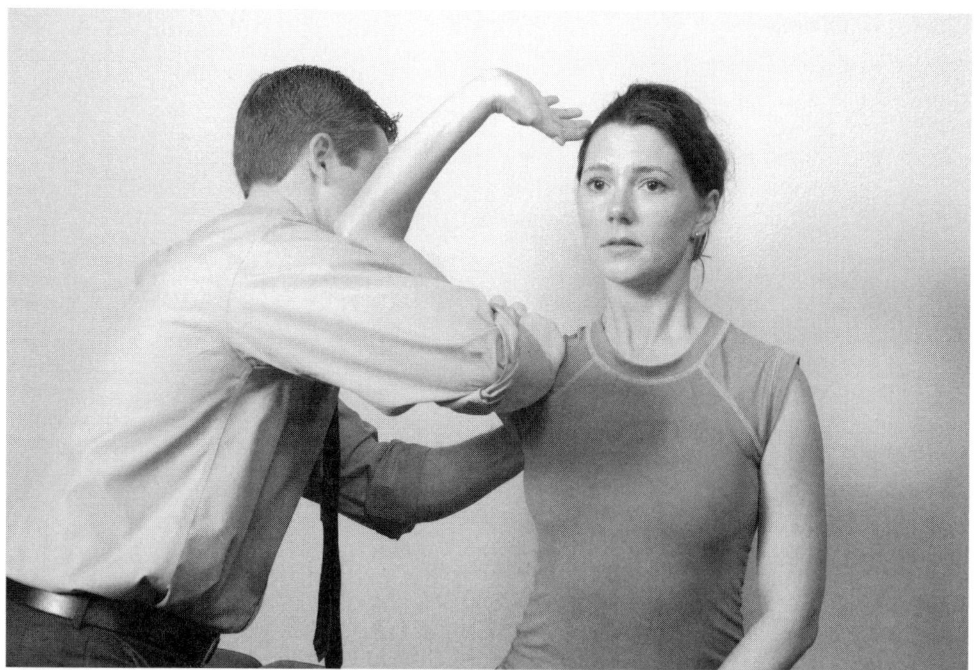

Fig. 19-16 Mulligan's mobilization with movement. Have the patient abduct the shoulder. If this is painful, apply anterior-posterior pressure to the head of the humerus. Reduction or elimination of pain when raising the arm while the pressure is applied indicates a positive test. Treat by repeating this maneuver ten times. Stop or change the vector of pressure if the patient experiences any pain.[182]

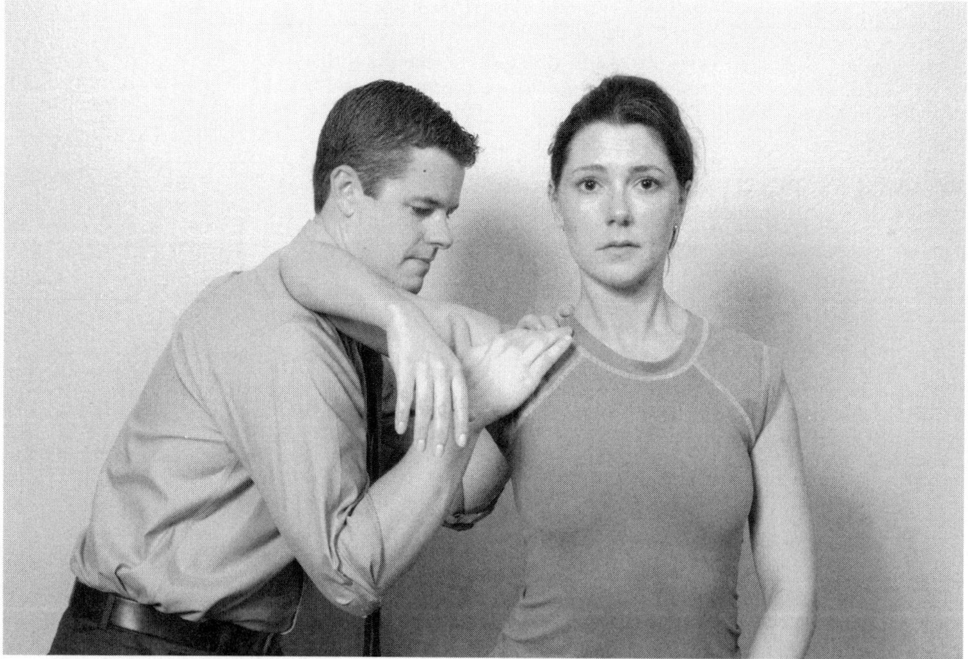

Fig. 19-17 Mobilization of the distal clavicle. With the patient's arm draped over the clinician's shoulder, contact the distal clavicle with the second and third fingers. Mobilize superior-inferior.

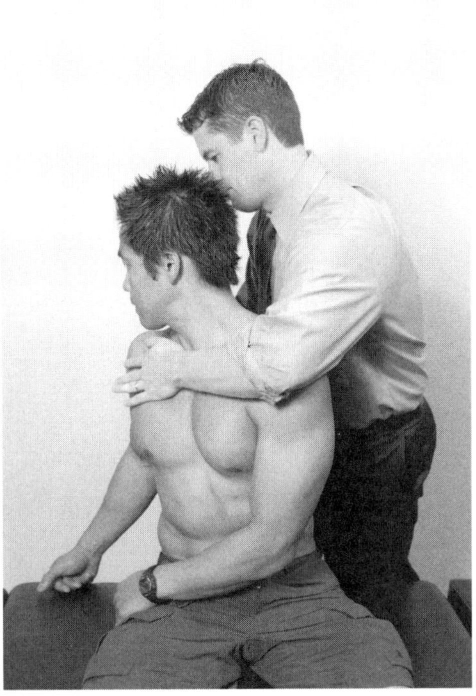

Fig. 19-18 Correction of anterior displaced proximal clavicle. Contact the proximal clavicle with the heel of the clinician's hand. Gently rotate the patient's torso to the affected side and then apply a posterior and inferior directed thrust to the clavicle.

referred pain mechanisms. Or, it can create shoulder problems by inhibiting the rotator cuff muscles, thereby changing biomechanics in this sensitive region. This in turn causes joint and muscle pathology. Please consult Chapter 11, The Cervical Spine, for details on cervical spine examination and treatment.

THORACIC SPINE

The thoracic spine should also be examined in the presence of shoulder dysfunction. This is because it directly influences the structure of the ribcage, which then influences the position of the scapula. Thus, faulty structure or altered motion of the thoracic spine will impact the function of the scapula.

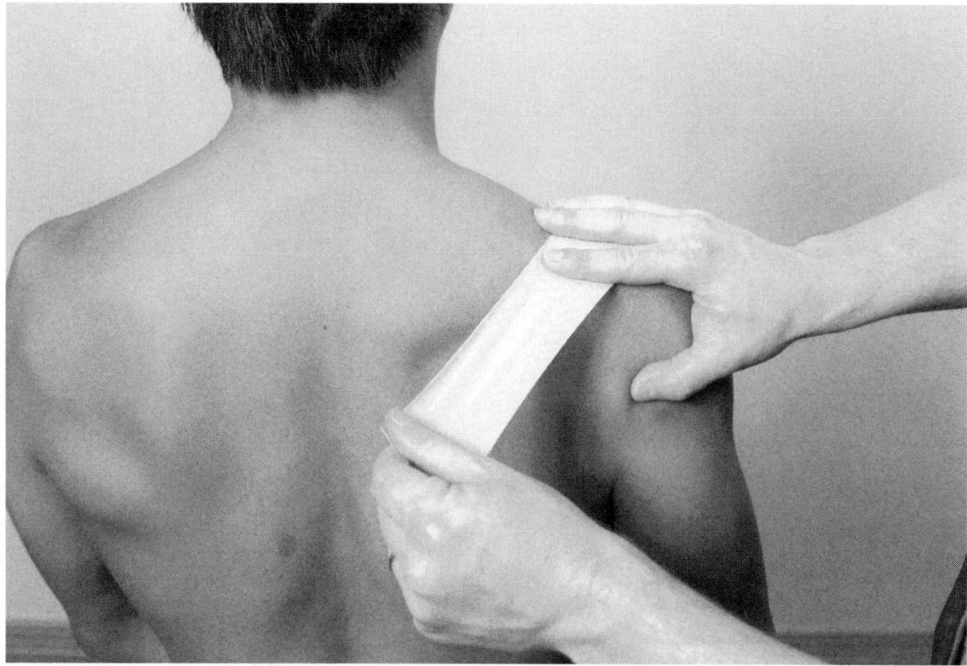

Fig. 19-19 Corrective taping of the scapula. Have the patient retract and depress the scapula first. Next, apply tape to the supraspinous fossa and pull inferior-medially to correct the structural fault. In cases involving anterior tilting of the scapula, apply the tape to the anterior proximal humerus and pull upwards, then down the back in the same direction.

The relationship between the thoracic spine and shoulder is evident in an excellent treatment technique used by physical therapists such as Partridge.[152] This technique is basically just an anterior mobilization of the middle and upper thoracic spine, with the goal being to improve thoracic extension (Fig. 19-20). Impressively, it often results in an immediate improvement of 10–15 degrees in shoulder elevation. The rationale behind its success is that the improved thoracic/ribcage extension allows the scapula to tilt posteriorly, thereby improving glenohumeral mechanics (while the author agrees with this rationale, remember that the thoracic spine is covered with neurolymphatic reflex zones as well as meridian-based Associated Reflexes. Stimulating these with manual pressure can facilitate an inhibited muscle, which will result in improved shoulder motion as well).

A more specific thoracic disorder to look for in the shoulder-pain population is 2nd rib dysfunction. In the strain-counterstrain literature, Jones reports that a depressed second rib will cause diminished shoulder abduction.[178] He suggests assessment and treatment with strain-counterstrain principles (Fig. 19-21 and 19-22).

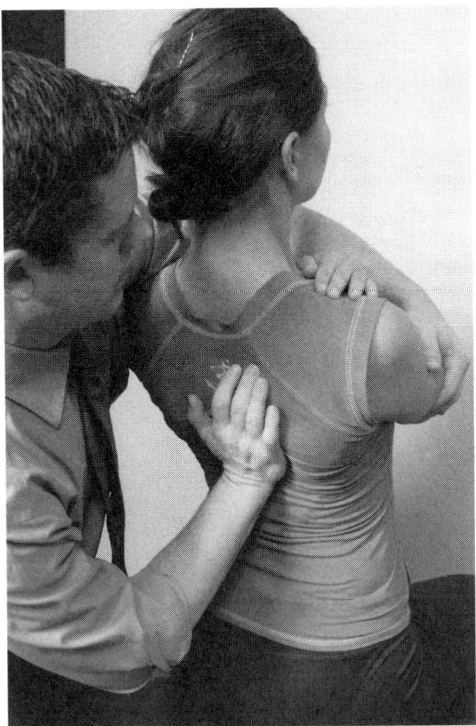

Fig. 19-20 General mobilization of the mid-thoracic spine.

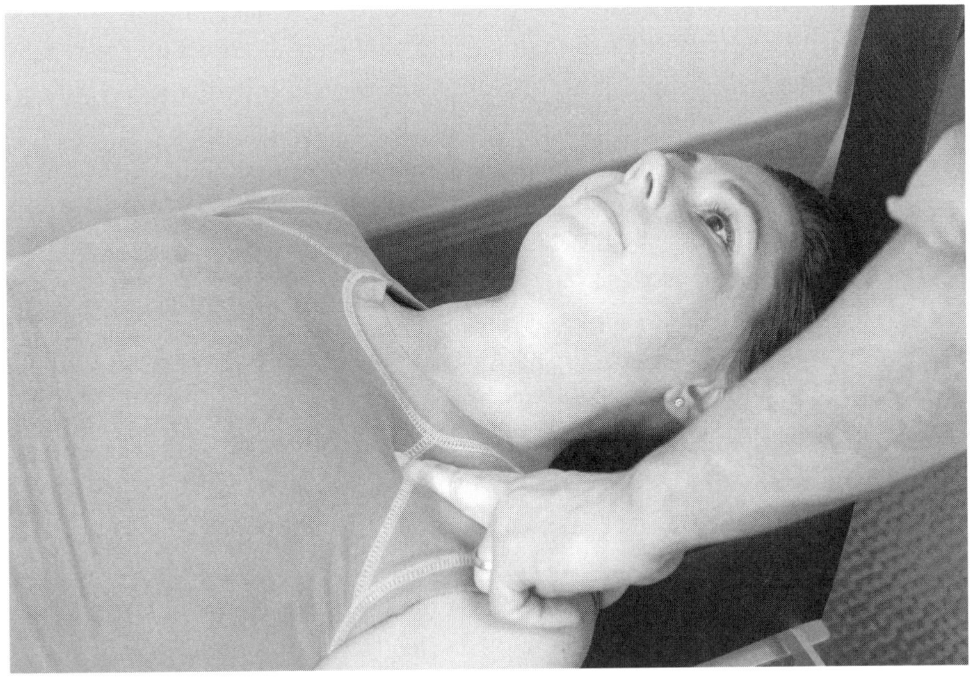

Fig. 19-21 Assessing for a depressed 2nd rib. Palpate for a tender point on the 2nd rib, one and a half inches inferior to the middle of the clavicle.

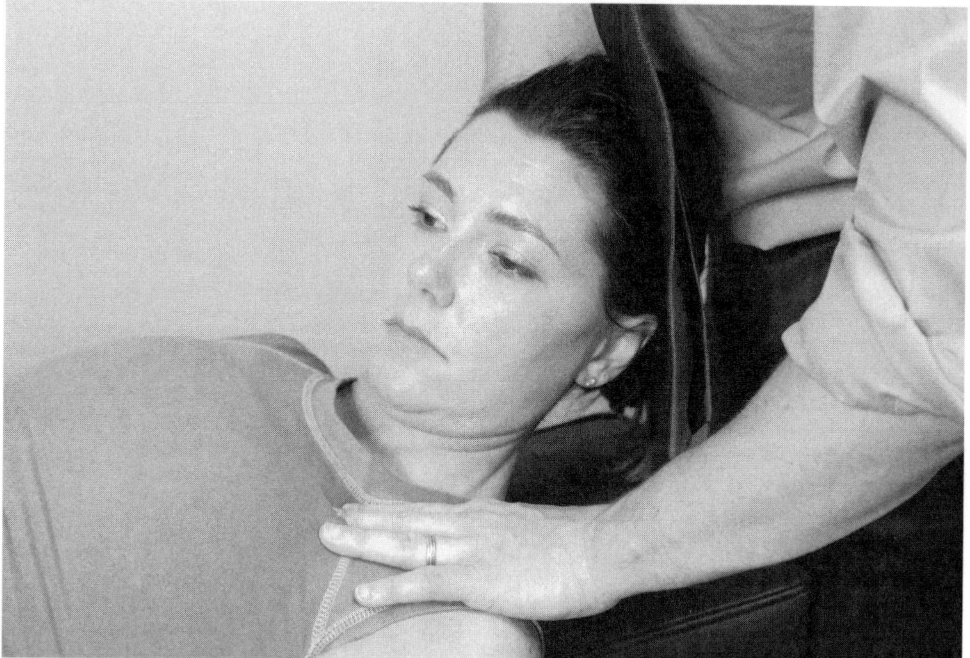

Fig. 19-22 Treatment of a depressed 2nd rib. The position of ease is found by flexion, ipsilateral sidebending and rotation.

Other manual therapists note this connection as well. Boyle presents two case reports of patients with shoulder pain who were successfully treated by mobilizing the 2nd rib in a posterior-anterior direction.[183] Not only did this therapy eliminate shoulder symptoms, but it also eliminated the positive shoulder orthopedic tests each patient demonstrated prior to treatment.

MOVEMENT PATTERNS

Assess the shoulder's quality of motion during abduction. Look for any signs of disharmony between the scapula and humerus. Also look for premature elevation of the scapula or even an excessive amount of scapular elevation (Fig. 19-23). This is often an attempt to elevate the arm without moving the glenohumeral joint the normal amount. These abnormal findings correspond with the upper crossed syndrome pattern; the scapular rhythm is altered and arm elevation is compromised as a result.

Correcting faulty movement patterns involves addressing muscle imbalances as previously described. It also requires changing the way the person is using his or her shoulder. This re-education should focus on having the person assume an Alexandrian posture before raising the arm. In addition to this, he/she must retract and depress the scapula before raising the arm. This helps inhibit the upper trapezius' dominance over the scapulothoracic rhythm. It also helps maximize clearance of the acromion from the humerus. This leads to less impingement, which leads to less pain (Fig. 19-24).

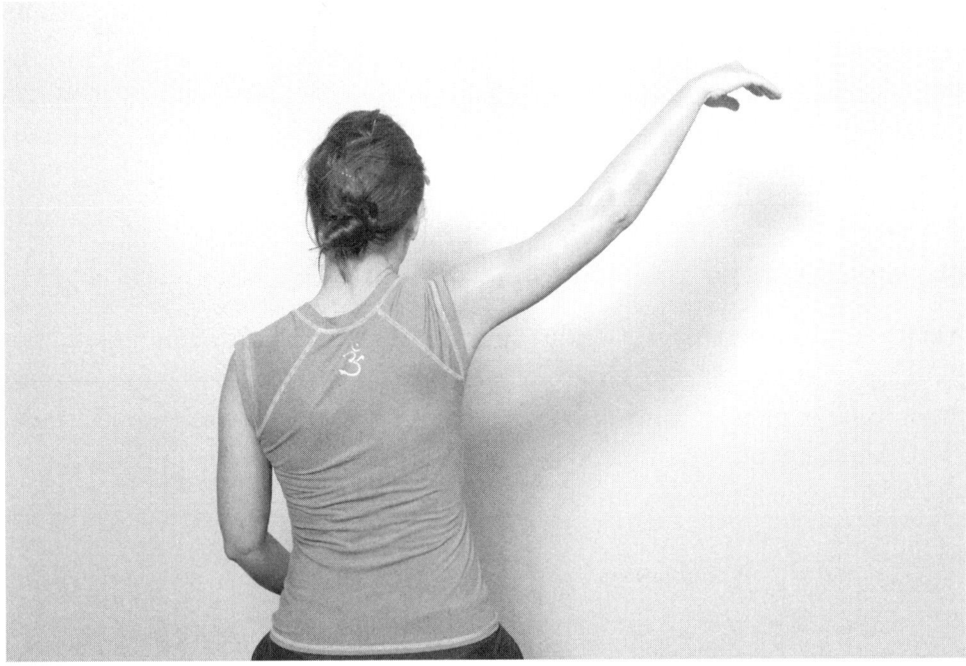

Fig. 19-23 Faulty arm elevation pattern.

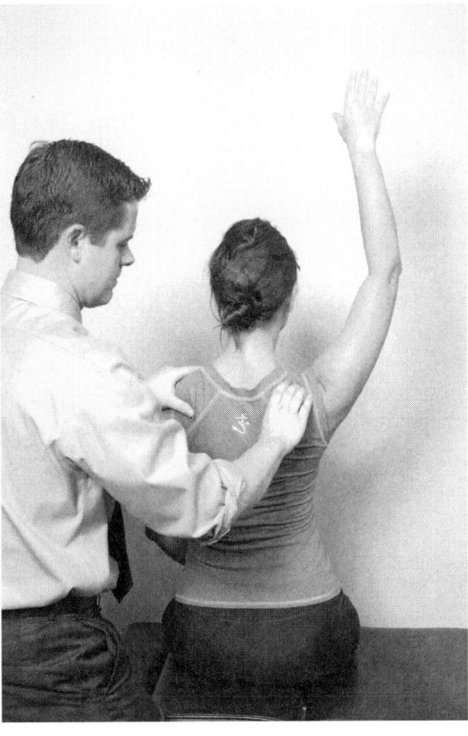

Fig. 19-24 Teaching the proper arm elevation recruitment pattern.

Another benefit of retraining the scapular stabilizers (especially the middle and lower traps, rhomboids) is that it activates the body's extensor synergy. This helps diminish the dominance of the upper crossed/common pattern while aiding in the recruitment of other extensor muscles. This is beneficial for obvious reasons.

ENERGY-BASED TECHNIQUES

Auricular Acupressure. Gently squeeze the point corresponding to the shoulder with two fingers. Hold for 5 seconds, then relax 5 seconds. Increase the amount of pressure with each cycle for a total time of one minute (6 cycles). Do this initially on the ear on the involved side only; treat the opposite ear as well if the patient does not improve.

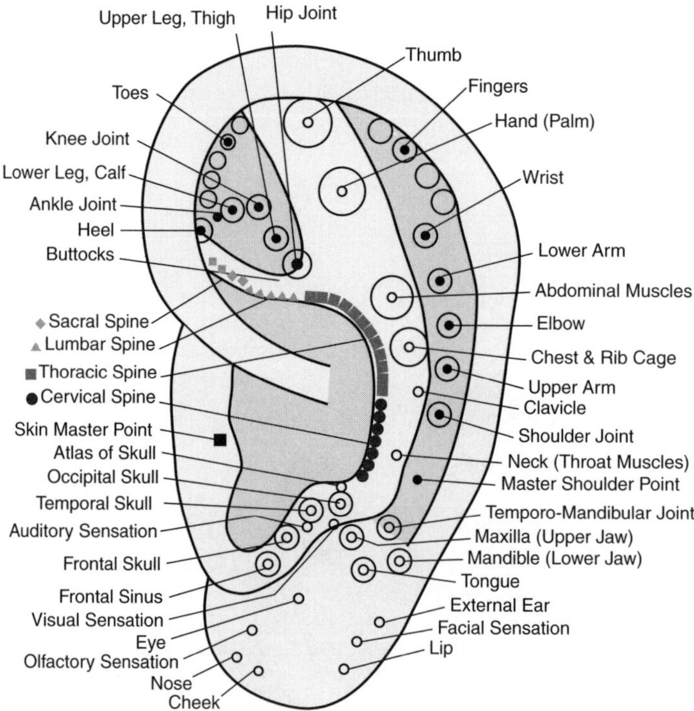

Fig. 19-25

Reflexology. Begin by massaging the entire foot. Walk up the foot with the thumbs along the five zones. Treat both the plantar and dorsal surfaces. Work the toes as well. Spend extra time on the medial border of the foot corresponding with the spine. Also, work on areas associated with different organs needing an extra "boost." Following this long warm-up, massage the area on the foot corresponding to the shoulder.

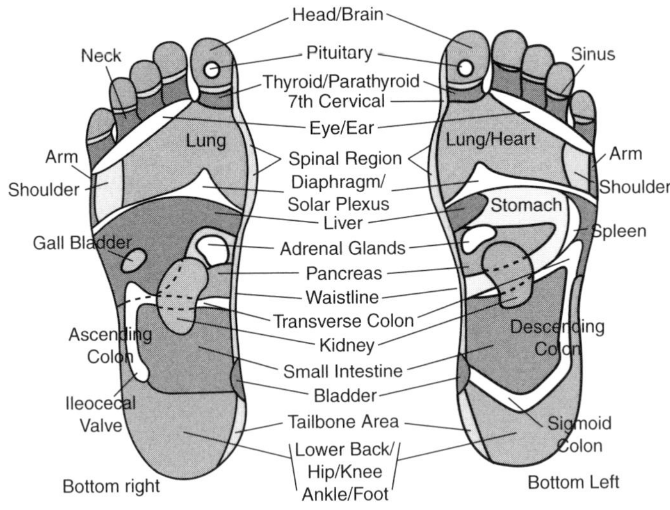

Fig. 19-26

HIGH-YIELD SCAN

Perform a scan of the high-yield elements of the body including:

- Gait
- Posture
- Sit-to-Stand
- Miniature Squat
- Respiration
- Romberg Test
- Fukuda's Test
- Upper Cervical Spine
- Middle Cervical Spine
- TMJ
- Pelvis
- Feet
- Stress Screen

EVALUATING AND TREATING THE SECONDARY FACTORS

Posture. Assess the patient's posture with the methods described. If the upper crossed pattern is present, there is a greater likelihood of shoulder dysfunction. Poor postural habits at work and home add to this, as the acromiohumeral space is usually compromised and the rotator cuff's leverage is altered. Taking steps to help the patient sit and stand up straight will improve his biomechanical status and reduce rotator cuff symptoms.

Sleeping. Many patients with shoulder dysfunction complain of increased pain with sleeping. This is usually from lying directly on the joint when they are in bed. Educate them of this stressor and urge them to lie on the other side. If this is not possible, place pillows under the ribcage so the shoulder's load is lessened.

The shoulder may also be aggravated even when it is not layed upon. Oftentimes, this is because it must hang down across the person's chest while they are asleep. To combat this strain, have the person place a body pillow in front of their torso so that they may rest the arm upon it.

Repetitive Motions. Oftentimes, elevation the arm or reaching backwards bother the shoulder. In the first case, remember that humeral internal rotation creates impingement when the arm is elevated. Keeping this in mind, teach the patient to place the arm in neutral or external rotation when they elevate it so that impingement is minimized.

In the latter case, expect this movement to cause anterior instability. Urge the patient to avoid repetitive movements involving extension or horizontal abduction. Teach him to rotate his torso towards the arm when it is retracting so that overall stress is decreased. There are many other activities which stress the shoulder joint that are not covered in this text. The reader must thoroughly question the patient in order to find out if he/she is doing things detrimental to their recovery, and then teach him or her ways to lessen or eliminate the stress.

20 The Elbow

EVALUATION AND TREATMENT OF THE PRIMARY FACTORS

Wrist Extensors. Palpate these muscles for hypertonicity, fascial adhesions, tenderness, and trigger points. Utilize soft tissue techniques including myofascial release, sustained pressure, strumming and ischemic compression to address the findings. Post-isometric relaxation useful in reducing tone and improving flexibility (Fig. 20-1).

The wrist extensors become inhibited as part of the common pattern. This compromises their peak strength and endurance, exposing them to strain and overuse injuries in a high percentage of people. This can cause wrist problems through altered joint mechanics and impaired stability. More commonly, however, dysfunction of this muscle results in lateral epicondyle pain. Conventional methods to address myofascial dysfunction, increase strength and increase flexibility are often helpful but they are not enough. The practitioner must also address the articulations of the wrist and elbow while working to combat the common pattern synergy. Additionally, the therapist must remember to inspect muscles including the scalenes which can activate trigger points in the wrist extensors.

Wrist Flexors. Palpate these muscles for hypertonicity, fascial adhesions, tenderness, and trigger points. Utilize soft tissue techniques including myofascial release, sustained pressure, strumming and ischemic compression to address the findings. Post-isometric relaxation is useful in reducing tone and improving flexibility (Fig. 20-2).

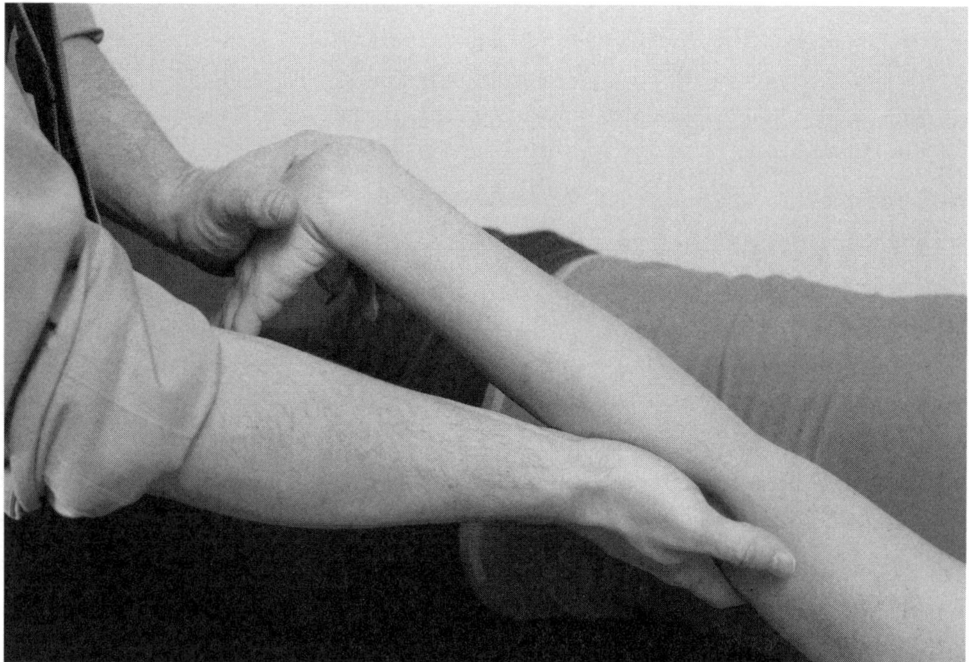

Fig. 20-1 PIR stretching of the wrist extensors. Stretch the wrist into further flexion after the patient gently contracts the wrist extensors.

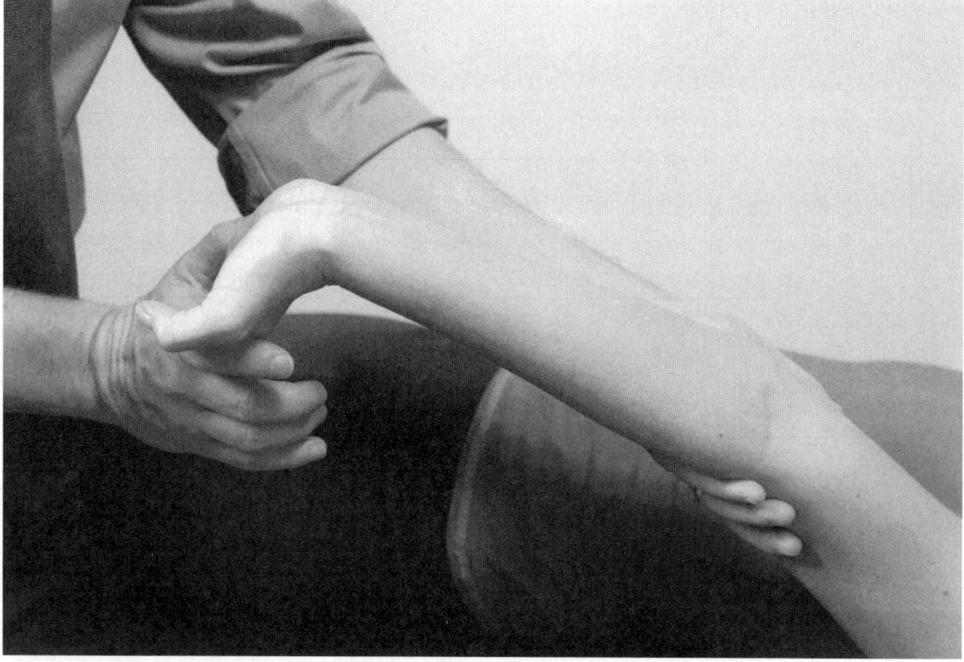

Fig. 20-2 PIR stretching of the wrist flexors. Stretch the wrist into further extension after the patient gently contracts the wrist flexors.

The wrist flexors are facilitated as part of the common pattern. This can lead to wrist problems by altering joint mechanics. More commonly it causes symptoms at the elbow. This may be a direct result of increased tension in this muscle, as seen with medial epicondylitis.

Supinator. Palpate the muscle for hypertonicity, fascial adhesions, tenderness, and trigger points. Utilize soft tissue techniques including myofascial release, sustained pressure, strumming and ischemic compression to address the findings. Post-isometric relaxation is useful for reducing tone and improving flexibility (Fig. 20-3).

Pay special attention to the supinator in patients with chronic elbow problems. In some individuals this muscle has the potential to entrap the deep radial nerve, thereby mimicking lateral epicondylitis.

Pronator Teres. Palpate the muscle for hypertonicity, fascial adhesions, tenderness, and trigger points. Utilize soft tissue techniques including myofascial

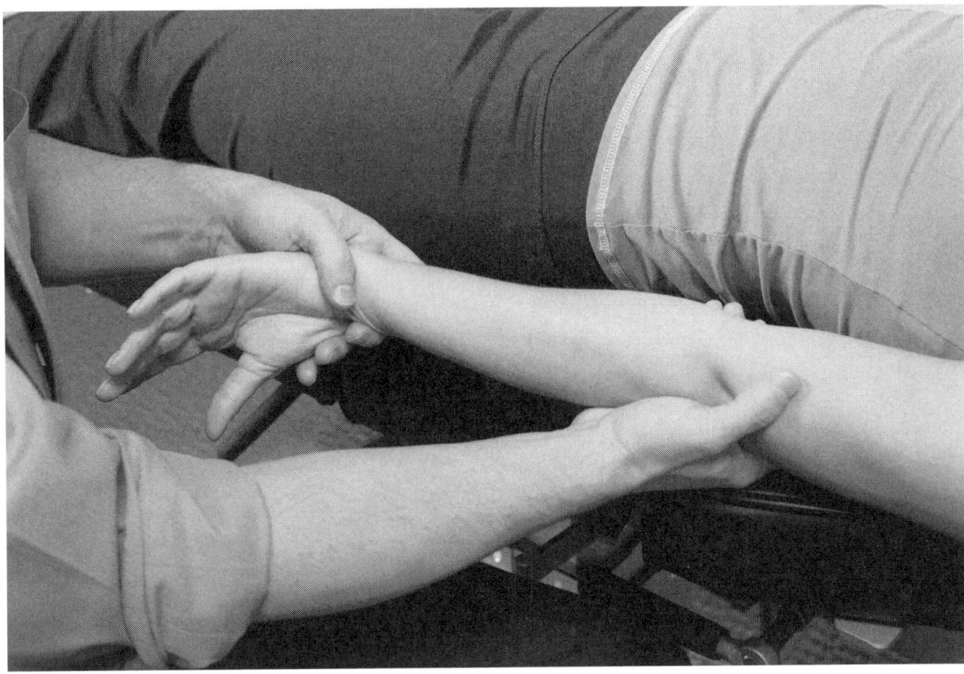

Fig. 20-3 PIR of the supinator. Stretch the forearm into further pronation after the patient gently contracts the supinator into resistance.

release, sustained pressure, strumming and ischemic compression to address the findings. Post-isometric relaxation is useful in reducing tone and improving flexibility (Fig. 20-4).

The pronator teres is best-known for its ability to compress the median nerve, which runs between the muscle's two heads. This will simulate carpal tunnel syndrome, though it can be distinguished as having sensory loss in the thenar region whereas carpal tunnel syndrome will not involve this area.

Biceps. Palpate the muscle for hypertonicity, fascial adhesions, tenderness, and trigger points. Utilize soft tissue techniques including myofascial release, sustained pressure, strumming and ischemic compression to address the findings. Post-isometric relaxation is useful in reducing tone and improving flexibility (See Fig. 19-7).

The biceps are facilitated as part of the common pattern. This alters the biomechanics of the elbow joint. It also leads to trigger point formation; expect these to refer pain to the anterior shoulder and elbow.

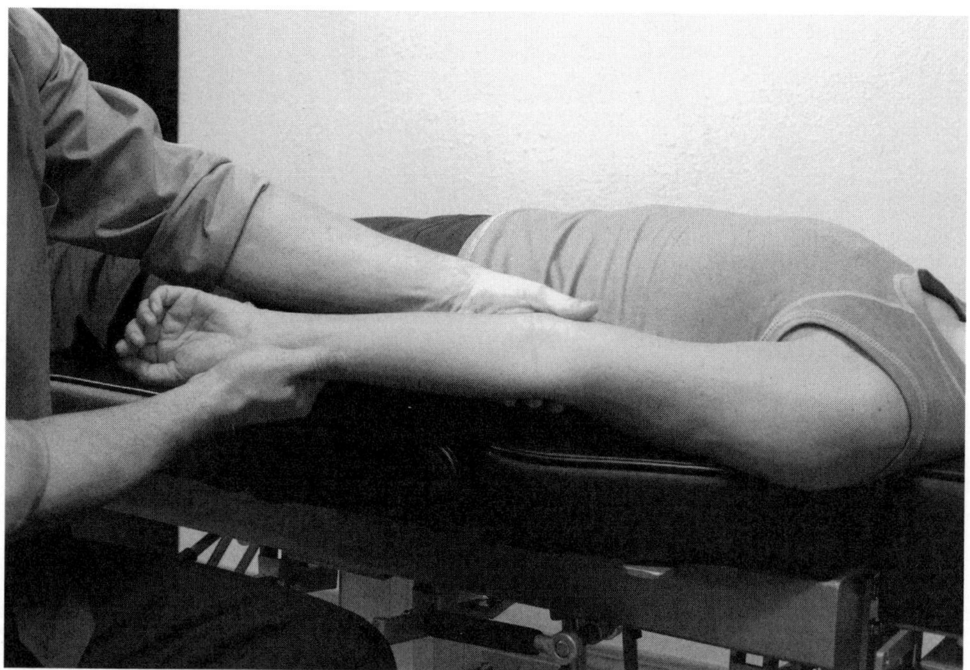

Fig. 20-4 PIR of the pronator teres. Stretch the forearm further into supination after the patient gently contracts into pronation. Be sure to have the elbow extended during this treatment.

Triceps. Palpate the muscle for hypertonicity, fascial adhesions, tenderness, and trigger points. Utilize soft tissue techniques including myofascial release, sustained pressure, strumming and ischemic compression to address the findings. Post-isometric relaxation is also useful in reducing tone and improving flexibility (Fig. 20-5).

The triceps are inhibited as part of the common pattern. They are easily overworked and can sometimes develop trigger points. When present, these trigger points can refer pain to the posterior shoulder, arm and forearm. They may also refer to the lateral epicondyle, so consider this in the differential diagnosis in cases of tennis elbow.

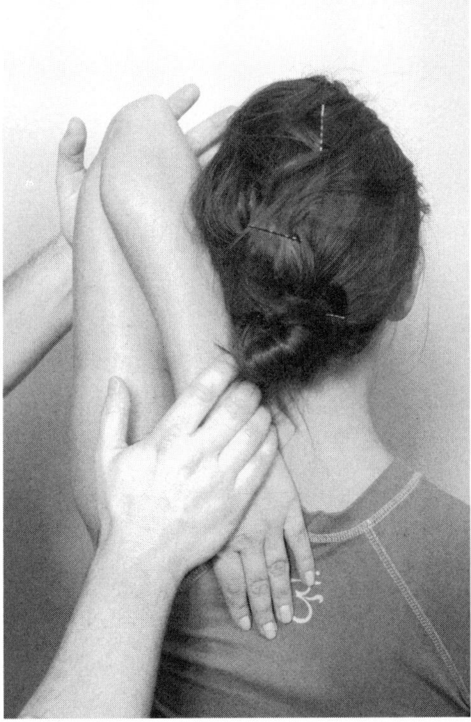

Fig. 20-5 PIR of the triceps. With the patient's arm elevated over her head, have her gently extend her elbow into resistance. Upon relaxation, stretch her further into flexion. If maximal elbow flexion is attained but the triceps is not adequately stretched, flex the shoulder further.

MUSCLE STRENGTH

Evaluate elbow strength with traditional methods. Make sure to assess both the ability to initiate a contraction as well as sheer strength. Most often, what we perceive as weakness is more a matter of inhibition. This will follow the common pattern and/or be due to local or segmental dysfunction. Treating the causative factor restores normal strength in these cases. In cases of true muscle weakness, such as those involving muscle atrophy, remedial strengthening is indicated. This is done with traditional strengthening techniques.

JOINT MOBILITY

Radial Head Mobility

Impaired radial head motion is implicated in cases of lateral epicondylitis and lateral elbow pain. Assess the radial head's motion with conventional methods and mobilize/thrust into the direction of restriction (Fig. 20-6). Take note that the radial head is most often malpositioned posteriorly.

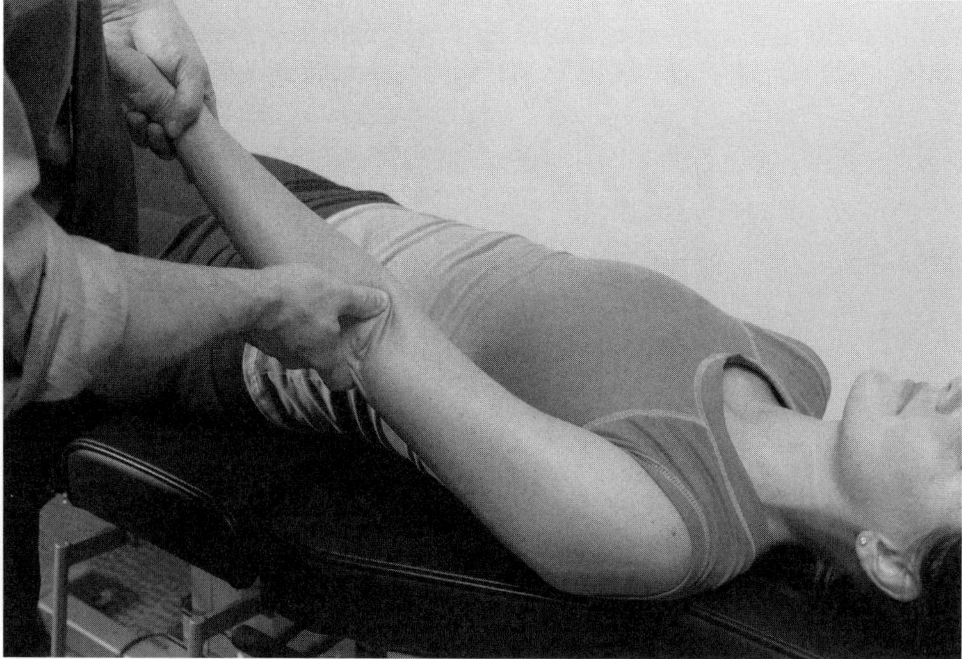

Fig. 20-6 Correction of posterior radial head displacement.

Ulnohumeral Mobility

Assess ulnohumeral mobility using conventional methods. Dysfunction most often involves medial subluxation of the olecranon with restricted lateral motion of the ulna on the humerus. This is consistent with findings that patients with excessive cubital valgus are more prone to elbow problems than those with normal elbow structure. Mobilization can be through direct, specific contact on the olecranon or with a broad contact on the medial or lateral aspect of the joint (Fig. 20-7 and Fig. 20-8). Mulligan's MWM is another excellent technique to address ulnohumeral dysfunction(Fig. 20-9).[28]

SEGMENTAL MOBILITY

Examine the lower cervical spine for signs and symptoms of vertebral dysfunction. The C6 level directly innervates the joint and can refer pain to the elbow. Dysfunction in the rest of the lower cervical spine contributes to elbow problems as well through patterns of facilitation and inhibition, thereby affecting its strength and flexibility. Vicenzino has shown the cervical lateral glide

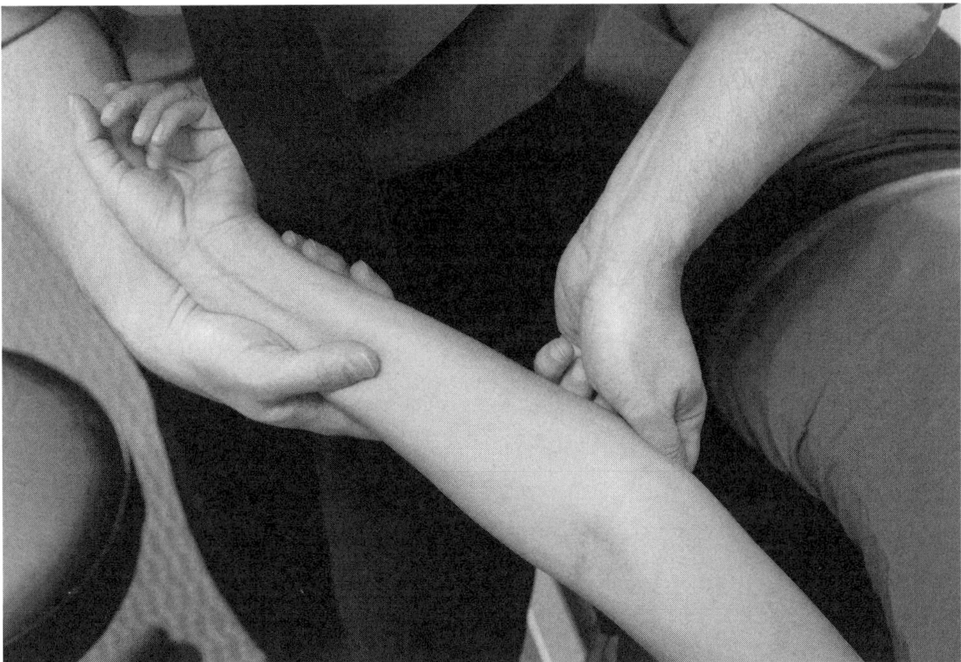

Fig. 20-7 Mobilization of the ulnohumeral joint: specific contact. Make contact on the medial aspect of the olecranon process and mobilize in a medial-lateral direction, taking care to stabilize the distal forearm.

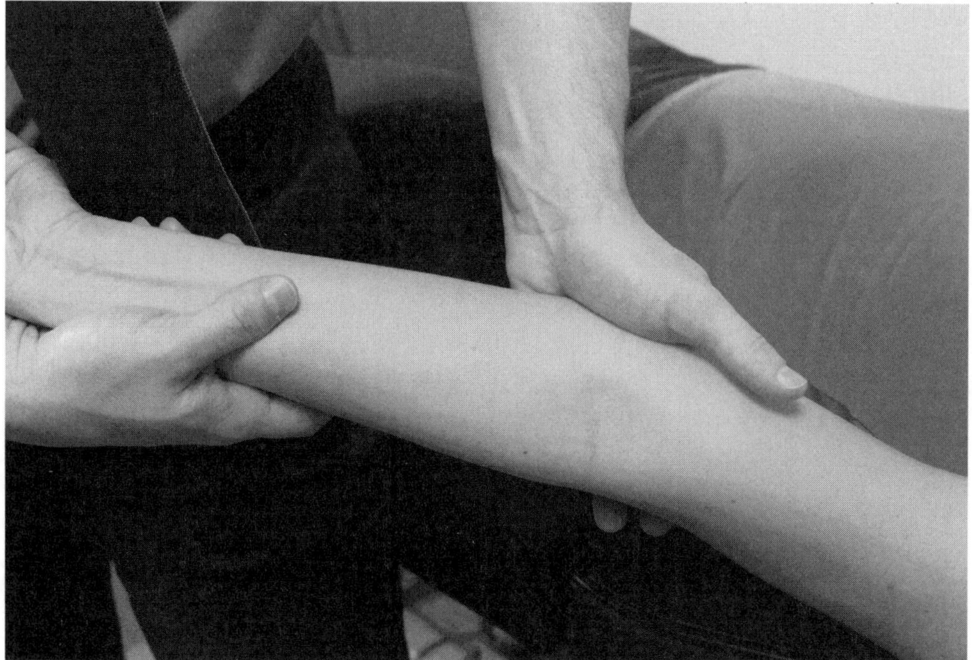

Fig. 20-8 Mobilization of the ulnohumeral joint: broad contact. Make contact on the medial aspect of the elbow and mobilize in a medial-lateral direction.

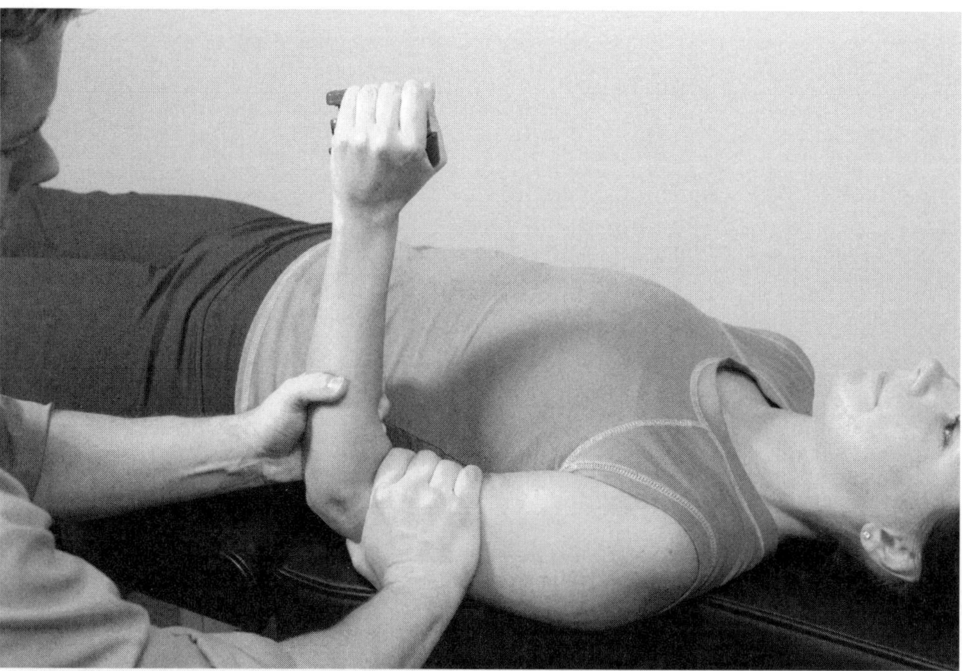

Fig. 20-9 Mulligan's MWM for lateral epicondylalgia. Stabilize the distal humerus while applying a sustained lateral glide to the proximal ulna. When indicated, this mobilization eliminates pain during an otherwise painful motion such as making a fist. As always, alter the direction of the pressure to maximize pain relief, then repeat 10 times as treatment.

mobilization (See Figure 11-21) to be especially effective in treating lateral epicondylalgia.

POSTURE OF THE UPPER EXTREMITY

Postural observation begins by examining the position of the entire extremity in space. Start by looking at the way the scapula rests on the ribcage. Expect to see scapular abduction, winging, and anterior tilting. Each of these components acts to de-stabilize the upper extremity. It will also contribute to other findings seen along with the common pattern including humeral internal rotation. Next, assess the elbow joint itself. Is the carrying angle greater or smaller than normal? Also, is the elbow pronated, supinated, or in neutral?

Each deviation from neutral places added stress on the elbow joint and the muscles controlling it. Take the effects of the common pattern, for instance. With the extremity internally rotated and the forearm already pronated, the person must actively externally rotate the arm and supinate the forearm just to bring the joint to neutral. This taxes the muscles and joints, not to mention depleting the system's energy reserves. Any activity requiring supination and external rotation beyond neutral places even greater stress on the extremity.

In essence, this situation makes it relatively easy to explain the overuse syndromes encountered at the elbow. Not only does this environment invite the development of problems, but it also makes it easy for them to remain. For these reasons be sure to address the patient's posture—from the feet and low back to the thorax and upper extremity—in order to reduce stress on the elbow.

MOVEMENT PATTERNS

Faulty movement patterns of the elbow and the entire upper quadrant are often responsible for generating and/or perpetuating elbow conditions. For this reason, the clinician should observe the way the entire upper extremity moves during all activities. Observe for qualities such as symmetry, smoothness of movement, and coordination as well as the presence of tremor, guarding, catching or locking. In short, any deviation from normal should be addressed with the goal being smooth, symmetrical motion.

Stressors such as poor alignment, improper recruitment patterns, and muscle imbalance due to the upper crossed syndrome/common pattern are present in most individuals and must be addressed. This is aided on a global scale using the methods described previously in this text. However, to achieve a much quicker change the patient should also be taught specific methods to alter his or her quality of movement right away. An easy way to implement this is by working on the person's scapular and shoulder recruitment patterns. Specifically, have her contract the scapular stabilizers and shoulder external rotators before using the affected extremity (Fig. 20-10). Not only does the pre-contraction stabilize the shoulder girdle, but it also activates the extensor synergy. This helps re-program the patient's motor patterns and aids in restoring normal muscle balance. In addition, this pre-contraction pulls the elbow out of the undesirable position of flexion, pronation, and humeral internal rotation prior to movement. This automatically lessens stress on the joint itself and lowers the demand on contractile tissues.

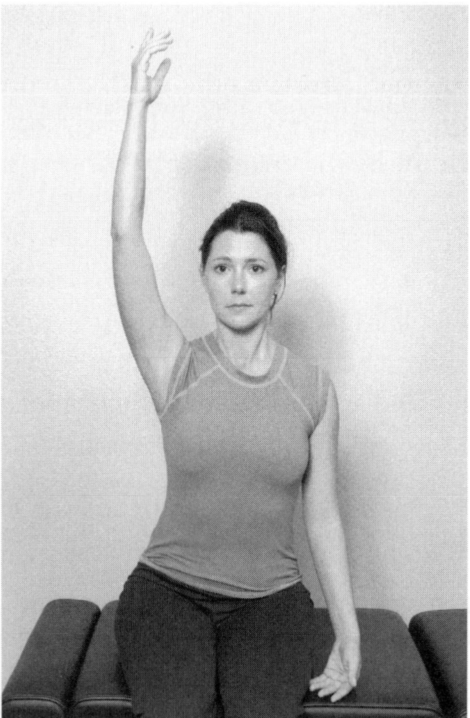

Fig. 20-10 Teach the patient to recruit the scapular stabilizers and external rotators prior to initiating movement with the elbow and wrist/hand.

ENERGY-BASED TECHNIQUES

Auricular Acupressure. Gently squeeze the point corresponding to the elbow with two fingers. Hold for 5 seconds, then relax 5 seconds. Increase the amount of pressure with each cycle for a total time of one minute (6 cycles). Do this initially on the ear on the involved side only; treat the opposite ear as well if the patient does not improve.

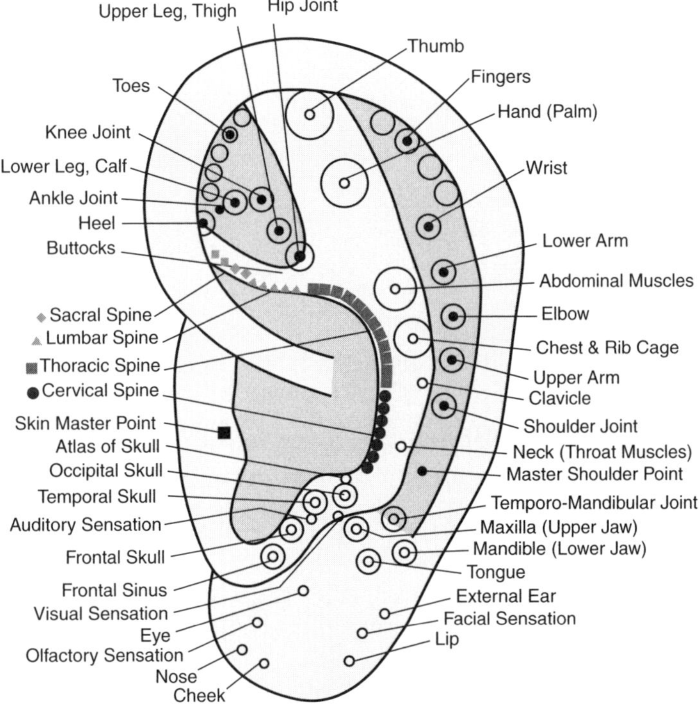

Fig. 20-11

Reflexology. Begin by massaging the entire foot. Walk up the foot with the thumbs along the five zones. Treat the plantar and dorsal surfaces. Work the toes as well. Spend extra time on the medial border of the foot corresponding with the spine. Also, work on areas associated with different organs needing an extra "boost." Following this long warm-up, massage the area on the foot corresponding to the elbow.

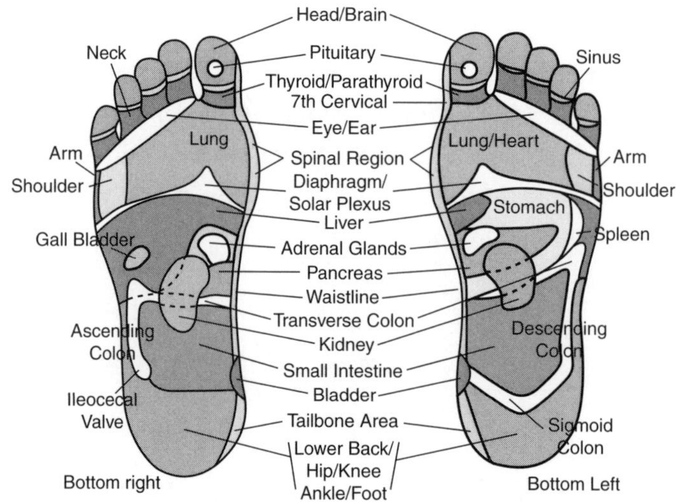

Fig. 20-12

HIGH-YIELD SCAN

Perform a scan of the high-yield elements of the body including:

- Gait
- Posture
- Sit-to-Stand
- Miniature Squat
- Respiration
- Romberg Test
- Fukuda's Test
- Upper Cervical Spine
- Middle Cervical Spine
- TMJ
- Pelvis
- Feet
- Stress Screen

EVALUATION AND TREATMENT OF THE SECONDARY FACTORS

The elbow is directly linked to the shoulder and wrist, and is affected by the same secondary factors which stress these two regions. Please review the secondary factors presented in Chapters 19 and 21 and apply each of these to the elbow joint.

21 The Wrist and Hand

EVALUATION AND TREATMENT OF THE PRIMARY FACTORS

Extensor Pollicis Longus and Abductor Pollicis Brevis. Palpate these muscles for hypertonicity, fascial adhesions, tenderness, and trigger points. Utilize soft tissue techniques including myofascial release, sustained pressure, and transverse friction massage to address the findings (Fig. 21-1).

Practitioners commonly apply transverse friction massage to these muscles in cases of DeQuervain's stenosing tenosynovitis. This is successful on some patients but not with everyone. In some cases it helps to work the muscle bellies in addition to the tendons. In other cases, it is wise to apply the radial nerve adverse neural tension test to determine if compression of this nerve at the wrist is responsible for the patient's symptoms (Fig. 21-2).

Intrinsic Muscles of the Hand

Palpate these muscles for hypertonicity, fascial adhesions, tenderness, and trigger points. Utilize soft tissue techniques including myofascial release, sustained pressure, strumming and ischemic compression to address the findings (Fig. 21-3).

In cases of local pain and joint dysfunction it is wise to search the hand intrinsics for trigger points or other forms of muscle dysfunction. These muscles alter joint mechanics and produce local symptoms just as other muscles do. In truth, they are probably more prone to dysfunction than other muscles because of the fact they are used so frequently. Therefore, be judicious in their examination. Do not rush through.

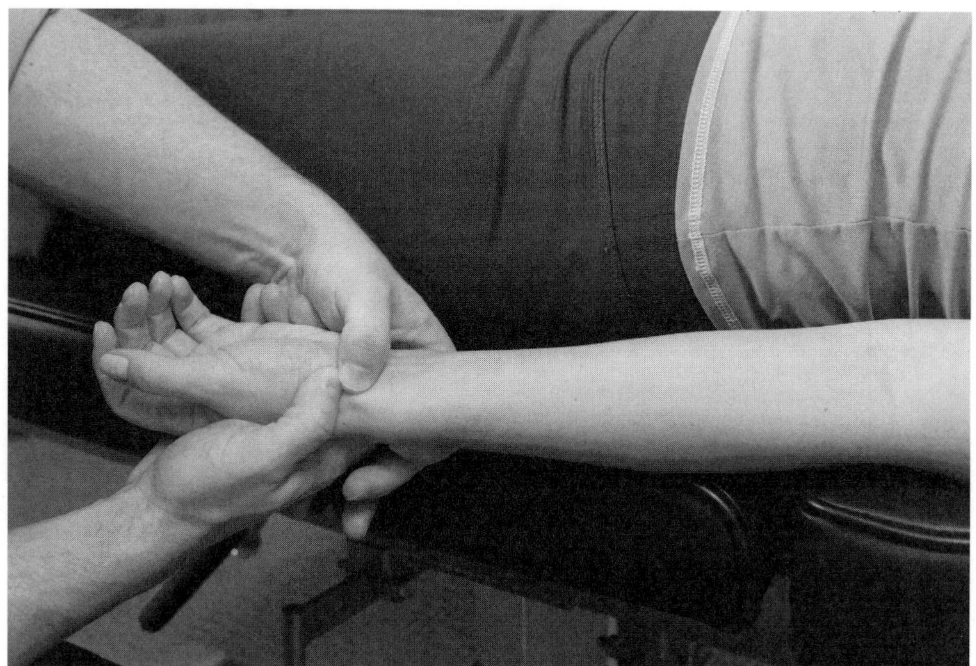

Fig. 21-1 The clinician can apply MFR, sustained pressure, and transverse friction massage in this position.

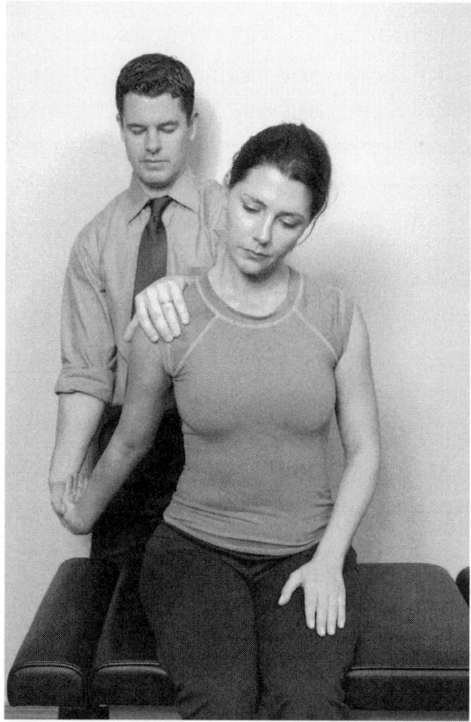

Fig. 21-2 Radial nerve adverse neural tension test.

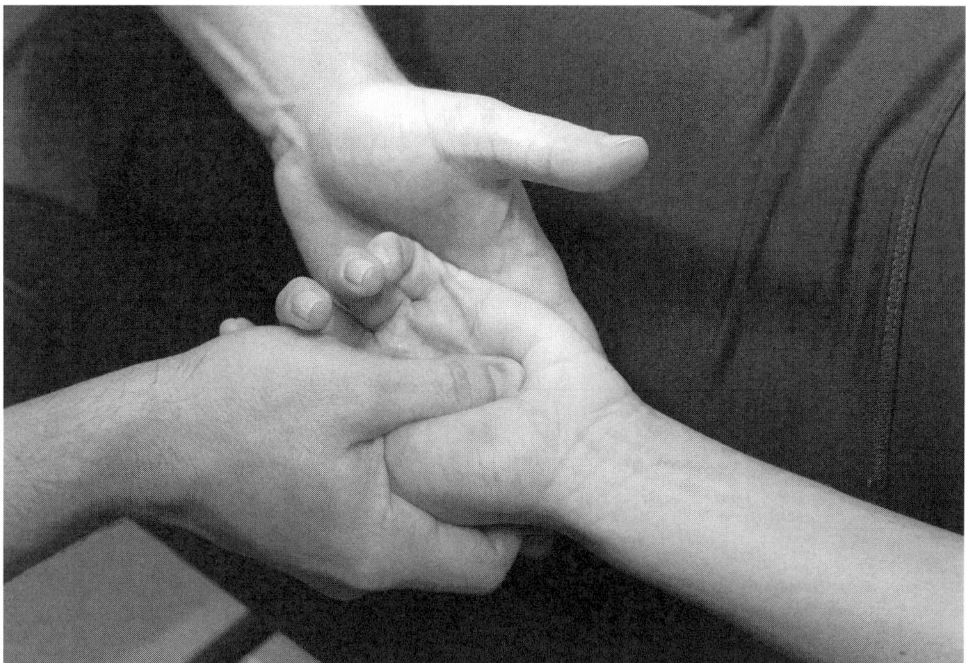

Fig. 21-3 The clinician can apply MFR, sustained pressure, strumming and ischemic compression in this position.

Wrist Flexors and Extensors

Palpate these muscles for hypertonicity, fascial adhesions, tenderness, and trigger points. Utilize soft tissue techniques including myofascial release, sustained pressure, strumming and ischemic compression to address the findings. Post-isometric relaxation is useful in reducing tone and improving flexibility (Fig. 20-1 and 20-2).

These muscles were covered in Chapter 20 due to their ability to create elbow symptomatology. However, they are also very important for proper wrist function. Patterns of facilitation and inhibition in these muscles often cause problems at the wrist. Conversely, problems such as hypomobile carpal motion will stress these muscles. Given this relationship, it is wise to investigate both joints when these muscles are problematic.

MUSCLE STRENGTH

Evaluate wrist and hand strength with traditional methods. Make sure to assess both the ability to initiate a contraction as well as sheer strength. Most often, what we perceive as weakness is more a matter of inhibition. This will follow the common pattern and/or be due to local or segmental dysfunction. Treating the causative factor restores normal strength in these cases. In cases of true muscle weakness, such as those involving muscle atrophy, remedial strengthening is indicated. This is done with traditional strengthening techniques.

JOINT MOBILITY

Distal Radioulnar Joint

Several sources find a relative separation of these two bones in cases of dysfunction.[14,184] This alters wrist mechanics while also compressing the median nerve, thus contributing to carpal tunnel syndrome. In applied kinesiology, work is applied to strengthen the pronator quadratus in order to facilitate the approximation of these bones. For the purposes of this text, the reader is urged to apply gentle mobilization and approximate the distal radius and ulna

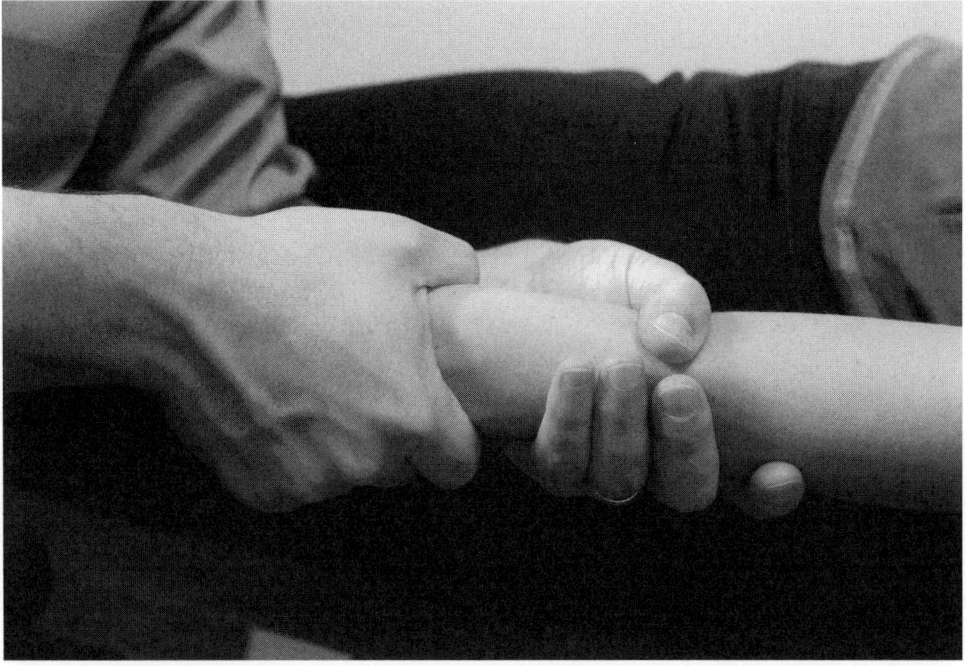

Fig. 21-4 Approximation of the distal radioulnar joint. Gently traction the wrist with one hand while squeezing the distal radius and ulna with the other.

in addition to addressing pronator quadratus dysfunction with soft-tissue work (Fig. 21-4).

THE CARPAL JOINTS

Impaired carpal motion is strongly associated with limited wrist motion. It is also associated with lateral epicondylitis[185] and carpal tunnel syndrome among other problems. Mulligan's mobilization with movement technique is extremely effective in treating limited mobility. In addition to Mulligan, there are other clinicians with valuable approaches for the wrist. One of the most popular in chiropractic is the Charrette protocol. Charrette has done extensive research on the subluxation patterns of the extremities and matches his adjusting technique to counter these patterns. At the wrist, he concurs with many other authors who find the lunate subluxates anteriorly (Fig. 21-5). He also finds the triquetrum and scaphoid subluxate dorsally and then approximate one another

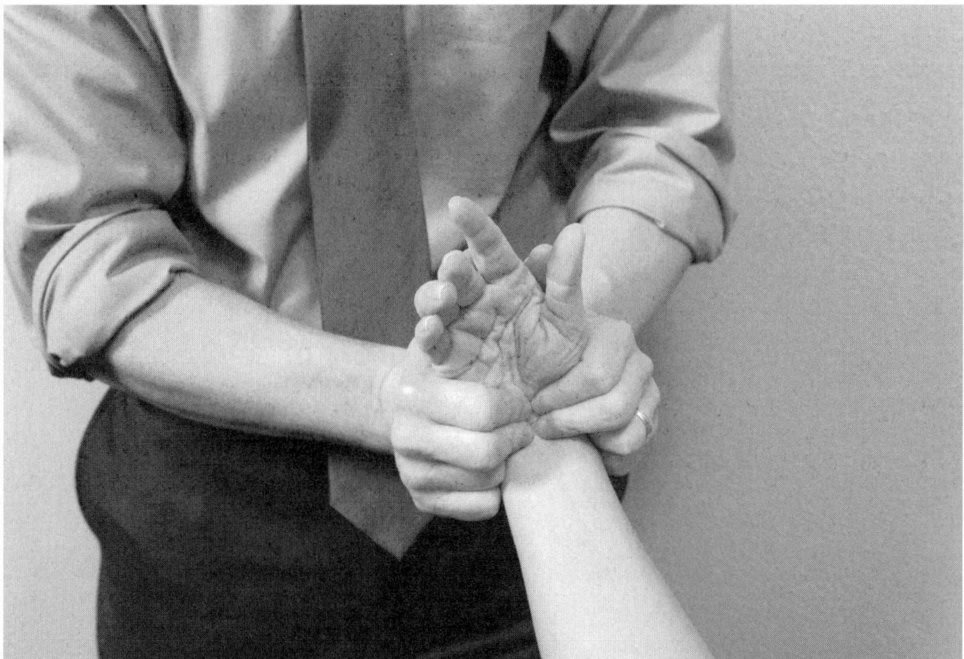

Fig. 21-5 Manipulation of an anteriorly-displaced lunate. Grasp the thenar and hypothenar eminences, gently rolling them inwards. Then, with the wrist in slight flexion, take out slack in the wrist, elbow, and shoulder. Next, drive the lunate dorsally with the tips of the 2nd and 3rd fingers. Take caution not to "yank" the entire extremity with this maneuver.

as they slide behind the lunate. Adjustment aims to drive the subluxated bones back into their normal position.

In cases where the two techniques presented above are not helpful, the clinician can fall back on traditional mobilizations taught by Maitland and Kaltenborn. In general, these involve finding the motion restriction and then applying the mobilization in this direction (Fig. 21-6 and 21-7). Be sure to stabilize the proximal end adequately so that intra-articular motion takes place.

Another point worth mentioning is that the reader must assess the elbow in cases of wrist joint dysfunction. This is because these two bodyparts directly influence one another. A case-in-point is that of the osteopathic ulnohumeral abduction lesion wherein a fall on an outstretched hand causes a valgus strain at the elbow.[187] This causes a valgus deformity at the elbow joint which changes the relationship between the radius and ulna. Of course, this has repercussions at the wrist, leading to abnormal forces upon the joint itself while forcing the wrist flexors and extensors on the radial side to work constantly in an attempt to realign the joint. This is just one documented sequelae of proximal joint dysfunction; look for others.

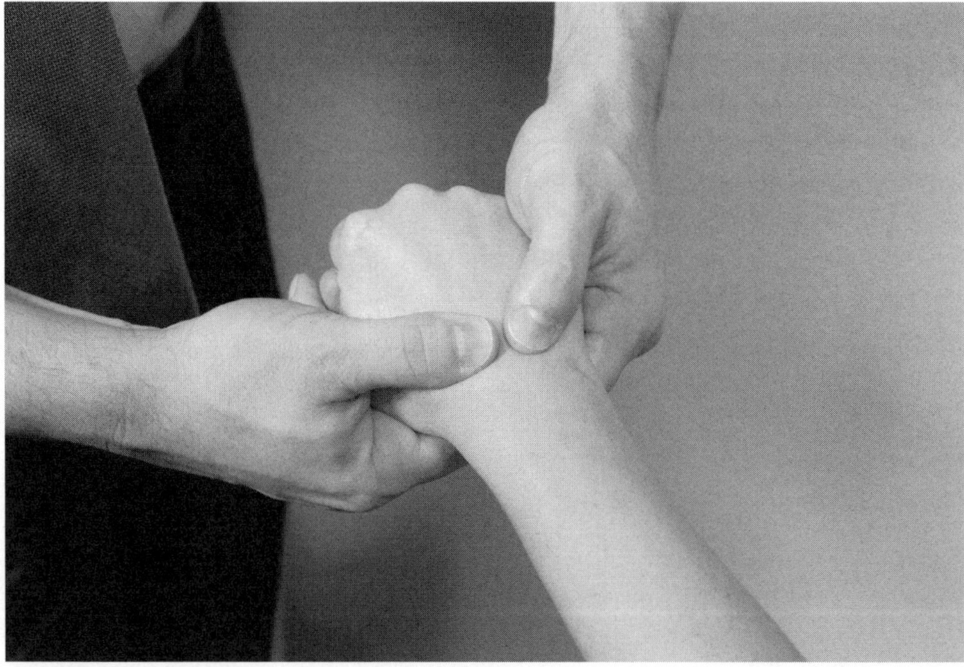

Fig. 21-6 Assessment of carpal motion. The clinician can quickly turn the assessment into repetitive mobilization when restriction is found.

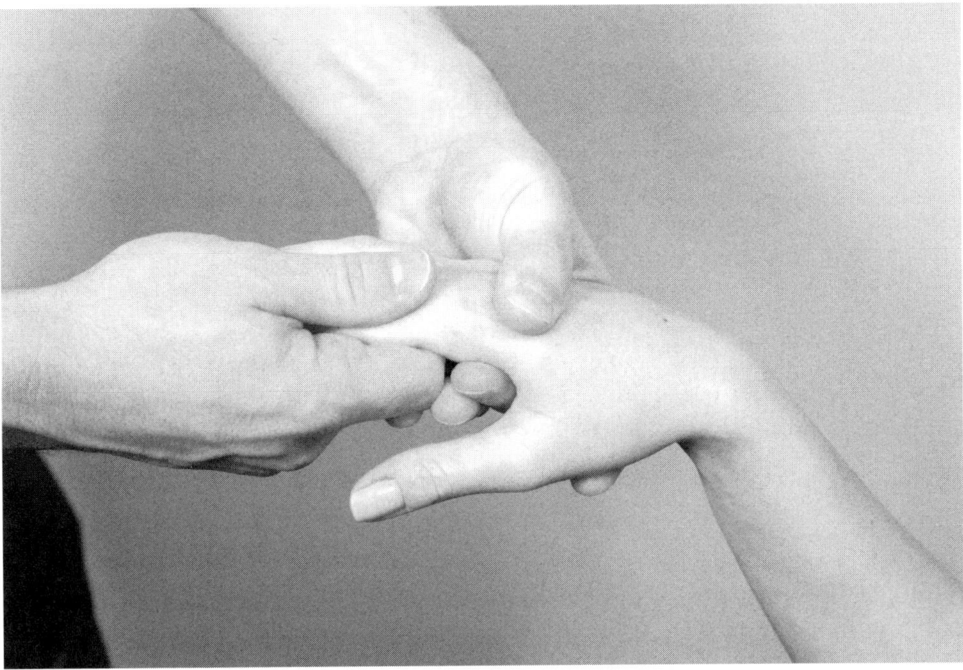

Fig. 21-7 Assessment of metacarpalphalangeal motion. Again, the clinician can quickly turn the assessment into repetitive mobilization if restriction is found.

SEGMENTAL MOBILITY

Examine the lower cervical spine for signs and symptoms of segmental dysfunction. The C6, C7, and T1 levels are most likely to refer pain to the wrist. Other levels nearby can affect surrounding musculature, thereby indirectly causing wrist dysfunction or referred pain. With this in mind, carefully palpate the muscles of the neck, shoulder and elbow for myofascial trigger points.

POSTURE AND MOVEMENT PATTERNS

Please refer to the corresponding sections in Chapter 20, The Elbow.

ENERGY-BASED TECHNIQUES

Auricular Acupuncture. Gently squeeze the point corresponding to the wrist and hand with two fingers. Hold for 5 seconds, then relax 5 seconds. Increase the amount of pressure with each cycle for a total time of one minute (6 cycles). Do this initially on the ear on the involved side only; treat the opposite ear as well if the patient does not improve.

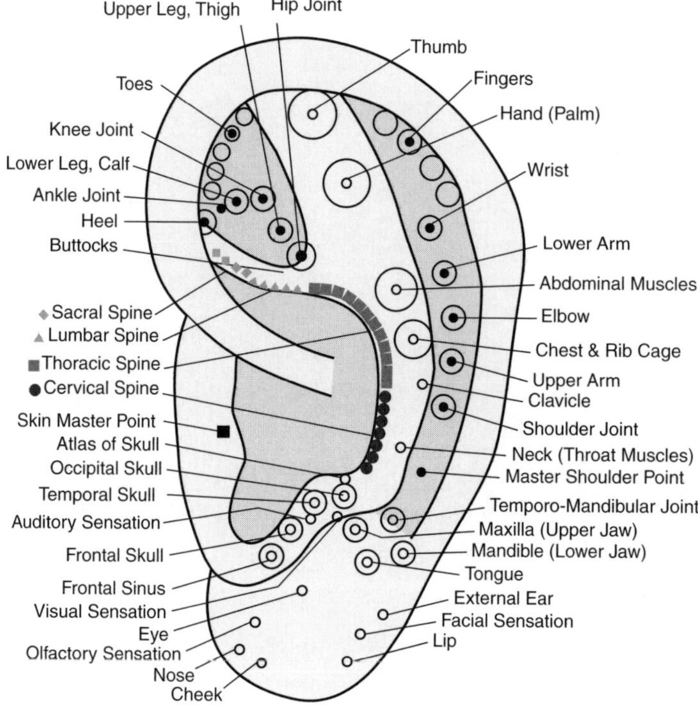

Fig. 21-8

Reflexology. Begin by massaging the entire foot. Walk up the foot with the thumbs along the five zones. Treat the plantar and dorsal surfaces. Work the toes as well. Spend extra time on the medial border of the foot corresponding

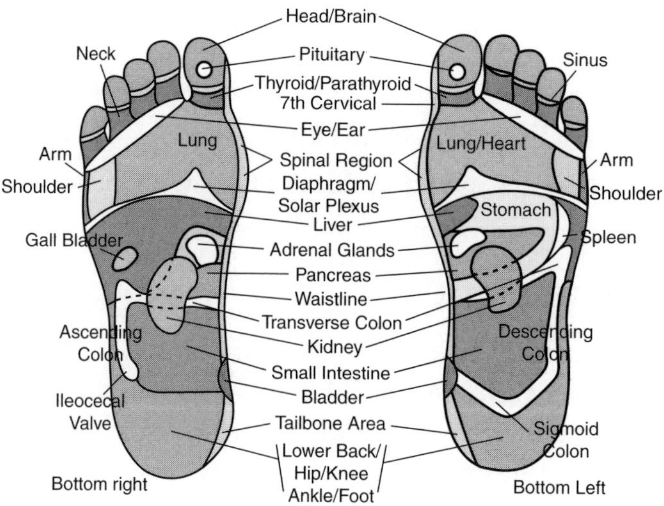

Fig. 21-9

with the spine. Also, work on areas associated with different organs needing an extra "boost." Following this long warm-up, massage the areas on the foot corresponding to the wrist and hand.

HIGH YIELD SCAN

Perform a scan of the high-yield elements of the body including:

- Gait
- Posture
- Sit-to-Stand
- Miniature Squat
- Respiration
- Romberg Test
- Fukuda's Test
- Upper Cervical Spine
- Middle Cervical Spine
- TMJ
- Pelvis
- Feet
- Stress Screen

EVALUATION AND TREATMENT OF THE SECONDARY FACTORS

Work Activities. There is an almost endless list of activities people do at work which stress the wrist and hand. With this in mind, the manual therapist's first job is to find out exactly what the patient does. For instance, if the patient sits at the computer all day long, find out how high the screen is and where it is placed, how high the keyboard is, what type of chair the patient uses and how much support it provides, whether or not the wrists are supported while the patient types, how long he sits at the computer at one time, how many hours he sits at the computer each day, as well as other questions.

A similar line of questioning must be applied to obtain details about any type of work. Take an assembly-line worker, for instance. Ask him what types of tools he uses. How heavy are the tools? What position is his hand/wrist/arm in when he is using the tools? What position is his entire body in while performing his tasks? What is the speed of the task? Are there any breaks? How long does he work continuously? How many hours per day and per week does he work? Do his tasks at work ever change?

The line of questioning should provide the practitioner with a mental picture of what the person's body goes through. From there, he can begin to suggest changes in both the environment and in the way the person performs his tasks. He can even predict which bodyparts are under excessive stress and implement exercises to prevent future injuries.

Home Activities. The clinician must also thoroughly question the patient to determine what activities he/she performs at home which may be stressing the wrist and hand. Probe for any activities—inside or outside—requiring repetitive motion, sustained muscle contraction, or forceful contraction. If an offending activity is found, use the principles described above to address it. Simply put, change the patient's surroundings to make things easier for the individual to perform.

22 The Mind-Body Connection

THIS CHAPTER WAS RESERVED FOR THE END OF THIS TEXT BECAUSE IT IS STILL SOMEWHAT controversial among manual therapists. While some therapists believe there is a strong connection between the mind and body, others believe these entities are entirely separate—and should stay that way. I must confess that for the first few years of my career as a physical therapist, I did not believe there was any connection between the mind/emotions and the physical body. Looking back, this is no surprise. This concept was *never* mentioned in my formal training. Besides that, no book or journal I owned ever mentioned the idea. It was not until coming across Thomas Hanna's *Somatics* did I begin to realize there was a viable connection between the mental and physical. Since that time my eyes have opened up to the potential influence of the emotions on the physical health of the body (and vice versa). In fact, the more I learn about this connection the more evident two facts become:

1. The mind can cause and/or perpetuate musculoskeletal/systemic problems.
2. The mind can heal/be used to heal musculoskeletal/systemic problems.

Now, this is not to say that all musculoskeletal problems have a basis in the mind. Nor are these statements an endorsement of, or consistent with the traditional psychological tenet which suggests the subconscious causes a musculoskeletal problem in order to distract the conscious from realizing there is some buried emotion it does not want to face. Instead, the connection alluded to is based on the mind's role in modulating the Stress Response. Once again, we find that the

Stress Response is activated when homeostasis is disrupted (this time in the case of anger, fear, anxiety, or other stress). Thus, the emotions can play the role of a stressor (either significant or minor) just as any physical stressor does. Likewise, by addressing this stressor we can bring the patient back to a balanced state.

In the sections that follow, this connection is explored in greater detail. First, we examine the work of several individuals who have brought the concept of the mind-body connection into widespread acceptance (even by traditional medicine). Second, we examine several approaches in manual therapy which have utilized this connection for some time (they did not wait for molecular biologists to tell them there was a connection). After this, we will end the chapter with a section on how the manual therapist can address the emotions with several non-invasive, non-traumatic methods.

TRENDS IN TRADITIONAL MEDICINE

For a long time, traditional medicine did not recognize a connection between the mind and body. Both were looked at as distinct and separate entities. However, due to the work of several pioneers this is slowly changing. There is even a relatively new field, psychoneuroimmunology, which has developed as a result of the advanced research being published on this topic. The reader is urged to peruse the latest periodicals to see what is being uncovered. Briefly, they are substantiating what common knowledge (and Hans Seyle's research) has told us for years: stress makes us sick. They are able to measure white blood cell counts, cytokine levels, hormone levels, etc., and confirm that the state of the mind *can* and *does* affect the function of multiple bodily systems.

Candace Pert, Ph.D.

Candace Pert is a researcher largely credited with starting the field of psychoneuroimmunology (PNI). Her breakthrough book, *Molecules of Emotion*, was the first to bring hardcore science and molecular biology into the mind-body connection equation.[188] Among her *many* findings was that macrophages actually have receptors for endorphins produced in the brain. This fact alone gives credence to the theory that our mental state affects immune function.

Besides this, Pert even found the reverse connection existed: the body can affect the mind. She discovered that interleukin-1, the cytokine released by macrophages, has receptors throughout the brain (not just in the hypothalamus). Thus, the immune system has the power to affect the mind and emotions.

Dr. Pert is responsible for discovering many other fascinating connections between the mind and body. The reader is urged to read her book to learn more about her research and the conception of the field of PNI.

Herbert Benson, M.D.

Herbert Benson's 1975 book, *The Relaxation Response*, was the first to prove that people could change their internal physiology through techniques such as meditation and other eastern-based methods.[189] Among his many findings were that practitioners using transcendental meditation could markedly reduce blood pressure, oxygen consumption (signifying decreased metabolism), and blood lactate levels.[189] These results, of course, substantiate the idea that the mind can influence our internal physiological function. In this case, we see how reducing the stress response and invoking parasympathetic action leads to several desirable benefits.

A funny side note to this story is that Benson's research was not well-received by his fellow professors at the Harvard Medical School. Nor was it well-received by many of his peers in the medical community. As he describes, the medical establishment did not like the notion that people could take care of their health on their own. Instead, patients needed to rely on drugs and surgery for that. This attitude might explain why such important research is not as well-publicized as one would assume.

Dean Ornish, M.D.

Dean Ornish is best known for his groundbreaking study in which he proved that intensive lifestyle changes can actually reverse heart disease. Most people are well-aware of the stringent diet he proposes in order to accomplish this. What many don't realize, however, is what Dr. Ornish believes is the true culprit in heart disease: emotional stress.

The emotional stress Dr. Ornish repeatedly describes comes from isolation—"from our feelings, our inner self, and inner peace. . .from others. . .from a higher force." To support this idea, he sites numerous studies linking this characteristic to heart disease. He also outlines the direct physiological effects stress has upon the cardiovascular system—all the way down to the intima of our blood vessels. He even ties-in emotional stress to the musculoskeletal system when describing how it can cause contraction-band necrosis: "This inability to relax and the resulting chronic constriction manifest themselves throughout the body, from the large muscles in the back down to the smallest fibers of the heart."[36]

Due to this influence, Dr. Ornish believes that treating the physical manifestations of heart disease (surgery, medicine) only provides temporary relief. For long-lasting results we must address the "fundamental causes" of disease. He refers to this as going far back in the causal chain of events (picture the wellness continuum). Therefore, in addition to changes in diet and exercise, he has his patients doing a great deal of work to reduce emotional stress each day. In a nutshell, this includes 20' of stretching, 15' of meditation, 15' of progressive relaxation techniques, 5' of deep breathing exercises, and 5' of directed or receptive imagery. Some of these techniques are described later in the section on treatment.

INFLUENCES FROM ALTERNATIVE MEDICINE

Unlike traditional medicine, alternative medicine has recognized the existence of the mind-body connection for a long time. Some approaches are practically based on the influence of the mind upon the body. Others respect this connection as well and have techniques to address its physical manifestations. By learning about each of them we can gain a greater understanding of the effects of the mind-body connection.

SOMATICS

Thomas Hanna did as much to help us understand the neuromuscular responses to stress as any other individual. In his text, *Somatics*, he begins by taking the two major types of stress and categorizing them. These are distress and eustress. Distress refers to negative stress—the kind of stress we usually think of when we hear that dreaded word. This activates the withdrawal response, which he calls the Red Light reflex. On the other hand, eustress refers to positive stress, which activates the action response. This response is called the Green Light reflex. The neuromuscular adaptation to distress occurs in the front of the body, while the adaptation to eustress occurs in the back of the body.

The Red Light Reflex

The Red Light Reflex is the postural manifestation of the withdrawal, or startle response. As detailed in Chapter 2, it was designed in the event we need to fight or escape from a dangerous situation. Unfortunately, it also becomes active when we are afraid or under stress. Consequently, it does not take a life-or-death situation to activate the startle response. Posturally, the startle response is identified by the following: closing the eyes, tensing the jaw and face, pulling the neck forward, elevating the scapulae, flexing the elbows, clenching the fists, flattening the chest, tightening the abdominals, diaphragm, and perineum. The gluteus minimus contracts (internally rotating the hips), the hips adduct, the hamstrings contract, and the feet flex and supinate.

The order of activation is clear. It goes from its origin in the brainstem directly to the skull and then downward towards the feet. As predicted by its location, this reflex is not under the control of the forebrain. Hanna points out that "it happens before we can perceive it or inhibit it."[17] He believes that this is where most of the problem lies. The body takes on the posture created by the Red Light Reflex without the person even knowing it. Hanna also points out that this is the exact posture most elderly people display. So common is this posture, in fact, that we accept it as a normal part of aging when it is not. Instead, it is merely the result of prolonged reflex activity. Hanna goes on to attribute many of the commonly-accepted "maladies of aging" to this reflex. Shortness of breath, constipation, frequent urination, and knee pain are just a few symptoms that can be linked mechanically to this stooped posture.

The Green Light Reflex

The Green Light Reflex is best described as the manifestation of the action response. Instead of withdrawing from a stimulus as seen in the Red Light Reflex, this reflex is our engrained motivation to do things. In the infant it is the Landau Reaction. This is seen when the prone-lying infant is picked up with one hand underneath its thorax. Not only will her head lift, but her back arches and legs extend. In essence, the infant is activating the muscles that will soon propel her through space.

The lumbar muscles are the first ones to become active in the Landau reaction. This is accompanied by the synergistic contraction of the muscles of the neck, shoulders, buttocks, and thighs. Again, all of these contractions take place on the posterior aspect of the body, whereas the Red Light Reflex contractions take place on the anterior aspect of the body. Contraction of the posterior musculature sets the stage for back pain, neck pain, headaches, and a sway-back posture.

Besides contraction of the spinal extensors, the Green Light reflex causes the following movements: opening the eyes, jaw and face, pulling the neck backwards, depressing the scapulae, extending the elbows, opening the hands, lifting the chest, lengthening the abdominals, relaxing the diaphragm and freeing breathing, relaxing the pelvic floor, contracting the gluteus maximus and minimus (externally rotating hips), abducting the thighs, contracting quadriceps, and extending and pronating the feet.

Hanna points out that all of this is activated by the eustress, or positive stress, we encounter so frequently in this modern world. We call on it every time we need to get something done. We have to take care of ourselves financially, and we constantly battle deadlines, calendars, and clocks in the process. Thus, the Green Light Reflex is still being triggered in the adult, although the thrill of being active has disappeared.

The Dark Vise

Hanna referred to the summation of all opposing reflexes as the Dark Vise. Instead of opposing sets of muscles working together and creating a balanced person, we find further dysfunction as these two reflexes come together. Typically, the spinal muscles in the Green Light reflex continue their pull on the spine, and the Red Light reflex continues to contract the abdominals and muscles of the anterior shoulder girdle. Thus, both reflexes are still present and the end result is a body in even greater disarray.

Hanna mentions that there may be countless varieties of the Dark Vise, some with a bias towards the Red Light reflex and others with a bias towards the Green Light reflex. Unfortunately, the clinical symptoms are often similar. Among these are reduced mobility, pain, fatigue, shallow breathing, and even high blood pressure.

The reader will note that Hanna's Dark Vise corresponds with the upper and lower crossed syndromes. This relationship is just further evidence of the frequency of this neurological synergy and its resultant posture. It is the reason why his work is presented here; so that the reader can further appreciate the role of the emotions and nervous sytem on our musculoskeletal system.

The Trauma Reflex

The final dysfunctional posture is due to the Trauma Reflex. Unlike the Red and Green Light Reflexes, the Trauma Reflex SMA is usually demonstrated in the coronal plane. It is best described as cringing or flinching when we are in pain or are threatened with pain. The body may contract in a protective pattern around the injured bodypart, or shift to the opposite side in order to avoid irritating an injury. The idea of this reflex is consistent with other approaches' beliefs that trauma changes the nervous system and leaves evidence of damage throughout the body. For this reason, old injuries (even surgical scars) must always be treated.

CHIROPRACTIC

Chiropractic has always recognized the connection between the mind and body. D.D. Palmer, the discoverer of chiropractic, taught that subluxations were caused by three things: thoughts (he called this autosuggestion), toxins, and trauma (micro- and macrotrauma). Since then, chiropractic views the state of the body in what is called the Triad of Health. This is a holistic way of viewing health in which structural, chemical, and mental factors are all considered important. In fact, the symbol for this concept is an equilateral triangle with each side composed of one of these three factors (see Fig. 22-1). Thus, the balance between these factors is imperative to the health of the individual. If one factor is not functioning properly, it affects the other two. Walther points out that one of the three factors is always involved when an individual experiences health problems.[14] When two or three of these factors are involved, the person is typically experiencing even greater health problems.[14]

APPLIED KINESIOLOGY

Applied Kinesiology (AK) can be used to examine and treat each component in the triad of health. In fact, the connection between emotion and the body can readily be observed in AK. For instance, a strong indicator muscle will turn weak if the patient concentrates on a subject damaging to his/her emotional state. This may be a powerful negative thought or a small stressor that will quickly resolve itself. In either event, the practitioner can gain valuable insight into the possible link between the patient's emotions and his or her symptomatology.

Neuro Emotional Technique (NET) is a brilliant off-shoot of AK developed by AK diplomate Dr. Scott Walker. In this approach, muscle testing is used to

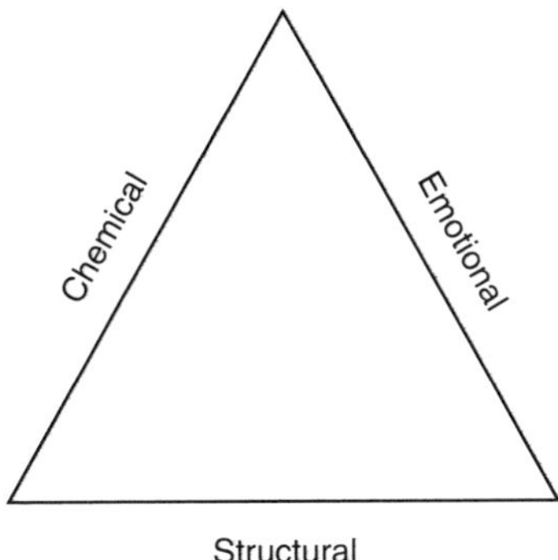

Fig. 22-1 The Triad of Health

determine the source of emotional discord and how it relates to the patient's symptoms. Through adjusting and homeopathic remedies, practitioners using NET relate remarkable results in patients who have responded poorly with more traditional techniques.

MYOFASCIAL RELEASE

The myofascial release approach recognizes the effects of the mind upon the body, especially following physical trauma. While it is well-known that the mind creates lasting memories of an accident or traumatic event, it is also believed the body does the same thing. However, the memories stored within the body are at a subconscious level. Therefore, the person is unaware of them and a form of "amnesia" results. Barnes refers to this as a reversible amnesia that is state or position dependent.[190] Thus, these memories can only be recovered when the person is in a specific position. Typically, this position is the position of the original injury.[70] Without outside assistance, this position is avoided due to subconscious fear that reinjury may occur. Over time, these protective patterns result in a shortening, or contraction, of the fascial tissue. This shortening may then create other structural or pathologic changes near or distant to the original site of injury.

This perspective is somewhat different than many of the others mentioned in this chapter. While it recognizes the presence of reflexive muscle contraction, it is really based on the concept of fascial shortening. This potential involvement of the fascial system is important to the practitioner, as it provides an extra means to help a patient with emotional involvement. Further discussion of the myofascial release approach in patients with an emotional component is presented in the Treatment section.

CRANIOSACRAL THERAPY

The fields of craniosacral therapy and myofascial release approach the mind-body connection in an almost identical fashion to one another. Their shared theories on trauma, emotions, and the body are discussed under the heading Myofascial Release above. Their approach to treatment is presented in the Treatment section.

ANATOMY TRAINS

Thomas Myers points out the similarity between the startle response and the Superficial Front Line.[162] In fact, shortening of the SFL mimics the movement occurring during part of the startle response. This is easy to picture, given the layout of this myofascial band. Briefly, this band encompasses the following tissues: toe extensors, ankle dorsiflexors, quadriceps, rectus abdominis, sternalis, sternocleidomastoid, and the fascia of the scalp.[162] Therefore, upon shortening, the body goes into flexion with the exception of the upper cervical spine. Due to the band's cross-over from anterior to posterior with the sternocleidomastoid, contraction causes occipital extension (when the person is standing, not supine).[162] This is consistent with the pattern that occurs during the startle response. Myers also notes that the muscles of the Superficial Front Arm Line participate in this reflex; this is seen when the elbows flex and the shoulders protract.[162]

Myers states that a postural version of the startle response can last for many years unless it is treated psychologically or structurally.[162] This is important, as problems may occur when this posture is maintained for prolonged periods of time. Most notably, Myers reports the patient's respiratory function is diminished. This is due to the loss of normal rib motion as well as the lack of reciprocal motion between the pelvic and respiratory diaphragms.[162]

ROLFING

Rolfing is yet another approach that recognizes the mind-body connection. In fact, it has been said that "the fascia is the emotional body."[191] In this regard, feelings are not only experienced in the mind, but in the entire body. We "interpret the physiological sensation as anger, affection, love, interest, and so forth."[191] Expanding from these concepts is the thought that true proprioception includes the physical component of emotion. We inhibit this physical proprioception when we do not want to face an emotion, energy, or structural event.[191] This behavior explains how an emotional problem transforms itself into a physical one.

Fear is specifically blamed for creating many holding patterns observed in children and adults. These holding patterns also create a muscular tightening out of fear that increased pain will be generated. Unfortunately, this contraction only leads to more pain.[191] Schultz notes that the fear of being unsteady also results in numerous modifications: locked neck, "sucked-in ass," flexed toes, high shoulders, and a clenched jaw.

Breathing is another movement pattern that suffers as a result of fear. In this case, it is believed that fear causes us to gasp air in and hold it there. This may be because we do not want to experience the sensation or emotion.[191] However, by doing this, we only create tension throughout the body and are unable to relax. This leads to the retention of pain instead of the elimination of pain. Like the restricted patterns mentioned above, the pattern of restricted respiration may become chronic.

Rolf also recognized the effects of the physical body upon the psyche.[192] She contended that behavior was the result of physiology, which is something we can change. In the patient with only minor emotional dysfunction, balancing the body can help tremendously. It can also be helpful in more complicated cases, including those with what Rolf refers to as "hang-ups." Normally, these hang-ups have a physiological component—glandular, visceral, or myofascial.[192] By releasing these physiologic factors, the potential for emotional change is greatly facilitated.

THE ALEXANDER TECHNIQUE

One of the most important concepts within the Alexander Technique is that of downward pull. It is the force we must consciously inhibit in order to facilitate optimal posture and function. But what creates the downward pull? Frank Jones, one of the primary researchers behind the Alexander Technique, considered downward pull to be habitual startle.[100] Conable notes several other reasons, each having an emotional component. These include fearfulness, a reaction to pain, a sense of worthlessness or defeat, and an attempt to reduce sensation or emotion. Other explanations involve self-survival strategies, including making oneself smaller as a means to prevent violence.[100] Whatever the exact reason, the Alexander Technique undoubtedly recognizes the importance of the mind-body connection.

The fact that F.P. Jones believed that downward pull was due to habitual startle tells us two things. First of all, it reinforces the importance of the startle response. Second, it demonstrates the incredible frequency of the startle response within the general population.

MYOFASCIAL TRIGGER POINTS

Psychological factors can function to perpetuate myofascial trigger points, according to Travell and Simons. These authors outline several common psychological profiles and describe how each condition can impact musculoskeletal rehabilitation. The five categories are as follows:[31]

1. Hopelessness—the patient in this category does not believe he or she can be helped. Consequently, he or she typically avoids any movement that may

irritate his or her condition. This behavior only perpetuates active trigger points, as the affected muscles are not worked at their end-range of motion. These patients must understand that their condition is treatable and reversible.

2. Depression—this condition is common in patients with chronic pain. The patient frequently has doubts he or she can be helped, is afraid that the condition may get worse, and does not understand why no one seems to know what causes the pain. These patients are helped with the addition of antidepressant medication along with standard trigger point therapy. Reducing the effects of the depression allows the patient to take a greater role in his/her recovery.
3. Anxiety and Tension—patients suffering from this condition display excessive muscle tone. Their posture and movement patterns appear to be stiff, and they do not seem to relax. Biofeedback and relaxation therapy are helpful to aid in general physical relaxation. However, if there is an emotional cause to this anxiety, it must be identified and dealt with accordingly.
4. The "Good Sport" Syndrome—this patient is very stoic and makes every effort to ignore pain. This may be because he or she looks at "giving-in" to pain as a sign of weakness. As expected, patients in this category also tend to irritate their condition by trying to overpower it. They return to normal duty too soon or perform activities that are likely to make their pain worse. These patients must be taught that "no pain, no gain" is not always an accurate expression. Instead of helping them, that notion has probably made them worse.
5. Psychological and Behavioral Aspects—this classification includes patients who demonstrate primary or secondary gain. These patients do not improve significantly with standard trigger point therapy for obvious reasons.

THE CRANIOMANDIBULAR JOINT

The craniomandibular (temporomandibular) joint is often recognized for its close relationship to both mental stress and psychological problems. In fact, the masseters are the only muscles in the body distinguished by Travell and Simons as specifically developing tension in people undergoing extreme emotional tension, determination or desperation. The relationship between psychological issues and TMD has been studied by many authors attempting to shed light on their close connection. One theoretical schema developed to demonstrate the relationship between the psyche and temporomandibular dysfunction is Gelb's Triad of Symptoms. It identifies three important factors contributing to TMD. These factors include tissue alteration, predisposition (physical qualities, not psychological), and psychological dependence. Within this schema, these three factors are equally weighted. Therefore, the issue of psychological dependence should not only be recognized, but placed at a high level of importance.[193,194,195]

Other research on this topic has attempted to classify the personality profiles of patients with TMD.[196] By using the MMPI (Minnesota Multiphasic Personality Inventory), researchers discovered that patients with head and facial pain demonstrate four distinct psychological profiles.[197] These profiles are as follows:

1. Psychophysiologic Reaction Profile: these patients demonstrate an elevated hypochondriasis and hysteria scale. As such, they are known to "somaticize their emotional problems."
2. Depression Reaction Profile: as expected, these patients show an elevated depression scale. Their depression symptoms may be the result of a specific incident or be the result of experiencing chronic pain.
3. Defense Reaction Profile: these patients show elevated scores in lying and correction on the MMPI. They often somaticize in order to control people and situations in the world around them.
4. No Diagnosis Profile: these patients are relatively normal and only somaticize in extremely stressful situations.

Despite recognizing this common relationship, Travell and Simons point out that the mind-body connection is not always a one-way street. Instead, there is also an inverse relationship that should not be ignored. That is, it is possible for the physical ailment to cause or contribute to psychological issues. This concept is also brought up by Rocabado, who urges the reader to avoid hastily blaming psychology for physical problems. He points out that the patient with TMD has been in pain for a long time. He or she was probably told many times that their pain is all in their head and that it is not as bad as they make it out to be. This frustrating experience would very likely cause emotional changes in any individual. Therefore, his or her psyche should only be considered as a cause when all other options are fully exhausted.

DAVID BUTLER, P.T.

Physical therapist David Butler is best-known for his excellent text, *Mobilisation of the Nervous System.*[198] This book, published in 1991, has been the authoritative text on diagnosing and treating peripheral nerve compression. However, despite this success, Butler has not settled into a life of complacency. Instead, he underwent a metamorphosis several years ago and now takes a different approach—more of a global one.

Now, Butler's focus is on measures to benefit the nervous system as a whole. Instead of limiting his work to mechanical issues (like neural compression and tension), he studies the physiology, biochemistry, and even the plastic changes occurring with neurological dysfunction. In *The Sensitive Nervous System,*[199] he spends a great amount of time describing these changes in peripheral and central sensitization. In *Explain Pain*, he reiterates the connection between the mind and body while delving into specific treatment options using this same connection. Indeed, he has gone from a paradigm limited to the mechanical system to an all-encompassing, global one. Bravo.

TREATMENT CONSIDERATIONS

Please note that it is not the author's intention to encroach upon the field of traditional psychology. However, the approaches covered thus far offer several basic treatment techniques that deserve to be mentioned here. Not only are they quick and easy-to-learn, but they are minimally invasive psychologically. In other words, they are unlike some approaches in classical psychology that propose the patient discuss old, painful memories. We will leave this to professionals. Instead, the techniques presented here involve the physical self in order to alter the patient's emotional status or in the least the influence of the subconscious mind upon the body.

SOMATIC TREATMENT

An important concept in the somatic approach is the theory of sensory-motor amnesia (SMA). Hanna describes this as a memory loss of how muscle groups feel and how to control them. In SMA, the person is not aware that his body is in a constant state of contraction. He likely does not remember what it was like to be "normal". Moreover, he probably does not remember when his posture became so terrible. He thinks it is the result of normal aging.

If he is unaware of this reflexive pattern, he is unable to defeat it. Trying to consciously "relax" the muscles is unsuccessful no matter how hard he tries. Indeed, this only causes more stress. Trying to treat each sore muscle individually will only bring temporary relief, as it will become symptomatic again in the near future.

With these concepts in mind, the goal of Somatic therapy is to make the person aware that his body is in a state of contraction. It is this awareness of the body, of movement, and of one's posture that is the key to addressing SMA. To do this, Hanna proposes that a form of indirect technique be used. But unlike strain-counterstrain, where the muscle is passively placed on slack, the Somatic approach brings the origin and insertion together with an active contraction. This creates proprioceptive feedback, thus causing reflexive inhibition of the agonist. It also gives sensory feedback to the brain, enhancing the patient's awareness of the contraction.

Dreaver developed a simplified version of Hanna's exercises.[200] They use the same theory that Hanna used, but in a format probably more familiar to the clinician. In fact, they are somewhat similar to certain PNF techniques many therapists use. For instance, let's look at the treatment of a chronically contracted cervical extensor group. First, the head is actively extended in order to shorten the affected muscle group. From this position, the patient extends the head against resistance given by the clinician's hand. After several seconds the patient is asked to allow the head to come forward into 1/3 of full flexion. It is important that the patient does not completely relax. Instead, he just lessens the strength of contraction. From this point, he is told to push into extension with greater force, and approximately one inch of concentric motion is allowed. This process is repeated for two more cycles until the head is in full flexion, then repeated from the start. The treatment ends with one final contraction into full extension followed by a contraction into full flexion.

This example is more simple than the description Dreaver gives, but it relays many of the concepts of Somatic therapy. As previously mentioned, the exercise starts in an actively shortened position. This position allows the muscles to relax, and the patient's voluntary contraction floods the CNS with afferent input. This causes reflexive inhibition of the cervical extensors. Moreover, it increases the patient's awareness of the state of contraction of these muscles. This is accentuated by the numerous changes in contraction intensity throughout the exercise. By then allowing the muscles to contract eccentrically, the Golgi tendon organs become excited. As a result, inhibitory interneurons become excited and the muscle is ordered to relax.

The last phase of most exercises, the antagonistic contraction, serves to further stimulate awareness. It also helps remind the brain where a bodypart belongs. In doing so, this technique reinforces the changes that have already occurred.

Hanna and Dreaver describe specific exercises in great detail in their respective texts. The reader is urged to review these for greater understanding of theoretical concepts and treatment techniques.

APPLIED KINESIOLOGY

A simple technique described in AK and Touch for Health uses Bennett's neurovascular reflexes to create emotional change. The specific reflexes used are the emotional neurovascular reflexes. These are located on the frontal bone eminence, which is on either side of the forehead at the mid-point of the eyebrow right-to-left and midway between the eyebrow and original hairline superior-to-inferior.

Treatment begins by first opening the conception vessel meridian. This is done by running the hand from the patient's pubic symphysis to the lower lip. Following this, contact is made with the emotional neurovascular points while the patient thinks of an emotional problem that may be perpetuating some of his or her symptoms.[14] This combination is continued for up to several minutes. The technique ends with closing the conception vessel meridian by passing the clinician's hand from the lower lip to the pubic symphysis. Success with this technique is demonstrated with negative therapy localization to this same thought.

MYOFASCIAL RELEASE/CRANIOSACRAL THERAPY

As previously mentioned, the treatment approaches taken by the fields of myofascial release and craniosacral therapy are strikingly similar. Each of them views the clinician's role as that of a facilitator of the body's inherent motions. With time, the patient's body will assume the position in which the injury occurred.[70] At this point, the craniosacral system will shut down.[70] This is called a still point.[190] During the still point, a reversible amnesia comes to the patient's conscious and is frequently accompanied by emotional outpouring, memories, and the physiologic responses which occurred at the time of trauma.[190] By bringing these emotions to the patient's attention, it is believed that their subconscious influence over the body will end.

One of the few appreciable differences in treatment is in patient positioning. In myofascial release, the patient is usually supine. Not only does this position allow for the elimination of gravity, but is reduces the influence of the body's righting reflexes.[190] As a result, the patient's body has minimal impedance to "unwinding" and a more natural movement can occur.

On the contrary, Upledger et al. describe two methods that are performed in weight bearing. The first of these two methods involves the patient in a sitting position. The clinician places one hand upon the patient's parietals and one hand on the posterior aspect of the upper thoracic spine.[70] Gentle pressure is given to the parietals in an inferior direction until slight motion is felt by the other hand. As soon as this pressure is perceived, the clinician waits for the unwinding process to begin. Body movements in all planes are likely, and the patient is allowed to perform any motion except for retracing his or her path. If this occurs, he or she should gently be led out of that tendency.

The other technique described takes place with the patient standing. The clinician places his or her hands on the anterior ilia and compresses medially. The patient's body will begin to move on its own. The operator is to follow this motion until all releases cease and the craniosacral system shuts down.

DEEP BREATHING EXERCISES

There are many different breathing exercises one can choose from to help his/her patients reduce stress and down-regulate the sympathetic nervous system. The common denominator between all of them seems to be the use of the diaphragm to generate "deep breathing." This is in direct contrast to the way most of us breathe, which is typically a shallow, inefficient method driven by accessory muscles of respiration (especially the scalene and sternocleidomastoids). Not surprisingly, this improper breathing style is the result of emotional stress.[36,201]

A simple, yet effective method one can teach patients is advised by Dr. Andrew Weil.[202] He suggests starting with a deep exhalation through the mouth, making a whoosh sound. Then, close the mouth and inhale slowly through the nose. This should take 4 seconds. Hold the breath in for 7 seconds. Next, slowly exhale through the mouth for 8 seconds (again making a whoosh sound). Repeat this cycle 3 times.

In his text, *Natural Health, Natural Medicine*, Dr. Weil urges the patient start by doing this exercise at least twice per day for best results. However, he cautions that one not do more than four breathing cycles per day for the first month. This can be extended to eight cycles in the future. Please see his and Dr. Ornish's texts for further information on different breathing exercises.

MEDITATION

As with deep breathing exercises, there are many different ways to meditate. Some methods take a lot of practice to master while others can be learned relatively quickly. The type of meditation described below is certainly one of the more basic versions. It is Dr. Benson's Relaxation Response technique—an effective, yet simple method to obtain the beneficial effects traditional meditation is known for.

Per Dr. Benson's instructions, there are really just two vital components to eliciting the Relaxation Response. The first is to repeat a word, sound, or phrase repetitively. The second is to try to ignore all thoughts entering one's mind; if they do just let them pass. Yes, that is the Relaxation Response in a nutshell. It can be done lying on the floor, sitting up, or even while performing a physical activity. Dr. Benson suggests doing this for 10–20 minutes at least twice per day. He gives other valuable pieces of advice to maximize the benefits of this technique in his books. The reader is urged to consult these for further information.

EXERCISE

Exercise is an excellent stress reducer. In a Duke University study it was shown that people who exercised for 30 minutes three or four times per week for 4 months experienced changes similar to those from prescription anti-depressants.[7] Improvement like this is not a surprise to most of us. We all know that exercise has a role in the production of dopamine and serotonin, two hormones known for their anti-depression and anti-anxiety effects. But this is not the only way exercise benefits us. As Chestnut points out, another powerful way motion influences our emotions is through stimulation of the cerebellum (especially the vermis).[15] The cerebellum, in turn, stimulates "pleasure centers located in the septal nuclei of the hypothalamus and corticomedial amygdala," while "simultaneously inhibiting adversive emotion centers located in the hippocampus and dorsolateral amygdala." This gives the exercise/emotional connection a neurological connection instead of just a hormonal one. At the same time, it also substantiates the importance of a subluxation-free spine, as most of the input going to this part of the cerebellum comes from the axial skeleton. Thus, proper vertebral motion appears necessary to maximize the benefits of motion.

PATIENT EDUCATION

Sometimes something as simple as patient education can make a world of difference to a person's recovery. This is especially true for the patient suffering from chronic pain, or central sensitization. Oftentimes these individuals do not want to move a bodypart because of the fact it hurts. This response to pain is normally a valuable instinct; it lets us know we can damage a bodypart by moving it in a specific manner. But in the patient with central sensitization these signals are constantly sending the person a "false alarm." They are screaming "pain" although further tissue damage is not imminent.

This is where patient education plays such an important role. Letting patients like these know that their pain does not indicate tissue damage gives them greater freedom to move without fear. This movement, of course, is absolutely vital for recovery and should be encouraged. It benefits the tissue on a local level by increasing circulation, restoring flexibility, and improving strength. More importantly, it bombards the CNS with afferent mechanoreception so critical to a full recovery.

Helping these patients understand that their tissues have healed and there *is* hope for the future also helps down-regulate the stress response. This is beneficial for many reasons as discussed throughout this text. But for the "sensitized" patient it is especially beneficial. That is because calming the stress response leads to a drop in epinephrine and norepinephrine, two substances largely responsible for sensitizing the nervous system in the first place.[199] Thus, by reducing the patient's fear and anxiety about their condition we can remove one of the biochemical culprits responsible for creating and perpetuating the patient's problem! For further information on the physiology of nerve sensitization as well as other treatment techniques, the reader is urged to read David Butler's *The Sensitive Nervous System.*

ENERGY-BASED APPROACHES

There are several non-invasive approaches which utilize acupuncture points to treat psychological conditions. Two such approaches, Emotional Freedom Technique and Roger Callahan's Thought Field Therapy, use the repetitive tapping of acupuncture points to achieve this goal. These methods are easily integrated into the manual therapist's repertoire. The reader is encouraged to learn either of these techniques to improve the patient's physical reaction to their respective emotional state.

In all cases the clinician is urged to remember that patients with significant psychological conditions should be referred out. However, he is urged to always be cognizant of the role the emotions play in the patient's musculoskeletal complaint.

23 References

1. Becker RO. *The Body Electric.* New York, NY: Quill; 1985.
2. Hocking BR. *ETPS Neuro-Mechanical Acupuncture Manual.* 11th edition. ETPS Neuro-Mechanical Acupuncture Seminars; 2002.
3. Guyton AC. *Textbook of Medical Physiology.* Philadelphia, PA: WB Saunders Company; 1991.
4. Martinke DJ, Dowling DJ. The philosophy of osteopathic medicine. In: Schiowitz S, Dowling D. *An Osteopathic Approach to Diagnosis and Treatment.* Second Edition. Philadelphia, PA: Lippincott-Raven; 1997.
5. Greenman PE. *Principles of Manual Medicine.* 2nd ed. Philadelphia, Pa: Lippincott Williams and Wilkins; 1996.
6. Weil A. *Spontaneous Healing.* New York, NY: Fawcett Books; 1995.
7. Talbott S. *The Cortisol Connection.* Alameda, CA: Hunter House; 2002.
8. Hestbaek L, Leboeuf-Yde C, Manniche C. Is low back pain part of a general health pattern or is it a separate and distinctive entity? A critical literature review of comorbidity with low back pain. *Journal of Manual & Manipulative Therapy.* 2003; 26(4): 243–252.
9. Chilton FH. *Inflammation Nation.* New York, NY: Fireside; 2005.
10. Sears B. *The Anti-Inflammation Zone.* New York, NY: Regan Books; 2005.

11. Seaman D. The diet-induced pro-inflammatory state: a cause of chronic pain and other degenerative diseases? *Journal of Manipulative and Physiological Therapeutics*. 2002; 25(3) 168–179.

12. Vasey C. *The Acid-Alkaline Diet for Optimum Health*. Rochester, VT: Healing Arts Press; 2003.

13. Cotran R, Kumar V, Robbins S. *Robbins Pathologic Basis of Disease.* 5th edition. Philadelphia, PA: WB Saunders; 1994.

14. Walther, DS. *Applied Kinesiology: Synopsis*. 2nd Edition. Pueblo, CO: Systems DC; 2000.

15. Chestnut JL. *The 14 Foundational Premises for the Scientific and Philosophical Validation of the Chiropractic Wellness Paradigm*. Victoria, BC. The Wellness Practice; 2003.

16. Levine PA. *Waking the Tiger: Healing Trauma*. Berkeley, CA: North Atlantic Books; 1997.

17. Hanna T. *Somatics*. Reading, MA: Perseus Books; 1988.

18. Brimhall J. *Solving the Health Puzzle with the 6 Steps to Wellness*. Orlando, FL: E2: Books; 2006.

19. Davis M. The mammalian startle response. In: Eaton R. *Neural Mechanisms of Startle Behavior.* New York, NY: Plenum Press; 1984.

20. Schmitt W. 100-Hour Applied Kinesiology Course. Course videos; 2004.

21. Ryerson SD. Hemiplegia. In: Umphred DA. *Neurological Rehabilitation*. 3rd Edition. St. Louis, MO: Mosby; 1995.

22. Janda V. Muscles and motor control in cervicogenic disorders. In: Grant Ruth. *Physical Therapy of the Cervical and Thoracic Spine.* 3rd Edition. New York, NY: Churchill Livingstone; 2002.

23. Tecco S, Colucci C, Calvisi V, Orso CA, Salini V, Festa F. Influence of knee pathology on body posture and muscle activity of head, neck and trunk muscles. *Minerva Stomatol.* 2005; 5411-12:611-33.

24. Tecco S, Colucci C, Caraffa A, Salini V, Festa F. Cervical lordosis in patients who underwent anterior cruciate ligament injury: a cross-sectional study. *Cranio*. 2007; 25(1):42–9.

25. Pierrynowski M, Tiidus P, Galea V. Women with fibromyalgia walk with an altered muscle synergy. *Gait and Posture*. 2005; 22(3)210–218.

26. Ekholm J, Eklund G, Skoglund S. On reflex effects from knee joint of cats. *Acta Physiologica Scandinavica*. 1960; 50: 167–174.

27. Jull G, Kristjansson E, Dall'Alba P. Impairment in the cervical flexors: a comparison of whiplash and insidious onset neck pain patients. *Manual Therapy*. 2004; 9:89–94.

28. Abbott JH. Mobilization with movement applied to the elbow affects shoulder range of movement in subjects with lateral epicondylalgia. *Man Ther*. 2001; 6(3): 170–177.

29. Beck RW. *Functional Neurology for Practitioners of Manual Therapy*. New York, NY: Churchill Livingstone; 2008.

30. Buskirk RL. Nociceptive reflexes and the somatic dysfunction: a model. *Journal of the American Osteopathic Association*. 1990; 9(90): 792–809.

31. Simons DG, Travell JG, Simons LS. *Travell & Simons' Myofascial Pain and Dysfunction, The Trigger Point Manual. Vol 1. Upper Half of Body*. Baltimore, MD: Williams & Wilkins; 1999.

32. Lucas KR, Polus BI, Rich PA. Latent myofascial trigger points: their effects on muscle activation and movement efficiency. *Journal of Bodywork and Movement Therapies*. 2004; 8, 160–166.

33. Lewit K. Clinical importance of active scars: abnormal scars as a cause of myofascial pain. *Journal of Manipulative and Physiological Therapeutics*. 2004; 27(6): 397–400.

34. Leboeuf-Yde, Axen I. et al. The types and frequencies of improved non-musculoskeletal symptoms reported after chiropractic spinal manipulative therapy. *JMPT*. 1999 Nov–Dec; 22(9): 559–64.

35. Ornish D et al. Intensive lifestyle changes for reversal of coronary heart disease. *JAMA*. 1998; 280(23): 2001–2007.

36. Ornish D. *Dr. Dean Ornish's Program for Reversing Heart Disease*. New York, NY: Ballantine Books; 1990.

37. Ornish D et al. Intensive lifestyle changes may affect the progression of prostate cancer. *Journal of Urology*. 2005; 174(3):1065–1070.

38. Batmanghelidj F. *Your Body's Many Cries for Water.* 2nd edition. Vienna, VA: Global Health Solutions, Inc.; 2004.

39. Chestnut JL. *Innate Physical Fitness & Spinal Hygiene.* Victoria, BC: The Wellness Practice; 2005.

40. Edgelow PI. Dysfunction, evaluation, and treatment of the lumbar spine. In: Donatelli R, Wooden M. *Orthopaedic Physical Therapy.* 2nd Edition. New York, NY: Churchill Livingstone; 1994.

41. Mladenoff E. *Stressed Out Headed for Burnout.* Overland Park, KS: MYA Publications; 2006.

42. Dvorak J, Dvorak V. *Manual Medicine, Diagnostics.* New York, NY: Thieme-Stratton Inc.; 1994.

43. Schafer RC, Faye LJ. *Motion Palpation and Chiropractic Technic.* 2nd Edition. Huntington Beach, CA: Motion Palpation Institute; 1998.

44. Rothbart BA. Medial column foot systems: an innovative tool for improving posture. *Journal of Bodywork and Movement Therapies.* 2002; 6(4): 37–46.

45. Buskilia D, Neuman L et al. Increased rates of fibromyalgia following cervical spine injury. *Arthritis and Rheumatism.* 1997; 40(3): 446–452.

46. Tracey KJ. The Inflammatory Reflex. *Nature.* 2002; 420: 853–859.

47. Peterson DH, Bergmann TF. *Chiropractic Technique: Principles and Procedures.* 2nd Edition. St. Louis, MO: Mosby; 2002.

48. Sandoz R. The natural history of a spinal degenerative lesion. *Ann Swiss Chiro Assoc.* 1989; 9:149.

49. Kirkaldy-Willis WH ed. Pathology and pathogenesis of low back pain; The three phases of the spectrum of degenerative disease. In: *Managing Low Back Pain.* 3rd Ed. New York, NY: Churchill Livingstone; 1992.

50. Kirkaldy-Willis WH et al. Pathology and pathogenesis of lumbar spondylosis and stenosis. *Spine.* 1978; 3(4):319.

51. Meadows JT. *Orthopedic Differential Diagnosis in Physical Therapy: A Case Study Approach.* New York, NY: McGraw-Hill; 1999.

52. Cyriax JH, Cyriax PJ. *Cyriax's Illustrated Manual of Orthopaedic Medicine.* 2nd Edition. Delhi, India: Butterworth-Heinemann; 2001.

53. Viti J, Paris, S. Use of multifidus isometric for a patient with acute neck pain: a case report. *Journal of Manual and Manipulative Therapy.* 2003; 11(2): 103–109.

54. Murphy D. Dysfunction of the cervical spine. In: Murphy D. *Conservative Management of Cervical Spine Syndromes.* New York, NY: McGraw-Hill; 2000.

55. Russek LN. Examination and treatment of a patient with hypermobility syndrome. *Physical Therapy*. 2000; 80(4): 386–398.

56. Beighton P, Solomon L, Soskolne CL. Articular mobility in an African population. *Ann Rheum Dis*. 1973; 32:413–418.

57. Keer R, Grahame R. *Hypermobility Syndrome: Recognition and Management for Physiotherapists*. London: Butterworth-Heinemann; 2003.

58. Lee D. *The Pelvic Girdle*. 2nd edition. Edinburgh: Churchill Livingstone; 1999.

59. Hruska R Jr. *Postural Restoration: An Integrated Approach to Treatment of Upper Half Musculoskeletal Dysfunction.* Course Manual, Postural Restoration Institute. Lincoln, NE. 2001.

60. Dixon A St. J, Campbell-Smith S. Long leg arthropathy. *Ann Rheum Dis.* 1969; 28: 359–365.

61. Gofton JP, Trueman GE. Studies in osteoarthritis of the hip: Part II, osteoarthritis of the hip and leg-length disparity. *Can Med Assoc J.* 1971; 104:791–799.

62. Rush WA, Steiner HA. A study of lower extremity length inequality. *Am J Roentgen Rad Ther.* 1946; 56: 616–623.

63. Hudson OC, Hettesheimer CA, Robin PA. Causalgic backache. *Am J Surg.* 1941; 52: 297–303.

64. Giles LGF, Taylor JR. Low-back pain associated with leg length inequality. *Spine.* 1982; 7: 159–162, 1982

65. Botte RR. An interpretation of the pronation syndrome and foot types of patients with low back pain. *J Am Podiatr Assoc.* 1981; 71: 243–253.

66. Schamberger W. *The Malalignment Syndrome*. Edinburgh: Churchill Livingstone; 2002.

67. Maigne R. *Diagnosis and Treatment of Pain of Vertebral Origin*. Baltimore, MD: Williams and Wilkins; 1996.

68. Travell JG, Simons DG. *Myofascial Pain and Dysfunction: The Trigger Point Manual. Vol 2. The Lower Extremities.* Philadelphia, PA: Lippincott Williams and Wilkins; 1993.

69. Harris RI, Beath T. The short first metatarsal: its incidence and clinical significance. *J Bone Joint Surg (Am).* 1949; 31:553–565.

70. Upledger J. *Craniosacral Therapy*. Seattle, WA: Eastland Press; 1983.

71. Michaud TC. Biomechanics of the foot and ankle. In: Hyde, TE, Gengenbach, MS. *Conservative Management of Sports Injuries*. Baltimore, MD: Williams and Wilkins; 1997.

72. Greenman PE. Clinical aspects of sacroiliac function in walking. *J Manual Med.* 1990; 5:125–130.

73. Donatelli RA. *The Biomechanics of the Foot and Ankle*. 2nd edition. Philadelphia, PA: F.A. Davis Company: 1996.

74. Danenberg HJ. Lower back pain as a gait-related repetitive motion injury. In: Vleeming A, Mooney V, Dorman T, Snijders C, Stoeckart R. *Movement, Stability, and Low Back Pain*. Edinburgh: Churchill Livingstone; 1997.

75. Lewit K. *Manipulative Therapy in Rehabilitation of the Locomotor System*. 3rd edition. London: Butterworth-Heinemann; 1999.

76. Bullock-Saxton JE. Local sensation changes and altered hip muscle function following severe ankle sprain. *Physical Therapy*. 1994; 74: 17–31.

77. Cooperstein R, Gleberzon B. *Technique Systems in Chiropractic*. New York, NY: Churchill Livingstone; 2004.

78. Kulkarni V, Chandy MJ, Babu KS. Quantitative study of muscle spindles in suboccipital muscles of human foetuses. *Neurol India*. 2001; 49(4): 355–359.

79. Hack GD et al. Anatomic relation between the rectus capitis posterior minor muscle and the dura mater. *Spine.* 1995; 20(23):2484–6.

80. Grostic JD. Dentate ligament-cord distortion hypothesis. *Chiropr Res J.* 1988; 1(1): 47–55.

81. Harrison DE, Cailliet R, Harrison DD, Troyanovich SJ, Harrison SO. A Review of Biomechanics of the Central Nervous System—Part II; Spinal Cord Strain from Postural Loads. *J Manipulative Physiol Ther.* 1999; 22(5): 322–332.

82. Bakris G, Dickholtz M Sr. et al. Atlas vertebra realignment and achievement of arterial pressure goal in hypertensive patients: a pilot study. *J Hum Hypertens*. 2007; 21(5): 347–52.

83. Selano JL, Hightower BC, Pfleger B, Collins KF, Grostic JD. The effects of specific upper cervical adjustments on the CD4 counts of HIV positive patients. *Chiropractic Research Journal.* 1994; 3(1): 32–39.

84. Elster EL. Eighty-one patients with multiple sclerosis and Parkinson's disease undergoing upper cervical chiropractic care to correct vertebral subluxation: a retrospective analysis. *J Vertebral Subluxation Research.* 2004; Aug 2: 1–9.

85. Pollard H, Ward G. The effect of upper cervical or sacroiliac manipulation on hip flexion range of motion. *Journal of Manipulative and Physiological Therapeutics.* 1998; 21(9): 611–616.

86. Pollard H, Ward G. A study of two stretching techniques for improving hip flexion range of motion. *J Manipulative Physiol Ther.* 1997; 20(7):443–447.

87. Robinson S, Collins KF, Grostic JD. A retrospective study: patients with chronic low back pain managed with specific upper cervical adjustments. *Chiropractic Research Journal.* 1993; 2(4): 10–16.

88. Kessinger RC, Boneva DV. The influence of upper cervical specific chiropractic care on lumbar range of motion. Abstracts from the 17th annual upper cervical spine conference, Life University, Marietta, GA, February 3–4, 2001, Chiropr Res J, 2000; 7(2):80)

89. Rochester, RP. Neck pain and disability outcomes following chiropractic upper cervical care: a retrospective case series. *J Can Chiropr Assoc.* 2009; 53(3):173–184.

90. Wiles MR. Observations on the effects of upper cervical manipulations on the electrogastrogram: a preliminary report. *J Manipulative Physiol Ther,* 1980; 3(4):226–228.

91. Amalu WC. Upper cervical management of primary fibromyalgia and chronic fatigue syndrome cases. *Today's Chiropr.* 200; 29(3): 76–86.

92. Weigel G, Casey KF. *Striking Back! The Trigeminal Neuralgia Handbook.* Published by the Trigeminal Neuralgia Association, 2000.

93. Whittingham W, Ellis WB, Molyneux TP. The effect of manipulation (toggle recoil technique) for headaches with upper cervical joint dysfunction: a pilot study. *J Manipulative Physiol Ther.* 1994; 17(6):369–375.

94. Maffetone P. *Complementary Sports Medicine.* Champaign, IL: Human Kinetics; 1999.

95. Orbach G. A neurophysiological basis for adjusting the extremities. In: Charrette MN. *Charrette Adjusting Protocols.* Mark Charrette; 2002.

96. Mitchell FL, Jr. *The Muscle Energy Manual. Vol. 2.* East Lansing, MI: MET Press; 1998.

97. Gray J. *The Alexander Technique.* New York, NY: St. Martin's Press; 1990.

98. Young R, Young S. *The pH Miracle for Weight Loss.* New York, NY: Warner Books; 2005.

99. Yang K. A review of yoga programs for four leading risk factors of chronic diseases. *Evid Based Complement Alternat Med.* 2007; 4(4): 487–91.

100. Conable B, Conable W. *How to Learn the Alexander Technique.* Portland, OR: Andover Press; 1995.

101. Austin J, Ausubel P. Enhanced respiratory muscular function in normal adults after lessons in proprioceptive musculoskeletal education without exercises. *Chest.* 1992; 102(2): 486–490.

102. Cottingham JT, Maitland J. A three-paradigm treatment model using soft tissue mobilization and guided movement-awareness techniques for a patient with chronic low back pain: a case study. *J Orthop Sports Phys Ther.* 1997; 26(3):155–167.

103. Miyashita K, Urabe Y et al. The role of shoulder external rotation during throwing for elbow injury prevention in baseball players. *Journal of Sports Science and Medicine.* 2008; 7: 223–228.

104. Volf N. Somatosensory evoked potentials in the investigation of auricular acupuncture points. *Acupuncture in Medicine.* 2000;18(1): 2–9.

105. Uchida Sae, Hotta H. Acupuncture affects regional blood flow in various organs. *eCAM.* 2008; 5(2): 145–151.

106. Yim Y, Lee H, Hong K, Kim Y, Lee B, Son C, Kim J. Electroacupuncture at acupoint ST36 reduces inflammation and regulates immune activity in collagen-induced arthritis mice. *Evidenced-Based Complementary and Alternative Medicine.* 2007; 4(1): 51–57.

107. Felhendler D, Lisander B. Effects of non-invasive stimulation of acupoints on the cardiovascular system. *Complement Ther Med.* 1999; 7(4):231–4.

108. Mori H, Ueda S, Kuge H, Taniwaki E, Tanaka TH, Adachi K, Nishijo K. Pupillary response induced by acupuncture stimulation—an experimental study. *Acupuncture in Medicine.* 2008; 26(2): 79–85.

109. Liu CF, Yu LF, Lin CH, Lin SC. Effect of auricular pellet acupressure on antioxidative systems in high-risk diabetes mellitus. *J Altern Complement Med.* 2008; 14(3): 309–314.

110. Ohnishi ST, Nishino K, Uchiyama S, Ohnishi T, Yamagushi M. Ki-energy (life-energy) stimulates osteoblastic cells and inhibits the formation of osteoclast-like cells in bone cell culture models. *eCAM.* 2007; 4(2): 225–232.

111. Ohnishi ST, Ohnishi T. The Nishino Breathing method and ki-energy (life-energy): a challenge to traditional scientific thinking. *Evid Based Complement Med.* 2006; 3(2):191–200.

112. Yamaguchi N et al. Acupuncture Regulates Leukocyte Subpopulations in Human Peripheral Blood. *Evid Based Complement Alternat Med.* 2007; 4(4):447–453.

113. Napadow V, Leu J, Li M, Kettner N, Ryan A, Kwong KK, Hui KK, Audette JF. Somatosensory cortical plasticity in carpal tunnel syndrome treated by acupuncture. *Hum Brain Mapp.* 2007; 28(3):159–71.

114. Inoue M, Kitakoji H, Yano T, Ishizaki N, Itoi M, Katsumi Y. Acupuncture treatment for low back pain and lower limb symptoms—the relation between acupuncture or electroacupuncture stimulation and sciatic nerve blood flow. *eCAM.* 2008; 5(2):133–143.

115. Gaponjuk PJ, Sherkovina TJ. The clinical and physiological foundation of auricular acupuncture therapy in patients with hypertensive disease. *Acupuncture in Medicine.* 1994; 12(1):2–5.

116. Karavis M. The neurophysiology of acupuncture: a viewpoint. *Acupuncture in Medicine.* 1997; 15(1): 33–42.

117. Oschman JL. Can electrons act as antioxidants? A review and commentary. *The Journal of Alternative and Complementary Medicine.* 2007; 13(9): 955–967.

118. Oschman JL. Perspective: assume a spherical cow: the role of free or mobile electrons in bodywork, energetic and movement therapies. *Journal of Bodywork and Movement Therapies.* 2008; 12: 40–57.

119. Cheralier G, Mori K, Oschman, J. The effect of earthing (grounding) on human physiology. Unpublished research.

120. Quinn F, Hughes CM, Baxter GD. Reflexology in the management of low back pain: a pilot randomized controlled trial. *Complement Ther Med.* 2008; 16(1):3–8.

121. Jensen R, Gothesen O, Liseth K, Baerheim A. Acupuncture treatment patellofemoral pain syndrome. *J Altern Complement Med.* 1999; 5(6): 521–7.

122. Haslam R. A Comparison of acupuncture with advice and exercises on the symptomatic treatment of osteoarthritis of the hip—a randomized controlled trial. *Acupuncture in Medicine.* 2001; 19(1):19–26.

123. Ebneshahidi NS et al. The effects of laser acupuncture on chronic tension headache—a randomized controlled trial. *Acupuncture in Medicine.* 2005; 23(1):13–18.

124. Johansson KM, Adolfsson LE, Foldevi MO. Effects of acupuncture versus ultrasound in patients with impingement syndrome: randomized clinical trial. *Physical Therapy.* 2005; 85(6):490–501.

125. Guerra de Hoyos JA, Andres Martin Mdel C, Bassas y Baena de Leon E, Vigara Lopez M, Molina Lopez T, Verdugo Morilla FA, Gonzalez Moreno MJ. Randomized trial of long term effect of acupuncture for shoulder pain. *Pain.* 2004; 112(3):289–98.

126. Vas J, Ortega C, Olmo V, Perez-Fernandez F, Hernandez L, Medina I, Seminario JM, Herrera A. Single-point acupuncture and physiotherapy for the treatment of painful shoulder: a multicentre randomized controlled trial. *Rheumatology (Oxford).* 2008; 47(6):887–93.

127. Barker R, Kober A, Hoerauf K, Latzke D, Adel S, Kain ZN, Wang SM. Out-of-hospital auricular acupressure in elder patients with hip fracture: a randomized double-blinded trial. *Acad Emerg Med.* 2006; 13(1):19–23.

128. Usichenko TI, Dinse M, Hermsen M, Witstruck T, Pavlovic D, Lehmann CH. Auricular acupuncture for pain relief after total hip arthroplasty—a randomized controlled study. *Pain.* 2005; 114(3):320–7.

129. Zhang ZL, Ji XQ, Zhang YH, Yu SH, Xue L. Controlled study on the needling method for regulating the spleen and stomach for treatment of diabetic retinopathy. *Zongguo Zhen Jiu.* 2006; 26(12):839–42.

130. Zhang ZL, Ji XQ, Zhang YH, Yu SH, Xue L. Controlled study on the needling method for regulating the spleen and stomach for treatment of diabetic retinopathy. *Zongguo Zhen Jiu.* 2006; 26(12):839–42.

131. Wang H, Qi H, Wang BS, Cui YY Zhu L, Rong ZX, Chen HZ; Is acupuncture beneficial in depression: a meta-analysis of 8 randomized controlled trials. *J Affect Disord.* 2008; 111(2-3): 125–134.

132. Stener-Victorin E, Humaidan P. Use of acupuncture in female infertility and a summary of recent acupuncture studies related to embryo transfer. *Acupuncture in Medicine*. 2006; 24(4): 157–163.

133. Chen LL, Su YC, Su CH, Lin HC, Kuo HW. Acupressure and meridian massage: combined effects on increasing body weight in premature infants. *J Clin Nurs*. 2008; 17(9):1174–81.

134. Oleson T, Flocco W. Randomized controlled study of premenstrual symptoms treated with ear, hand, and foot reflexology. *Obstet Gynecol*. 1993; 82(6):906–11.

135. Haack M, Mullington JM. Sustained sleep restriction reduces emotional and physical well-being. *Pain*. 2005; 119(1-3):56–64.

136. Ayas et al. A prospective study of sleep duration and coronary heart disease in women. *Arch Intern Med*. 2003; 163(2):2005–9.

137. Kundermann B et al. The effect of sleep deprivation on pain. *Pain Res Manag*. 2004; 9(1):25–32.

138. Meier-Ewert HK et al. Effect of sleep loss on c-reactive protein, an inflammatory marker of cardiovascular risk. *J Am Coll Cardiol*. 2004; 43(4):678–83.

139. Haack M, Sanchez E, Mullington JM. Elevated inflammatory markers in response to prolonged sleep restriction are associated with increased pain in healthy volunteers. *Sleep*. 2007; 30(9):1145–52.

140. Hutchinson J. *Soft Tissue Management of the Shoulder Girdle and Upper Extremity*. Course Manual. 2001.

141. McKenzie RA. *The Cervical and Thoracic Spine*. Waikanae, New Zealand: Spinal Publications; 1990.

142. Mulligan B. *Manual Therapy "Nags", "Snags", "MWMs" etc.* 4th Ed. Wellington, New Zealand: Plane View Services; 1999.

143. McKenzie RA. *7 Steps to a Pain-Free Life*. New York, NY: Plume; 2001.

144. Hruska R Jr. *Myokinematic Restoration: An Integrated Approach to Treatment of Musculoskeletal Dysfunction*. Course Manual, Postural Restoration Institute. Lincoln, NE. 2002.

145. Huang ST, Chen GY, Wu CH, Kuo CD. Effect of disease activity and position on autonomic nervous modulation in patients with systemic lupus erythematosus. *Clin Rheumatol*. 2008; 27(3);295–300.

146. Chen GY, Kuo CD. The effect of the lateral decubitus position on vagal tone. *Anaesthesia.* 1997; 52(7): 653–7.

147. Miyamoto S, Fujita M, Sekiguchi H, Okano Y, Nagaya N, Ueda K, Tamaki S, Nohara R, Eiho S, Sasayama S. Effects of posture on cardiac autonomic nervous activity in patients with congestive heart failure. *J Am Coll Cardiol.* 2001; 37(7):1788–93.

148. Hall M. *Advanced Clinical Diagnosis.* Course Notes. Parker College of Chiropractic; 2007.

149. Iams J. *Stress Relief Beyond Belief.* Poway, CA: Superspine Inc; 1998.

150. Augustine C, Makofsky HW, Britt C et al. Use of the Occivator for the correction of forward head posture, and the implications for temporomandibular disorders: a pilot study. *Cranio.* 2008 26(2): 136–43.

151. Menezes A. *The Complete Guide to Joseph H. Pilates' Techniques of Physical Conditioning.* Alameda, CA: Hunter House Publishers; 2000.

152. Partridge D. Treating and Beating Adhesive Capsulitis. Seminar Notes. San Antonio, Texas. 2002.

153. Biddinger A. Functional Anatomy of the Elbow. In: Placzek J, Boyce D. *Orthopaedic Physical Therapy Secrets.* Philadelphia, PA: Hanley and Belfus; 2001.

154. Liebenson C. Self-treatment of mid-thoracic dysfunction: a key link in the body axis. *Journal of Bodywork and Movement Therapies.* 2001; 5(2): 90–98.

155. DonTigny RL. Anterior dysfunction of the sacroiliac joint as a major factor in the etiology of idiopathic low back pain syndromes. *Phys Ther.* 1990; 70(4); 250–65.

156. Muscolino J, Cipriani S. Pilates and the "powerhouse"—1. *Journal of Bodywork and Movement Therapies.* 2004; 8(1):15–24.

157. Cottingham JT, Porges SW, Richmond K. Shifts in pelvic inclination angle and parasympathetic tone produced by rolfing soft tissue manipulation. *Physical Therapy.* 1988; 68(9); 1364–1370.

158. Ireland JL et al. Hip strength in females with and without patellofemoral pain. *J Ortho Sports Phys Ther.* 2003; 33: 671–676.

159. Mascal CL et al. Management of patellofemoral pain targeting hip, pelvis, and trunk muscle function: 2 case reports. *J Ortho Sports Phys Ther.* 2003; 33: 642–660.

160. Ernst G et al. Patellofemoral disorders. In: Placzek J, Boyce, D. *Orthopaedic Physical Therapy Secrets.* Philadelphia, PA: Hanley and Belfus; 2001.

161. Willard FH. The muscular, ligamentous and neural structure of the low back and its relation to back pain. In: Vleeming A, Mooney V, Dorman T, Snijders C, Stoeckart R (eds). *Movement, Stability and Low Back Pain.* Edinburgh: Churchill Livingstone; 1997.

162. Myers T. *Anatomy Trains: Myofascial Meridians for Manual and Movement Therapists.* Edinburgh: Churchill Livingstone; 2001.

163. Evjenth O, Hamberg J. *Muscle Stretching in Manual Therapy: Vol II.* Alfta, Sweden: Alfta Rehab; 1997.

164. D'Ambrogio K, Roth G. *Positional Release Therapy: Assessment and Treatment of Musculoskeletal Dysfunction.* St. Louis, MO: Mosby; 1997.

165. Hall T, Chan HT, Christensen L, Odenthal B, Wells C, Robinson K. Efficacy of a C1-C2 Self-Sustained Natural Apophyseal Glide (SNAG) in the Management of Cervicogenic Headache. *J Ortho Phys Ther.* 2007; 37(3): 100–107.

166. Maitland GD. *Vertebral Manipulation.* 5th Edition. Boston, MA: Butterworth-Heinemann; 1996.

167. Murtagh J, Kenna C. *Back Pain and Spinal Manipulation.* 2nd edition. Boston, MA: Butterworth Heinemann; 1997.

168. Coppieters M et al. The immediate effects of a cervical lateral glide treatment technique in patients with neurogenic cervicobrachial pain. *J Ortho Sports Phys Ther.* 2003; 33(7): 369–378.

169. Vicenzino B et al. The initial effects of a cervical spine manipulative physiotherapy treatment on the pain and dysfunction of lateral epicondylalgia. *Pain.* 1996; 68:69–74.

170. Exelby L. The Mulligan concept: Its application in the management of spinal conditions. *Man Ther.* 2002; 7(2): 64–70.

171. Bergamini M, Pierleoni F, Gizdulich A, Bergaminini C. Dental occlusion and body posture: a surface EMG study. *Cranio.* 2008; 26(1): 25–32.

172. Sforza C, Tartaglia GM et al. Occlusion, sternocleidomastoid muscle activity, and body sway: a pilot study in male astronauts. *Cranio.* 2006; 24(1): 43–9.

173. Walther DS. *Applied Kinesiology, Vol II: The Stomatognathic System.* Pueblo, CO: Systems DC; 1983.

174. Makofsky HW. *Spinal Manual Therapy: An Introduction to Soft Tissue Mobilization, Spinal Manipulation, Therapeutic and Home Exercises.* Thorofare, NJ: Slack Incorporated; 2003.

175. Liebenson C. Self-treatment of mid-thoracic dysfunction: a key link in the body axis. Part two: treatment. *Journal of Bodywork and Movement Therapies.* 2001; 5(3): 191–195.

176. Koch L. *The Psoas Book.* Second Edition. Felton, CA: Guinea Pig Publications; 1997.

177. Johnson J. *The Multifidus Back Pain Solution.* Oakland, CA: New Harbuger Publications; 2002.

178. Jones, L. *Jones Strain-Counterstrain.* Boise, ID: Jones Strain-Counterstrain, Inc.; 1995.

179. Schafer RC, Faye LJ. Motion Palpation and Chiropractic Technic. Huntington Beach, CA: Motion Palpation Institute; 1998.

180. O'Sullivan PB, Beales DJ. Changes in pelvic floor and diaphragm kinematics and respiratory patterns in subjects with sacroiliac joint pain following a motor learning intervention: A case series. *Manual Therapy.* 2007; 12: 209–218.

181. McConnell J. Management of patellofemoral problems. *Manual therapy.* (1996) 1, 60–66.

182. Exelby L. Peripheral mobilisations with movement. *Man Ther.* 1996; 1: 118–126.

183. Boyle JW. Is the pain and dysfunction of shoulder impingement lesion really second rib syndrome is disguise? Two case reports. *Manual Therapy.* 1999; 4(1): 44–48.

184. Charrette MN. *Charrette Adjusting Protocols.* Mark Charrette; 2002.

185. Struijs P et al. Manipulation of the wrist for management for lateral epicondylitis: a randomized pilot study. *Physical Therapy.* 2003; 83(7): 608–616.

186. Backstrom KM. Mobilization with movement as an adjunct intervention in a patient with complicated de Quervain's tenosynovitis: a case report. *J Ortho Sports Phys Ther.* 2002; 32(3): 86–94.

187. Reid DC, Kushner S. The elbow region. In: Donatelli RA, Wooden, MJ. *Orthopaedic Physical Therapy*. 2nd edition. New York, NY: Churchill Livingstone; 1994.

188. Pert CB. *Molecules of Emotion*. New York, NY: Scribner; 1997.

189. Benson H. *The Relaxation Response*. New York, NY: Harper Collins; 2000.

190. Barnes JF. *Myofascial Release*. Paoli, PA: MFR Seminars; 1990.

191. Schultz RL, Feitis, R. *The Endless Web*. Berkeley, CA: North Atlantic Books; 1996.

192. Rolf IP. *Rolfing*. Rochester, VT: Healing Arts Press; 1989.

193. Gelb H. *Clinical Management of Head, Neck, and TMJ Pain and Dysfunction: A Multidisciplinary Approach to Diagnosis and Treatment*. Philadelphia, PA: WB Saunders Co.; 1977.

194. Gelb H, Bernstein IM. Clinical evaluation of two hundred patients with temporomandibular joint syndrome. *J Prosthet Dent*. 1983; 49: 234–243.

195. Gelb H, Bernstein IM. Comparison of three different populations with temporomandibular joint pain-dysfunction syndrome. *Dent Clin North Am*. 1983; 27:495–503.

196. Holmes-Johnson E, Terezhalmy G, Ross G. Personality profiles of TMJ-MPDS patients. *Ear Nose Throat*. 1982; 61: 76–82.

197. Rocabado M, Iglarsh ZA. *Musculoskeletal Approach to Maxillofacial Pain*. New York, NY: J.B. Lippincott Co.; 1991.

198. Butler DS. *Mobilisation of the Nervous System*. Melbourne: Churchill Livingstone; 1991.

199. Butler DS. *The Sensitive Nervous System*. Adelaide: NOI Group Publications; 2000.

200. Dreaver J. *Somatic Technique*. Sebastopol, CA: Wild Goose Press; 2000.

201. Benson H. *The Wellness Book*. New York, NY: Simon and Schuster; 1992.

202. Weil A. *Natural Health, Natural Medicine*. Boston, MA: Houghton Mifflin; 1998.